ONSEN AND RYOKAN OF JAPAN

Traditional Spa and Bathing Culture

gestalten

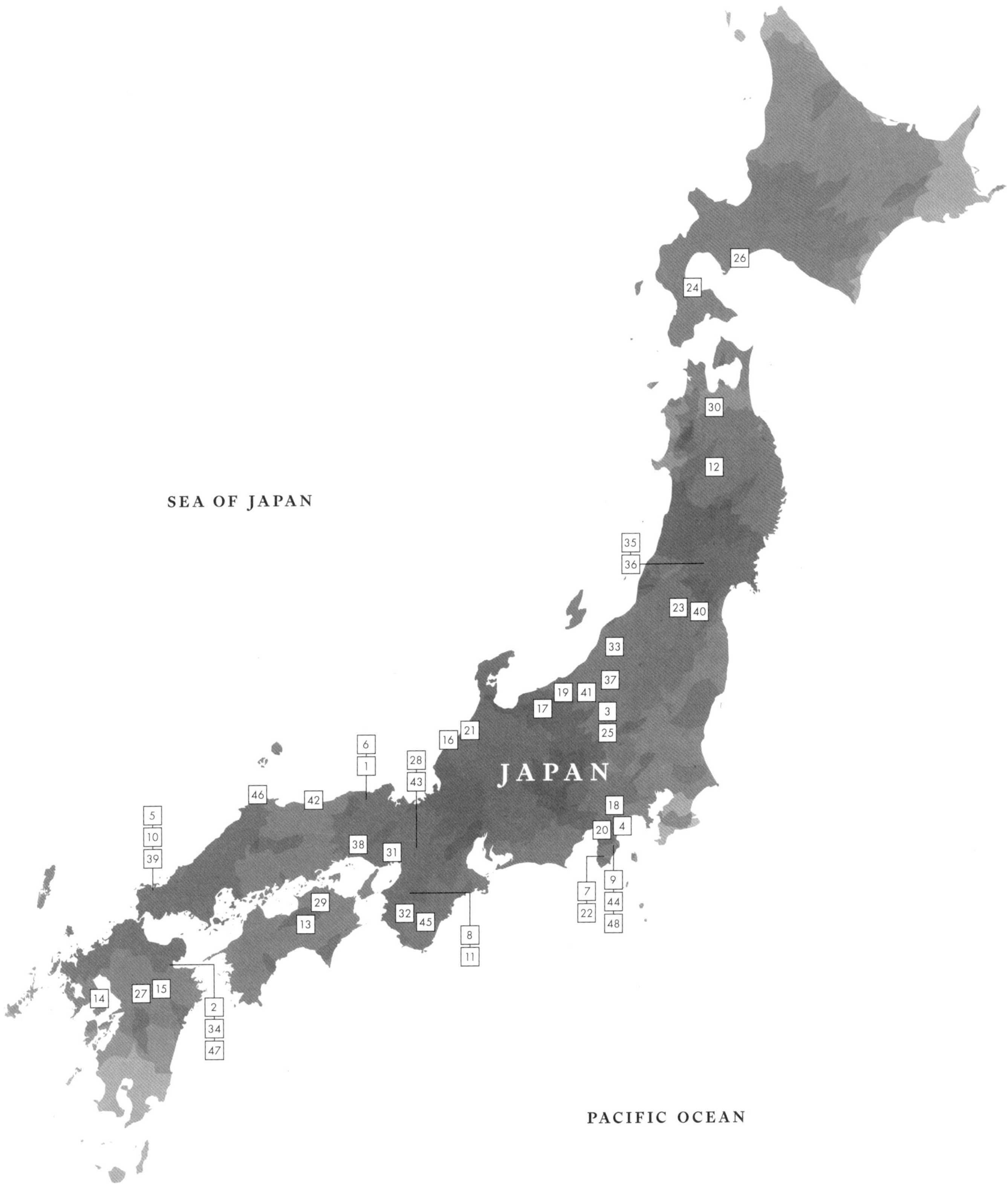
SEA OF JAPAN
JAPAN
PACIFIC OCEAN
26
24
30
12
35
36
23
40
33
37
19
41
17
3
25
16
21
6
1
28
43
46
42
5
10
39
18
4
20
38
31
9
44
48
7
22
29
13
32
45
8
11
14
27
15
2
34
47

THE ENDURING ENCHANTMENT OF JAPANESE ONSEN

Discover the culturally rich, restorative wonders of onsen bathing, a timeless practice embraced in both ancient and modern times.

The Way of Onsen

Deeply ingrained in Japanese culture for centuries is a love of onsen. The country's hot springs, bathing facilities, and the inns and hotels connected to them, remain places of sublime beauty and spiritual significance. Japan's volcanic archipelago is blessed with an abundance of these therapeutic sites—today the country is estimated to have some 27,000 hot spring sources and over 3,000 onsen accommodations.

Communal bathing in these geothermally heated waters can be traced back to the 6th century, the Asuka period, a time when Buddhism was introduced to the country, and the ideas of purification and cleanliness were highly valued. Many of today's oldest onsen were discovered by monks traveling through the land on pilgrimages. Known as *shinyu* (神湯—divine hot springs), these sites continue to hold sacred status.

The first buildings to house these purifying baths were known as *shukubo* (宿坊—temple accommodation). By bathing in the nearby onsen, Buddhist monks would cast off the seven ailments and receive in turn the seven blessings. It was these early *shukubo*, in fact, that would eventually evolve into today's ryokan (旅館—traditional inn), the lodgings now integral to Japan's bathing culture.

In the centuries that followed their discovery, onsen became more prominent in the everyday social life of the country, embraced by the samurai class during the feudal era. Many *daimyo* (大名—feudal lords) kept the location of their favored onsen secret for security reasons. The practice of bathing together with one's samurai and vassals, stripped of one's armor and weapons, strengthened both trust and camaraderie between the daimyo and his men—wounds were healed in the onsen, and battle strategies were discussed.

During the Edo period, *konyoku* (混浴—mixed bathing) onsen were commonplace, with both men and women relaxing together in the same baths. Few of these *konyoku* onsen remain today, but those that do can be found in the remote northern and southern mountainous reaches of the country.

Any hot spring which is difficult, even dangerous to reach, is beloved by onsen enthusiasts—these secret spots are known as *hitou* (秘湯). Travelers must commit to taking multiple forms of transport, and perhaps hike for several hours, but the journey often culminates in a restorative soak amid the most pristine, stunning landscapes.

Travelers from far and wide also visit onsen ryokan to partake in the healing therapy of *toji* (湯治), a practice where one stays at the site or an extended period of time in order to bathe, rest, and rejuvenate, drawing out the body's innate natural healing abilities. Historically, *toji* was practiced mainly by farmers and fishermen in their seasonal downtime to recover from their physically demanding work. They would often bring their own bedding to the simple inns, as well as cookware in order to prepare meals themselves.

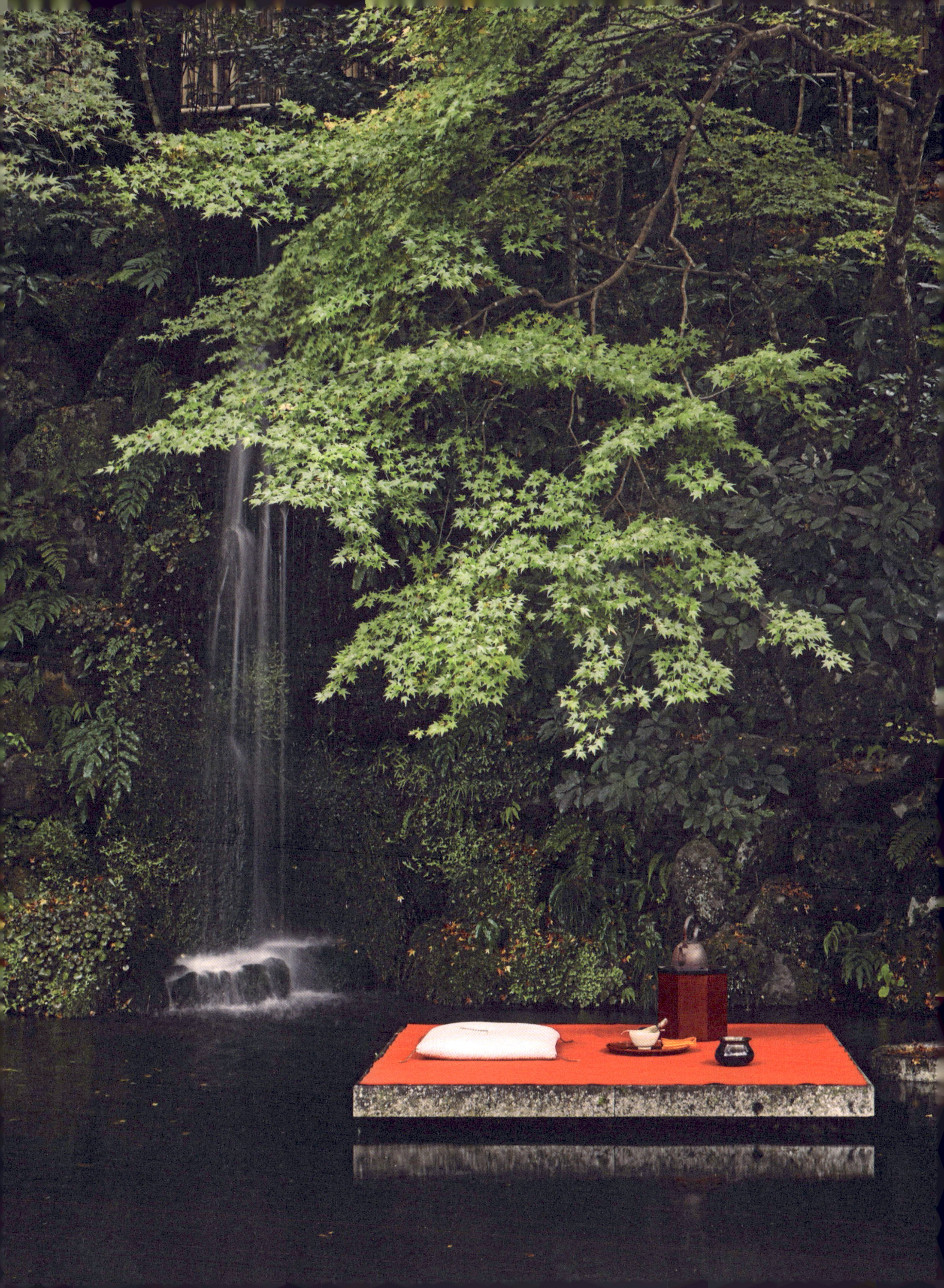

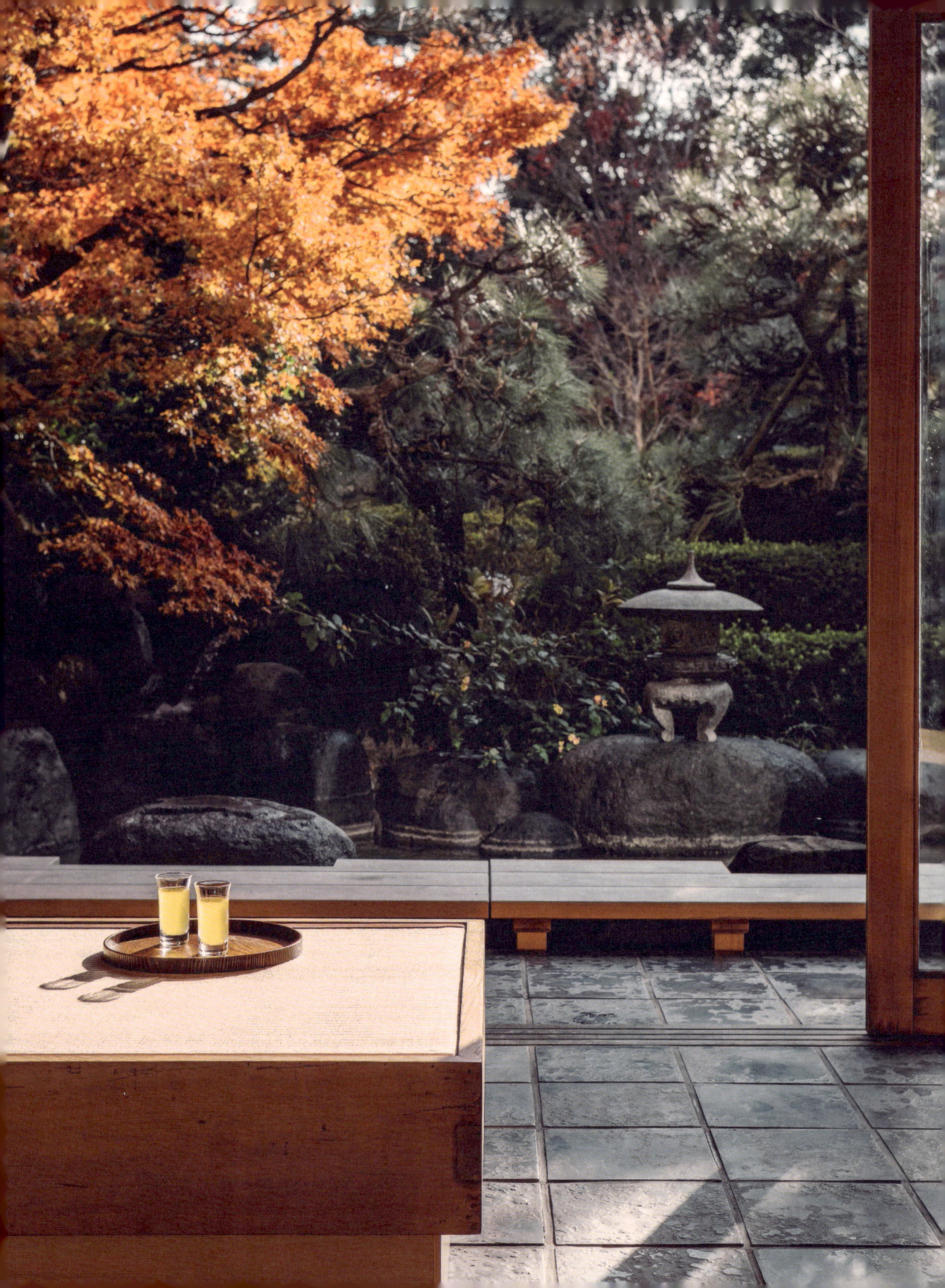

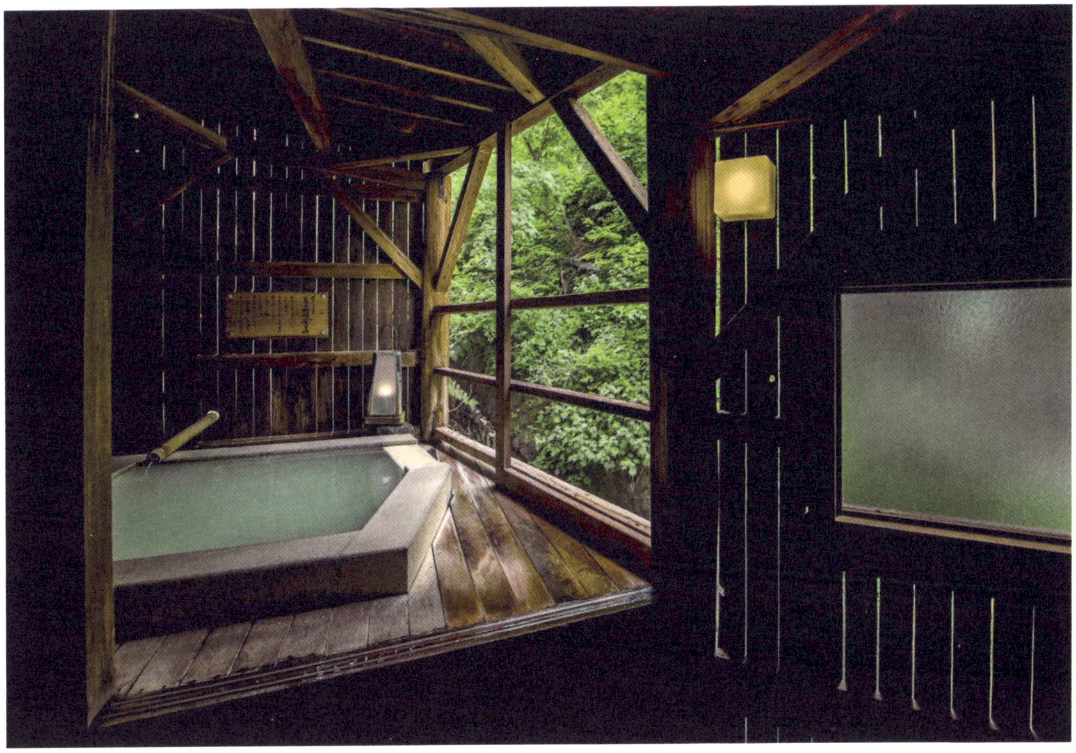

ABOVE Immerse yourself in the healing practices of onsen and *shinrin-yoku* (forest bathing).

Modern Onsen

With the frenetic pace of modern life and its increasing hunger for variety, the practice of *toji* has declined. The love of onsen, however, has not diminished, and many visitors now choose shorter getaways, often as part of an onsen *meguri* (温泉めぐり—onsen pilgrimage). Otherwise known as onsen-hopping, this sees the visitor bathing at multiple onsen over a short period of time, in a concentrated area like a single town.

According to Japan's Hot Springs Law, in order to qualify as an onsen, a hot spring must contain a certain amount of mineral components, originate at a depth of over 0.93 miles (1.5 kilometers) underground, and have a water temperature of 77 °F (25 °C) or higher at the outlet. Further categorization separates them into "volcanic hot springs" and "non-volcanic hot springs," or due to characteristics such as color, temperature, odor, and mineral composition.

Onsen waters typically fall into simple alkaline or slightly acidic categories, with waters at pH 8 and above known as *bijin-no-yu* (美人の湯—hot spring of beauty). This particular type of onsen is extremely popular with the beauty-conscious, as the thick, viscous quality of the water is said to result in lovely, smooth skin. *Gensen kakenagashi* (源泉掛け流し—free-flowing spring) is widely regarded as the most sought-after and purest onsen form, as it flows continuously and directly from the natural source into the bath without treatment (adding normal water to control temperature) or recirculation (when the water is recycled back and treated).

The Ryokan Experience

There is simply no better way for visitors to immerse themselves fully in onsen culture than a stay in a ryokan. In its simplest terms, a ryokan is defined as a traditional

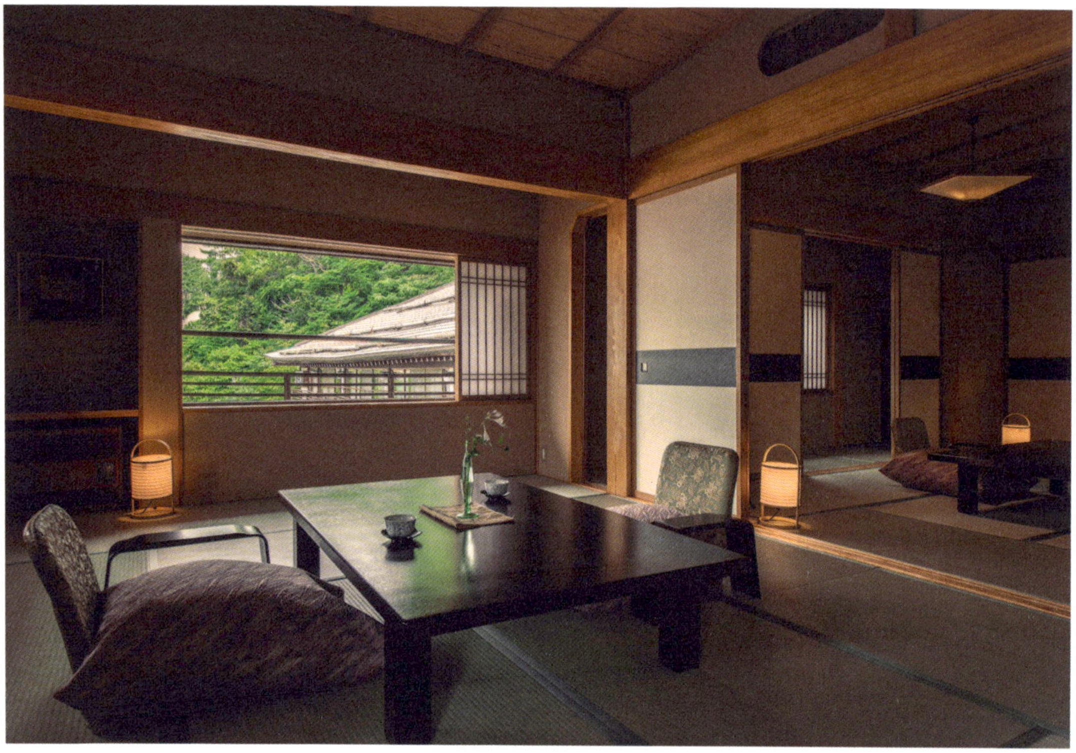

ABOVE Experience the beauty of traditional Japanese rooms at Takamiya Ryokan Miyamaso.

inn built with mainly Japanese architectural elements, as seen in its elegant structure, facilities, and equipment. Onsen ryokan are all the more special because their waters are drawn through pipes from naturally occurring hot springs whilst a ryokan will simply use normal water.

These dwellings can range from the simplest, most rustic wooden inns—with cozy, tatami-laden rooms and shared bathrooms—to luxurious private onsen and spaces whose design aesthetics might display influences of the romantic Taisho Roman era, modern Japanese minimalism, and new Western style. These ryokan can be found in picturesque onsen towns, remote mountain valleys, or craggy peninsulas, and might feature a multitude of baths: *uchiburo* (内風呂—indoor bath), *rotenburo* (露天風呂—outdoor bath), *mizuburo* (水風呂—cold bath) and perhaps even multiple *kashikiri/kazuko buro* (貸し切り風呂/家族風呂—private/family bath), making for a truly splendid and multifaceted experience.

Making the Most of an Onsen Experience

Easing into the soothing waters of an onsen is a calming, restorative experience. The first step is to disrobe completely, placing clothes and towels in a small cubicle or basket, and cleaning the body in the shower area. If there is no shower area, fill the small *yu-oke* (湯桶—the wooden/plastic bucket) with onsen water and pour it over yourself—traditionally at least three times, as it ensures that your body is purified. Place your small, folded towel on your head or by the side of the onsen and tie up any hair that falls below the shoulders, taking care not to drop your hair or towel into the water, as this is considered unhygienic. Slowly submerge yourself, take a moment to breathe in the onsen vapors, and let your mind focus on the restful present.

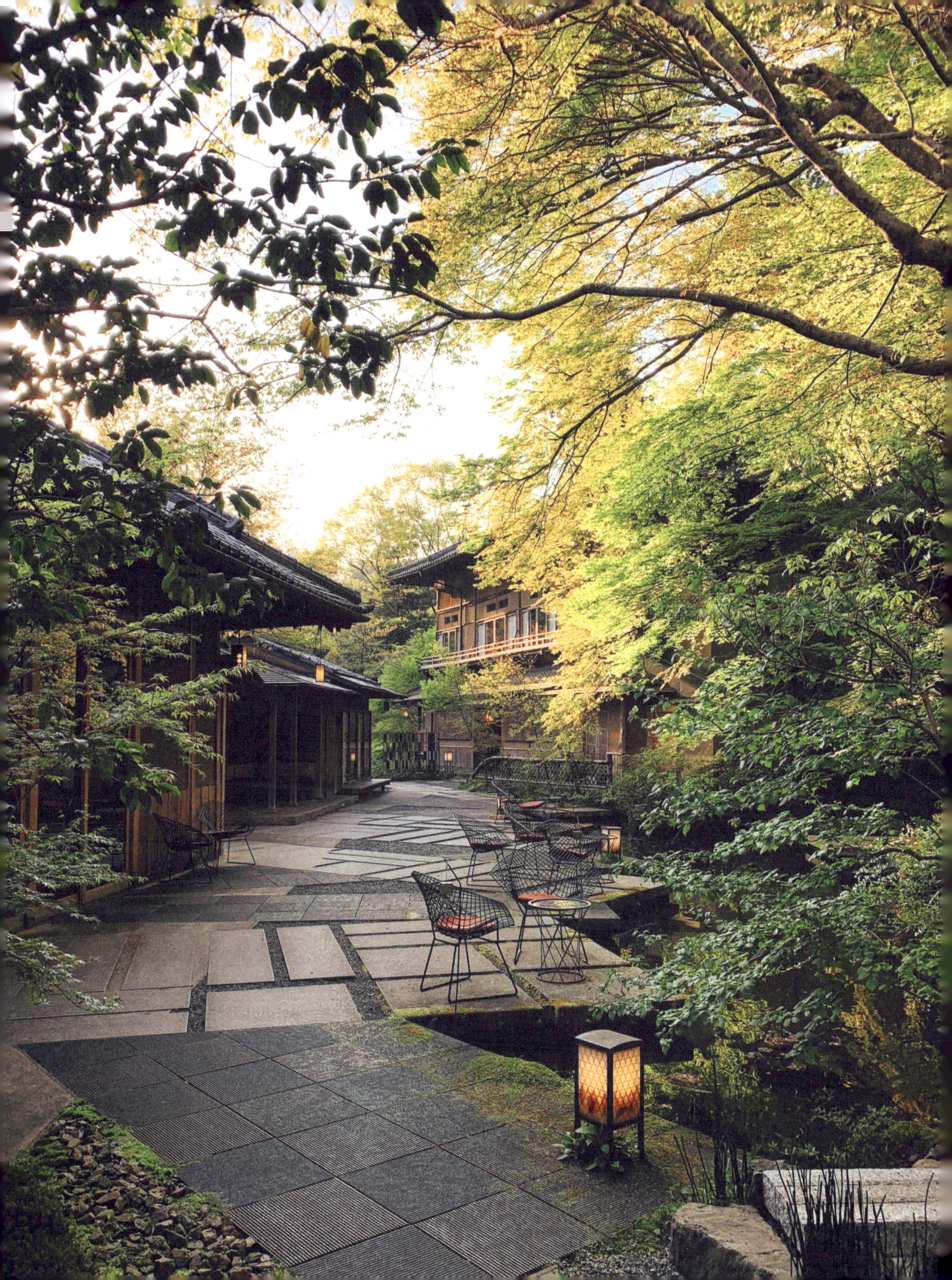

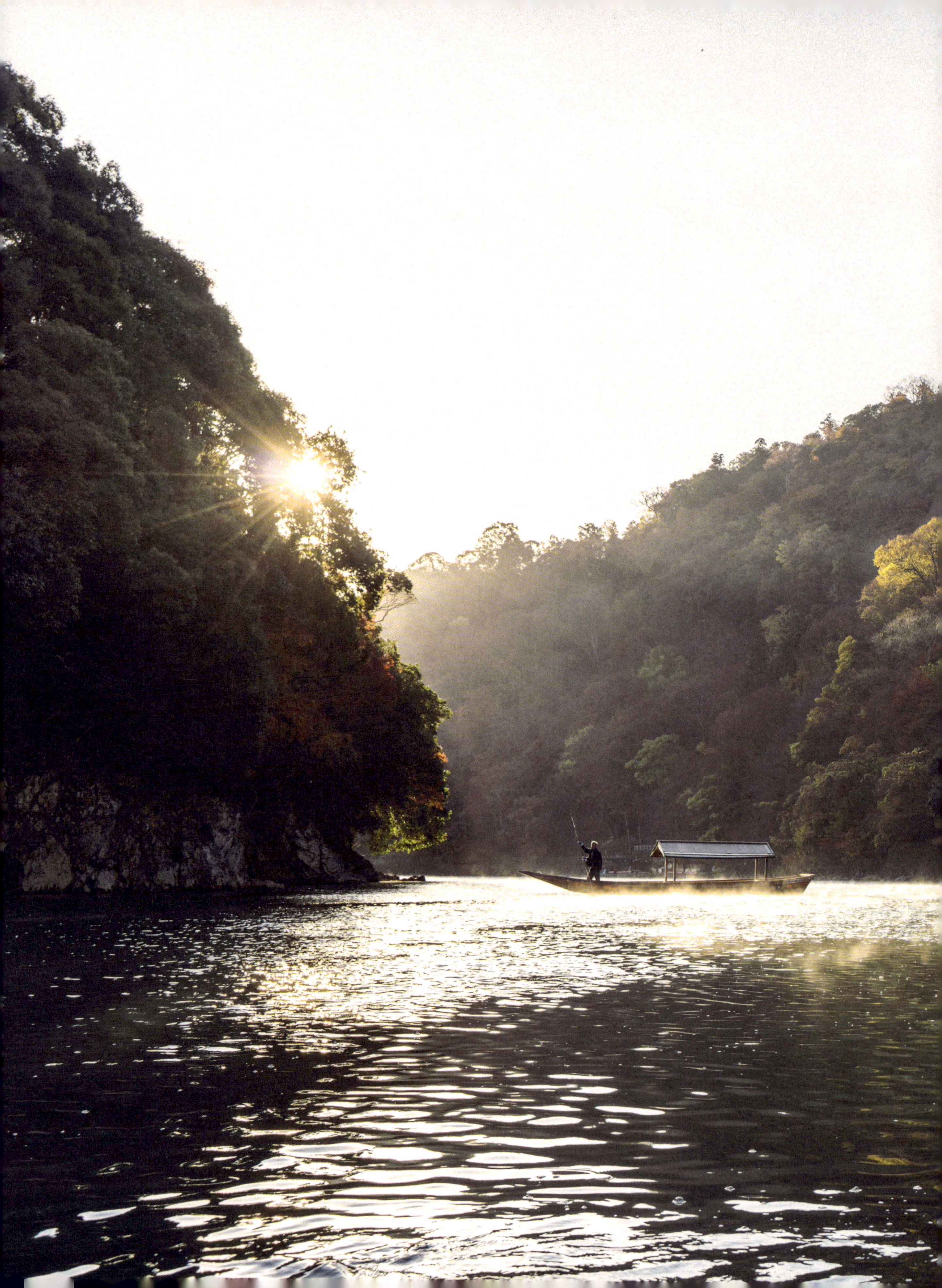

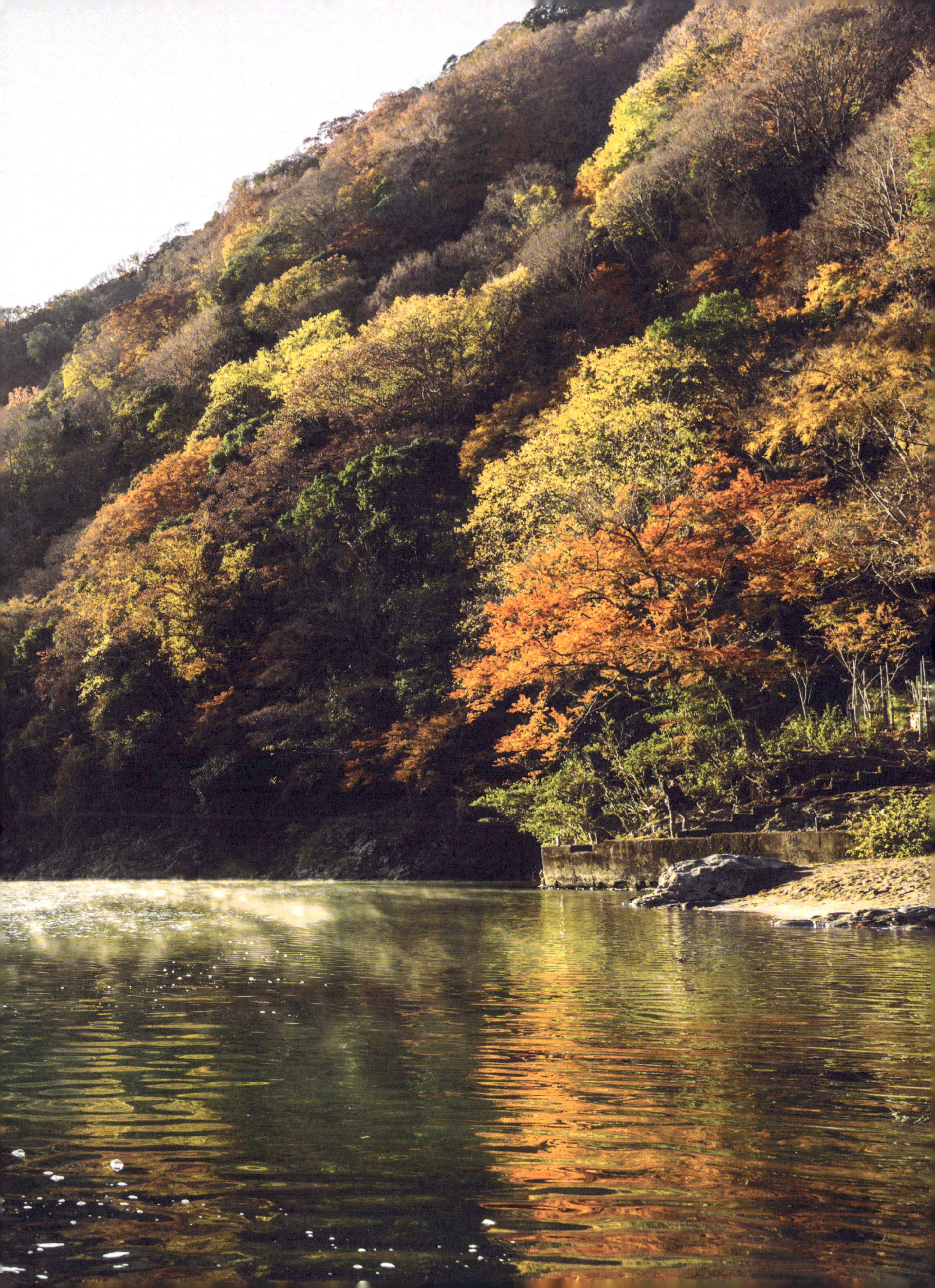

Nishimuraya Honkan
Toyooka ● Hyogo Prefecture

EXPERIENCE A QUINTESSENTIAL JAPANESE *OMOTENASHI* STAY

Perfect for a special occasion, a trip to this gorgeous, traditional onsen ryokan embodies the essence of ancient onsen culture and customs.

The onsen town of Kinosaki is home to one of Japan's most historic and iconic ryokan. Having recently celebrated its 165th anniversary, Nishimuraya Honkan is the longest-running ryokan in Kinosaki. It is currently helmed by the *nanadaime*, or seventh-generation family head, Nishimura Soichiro.

Since the ryokan's inception, the Nishimura family has been instrumental in Kinosaki's history: Nishimura Sahei, the *yondaime* (fourth-generation owner), was the town mayor when the great 1925 earthquake struck. He led the rebuilding of Kinosaki and proclaimed that "so long as there is onsen running in this town, Kinosaki will recover and will thrive." Through his vision, and with support from the community, the town was successfully rebuilt and the commitment to Kinosaki uniting as "one town, one ryokan" was strengthened.

Simply walking the large stone pathway through the entrance gate of Nishimuraya has an immediate effect—you sense that you have entered an ethereal world, steeped in history and stories. As staff in traditional garments bow low to greet you, assisting you in exchanging your shoes for indoor slippers, your gaze will be drawn to the extensive glass windows showcasing the immense garden Nishimuraya encircles. In whichever season one comes to stay, Nishimuraya's gardens will always offer a delicate tableau of natural beauty, from blooming sakura and striking greenery in spring, warm hues in summer and fall, and the white frost of winter.

Many of Nishimuraya's 34 rooms feature gorgeous views of the Japanese garden from their wooden balconies, all offering slightly different perspectives and angles. Relax in the wonderfully spacious living quarters with warm tatami floors, deep wooden beams, and sliding shoji doors. Several of the rooms have picturesque open-air baths; however, in accordance with Kinosaki's town standards, these baths are not technically onsen. The Matsu Suite at Nishimuraya is one of its most stunning rooms; a place where celebrities, politicians, and writers have been known to stay, while Kangetsu no Ma and the annex Hiratakan are renowned as outstanding examples of Sukiya architecture. These structures were built in the 1960s by the famed architect Hirata Masaya, a Sukiya-zukuri master craftsman.

At Nishimuraya, guests can enjoy Kinosaki's renowned onsen culture through the ryokan's public baths, Fuku no Yu and Ichi no Yu. While both have indoor and outdoor onsen, Ichi no Yu is set in a mini bamboo grove with hinoki baths, whereas Fuku no Yu draws from Chinese design, with its use of square stone tiling and rocks. The Hiratakan annex has its own indoor onsen called Shou no Yu, which offers views of Hiratakan's lovely garden.

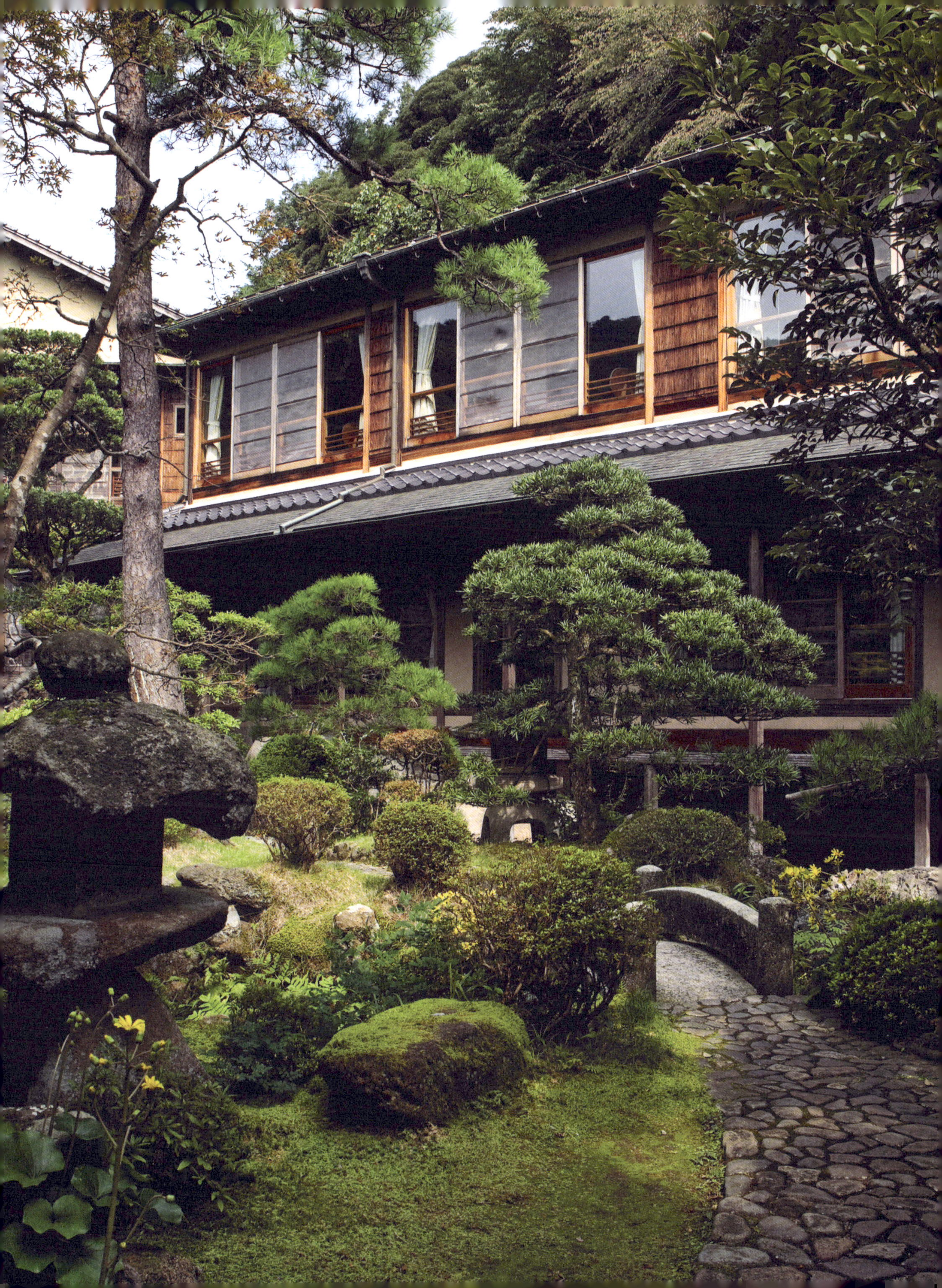

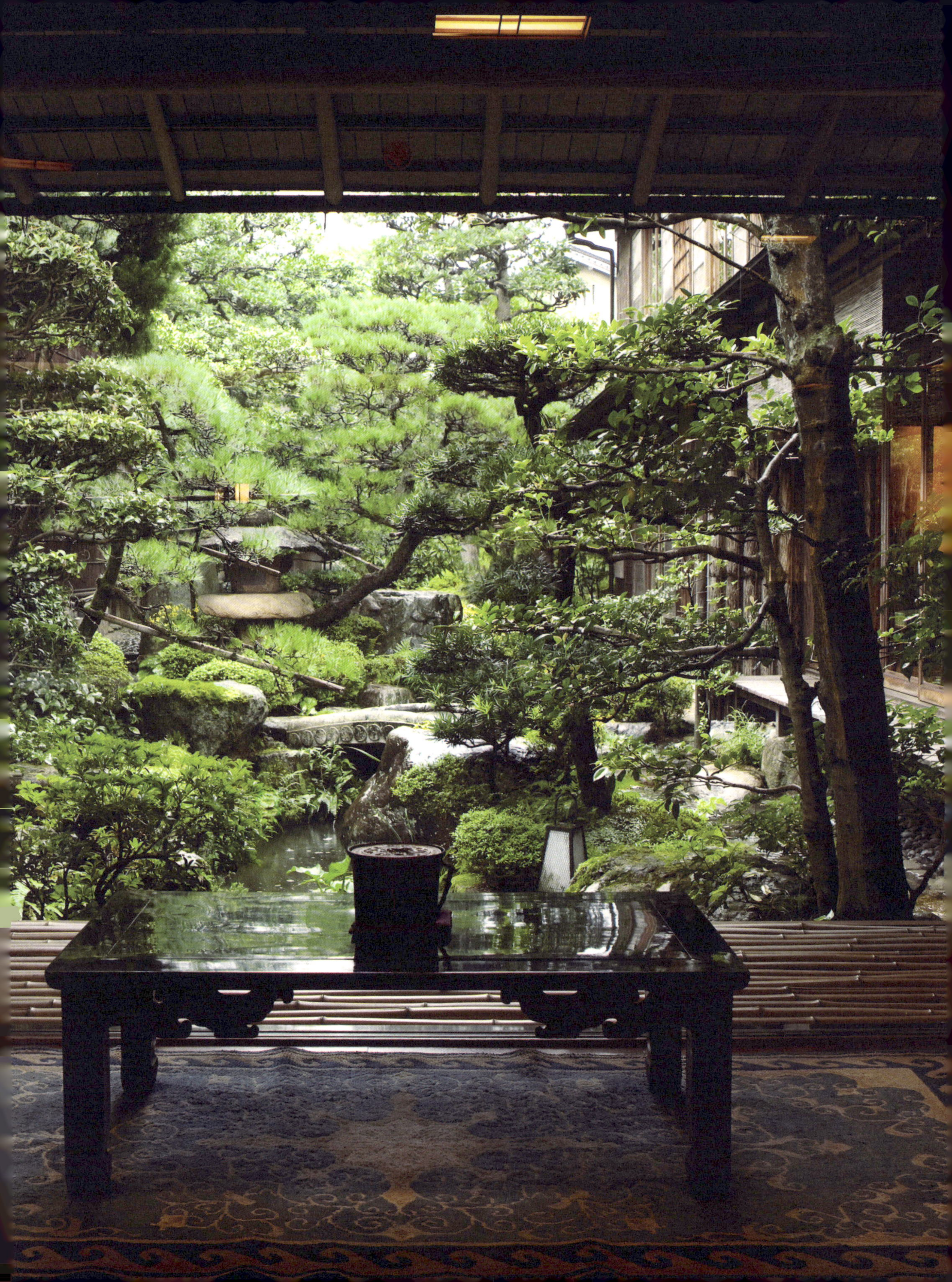

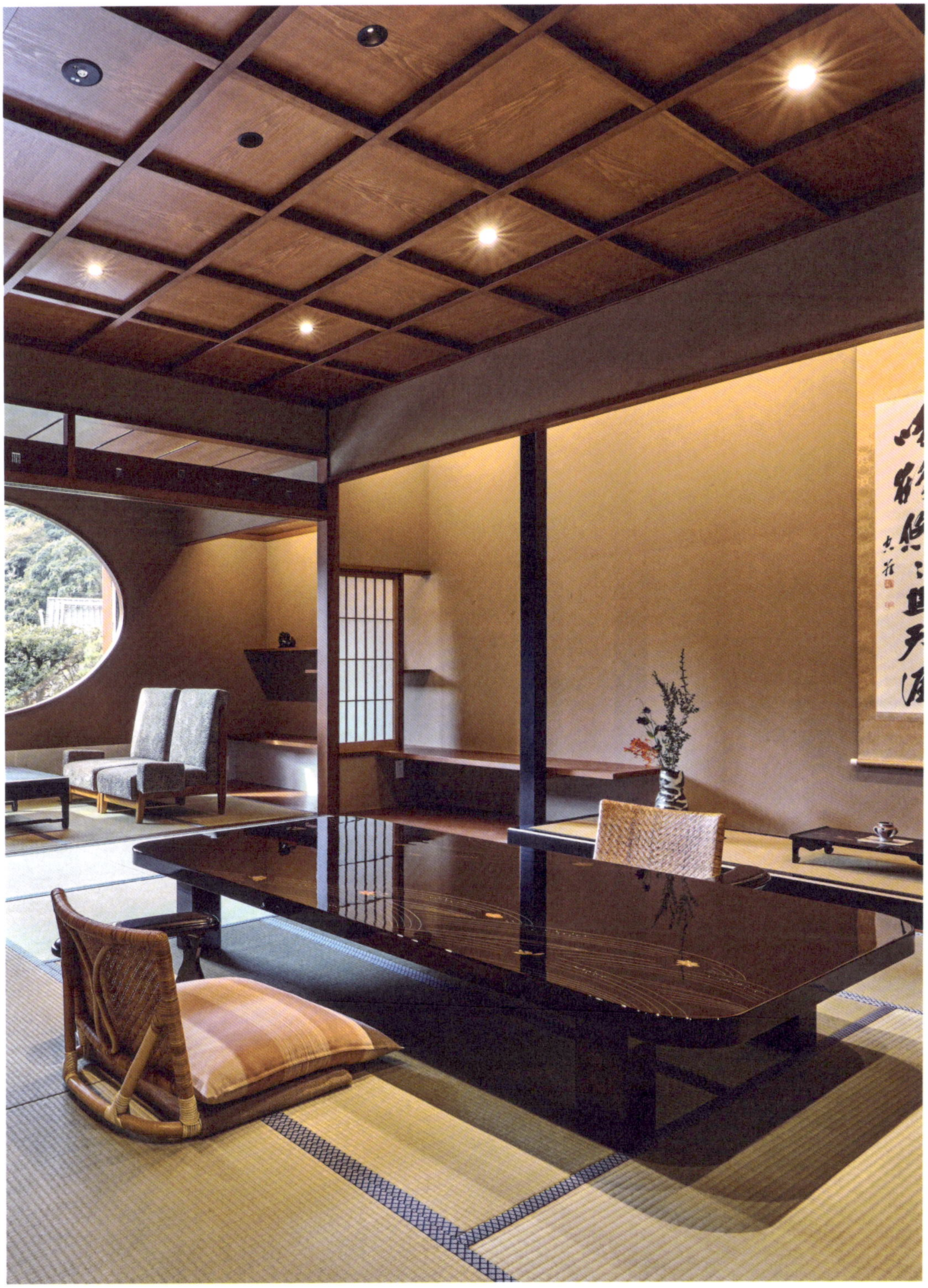

ABOVE Tatami rooms at Nishimuraya Honkan offer a luxurious take on the traditional Japanese stay.

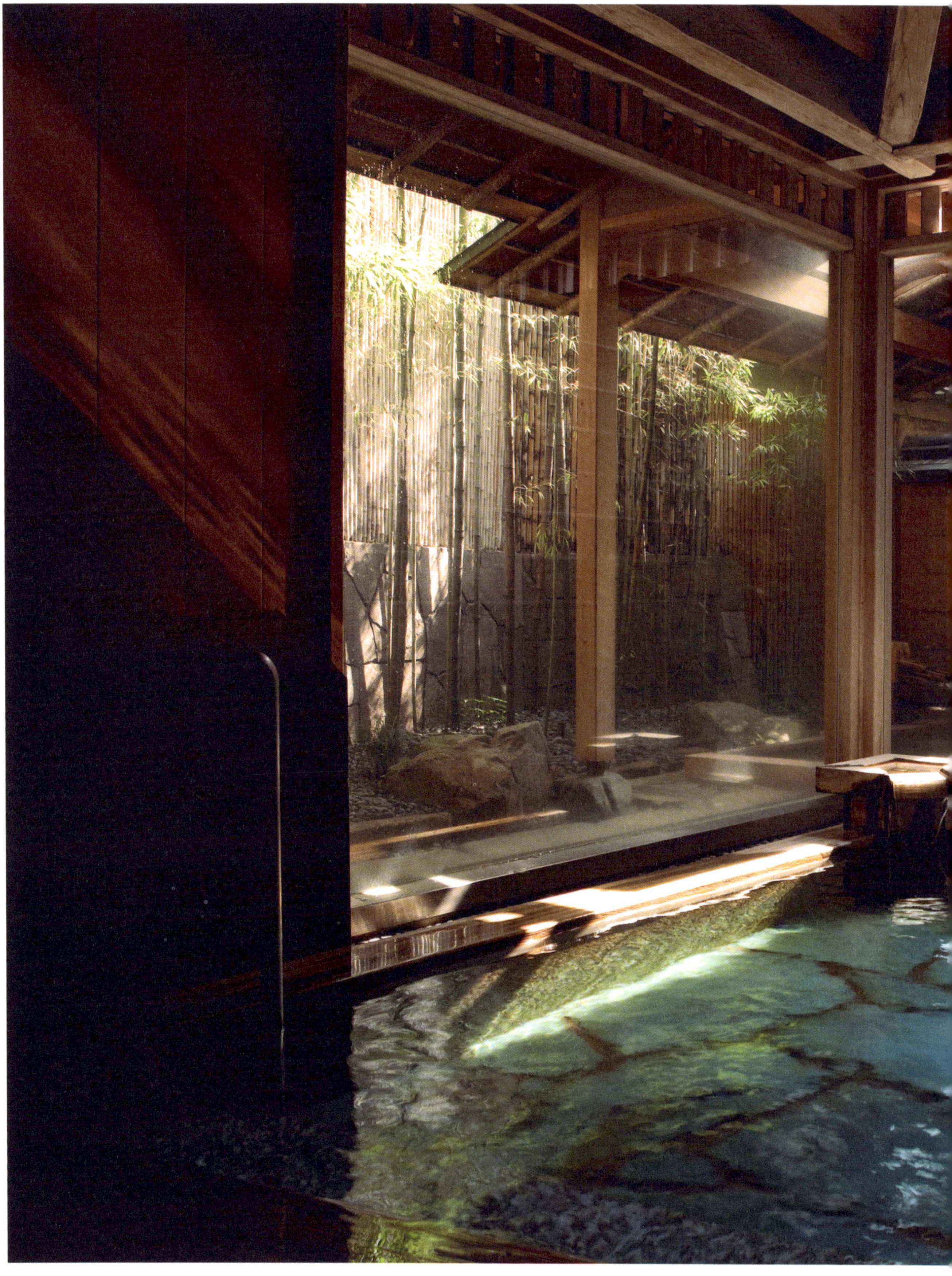

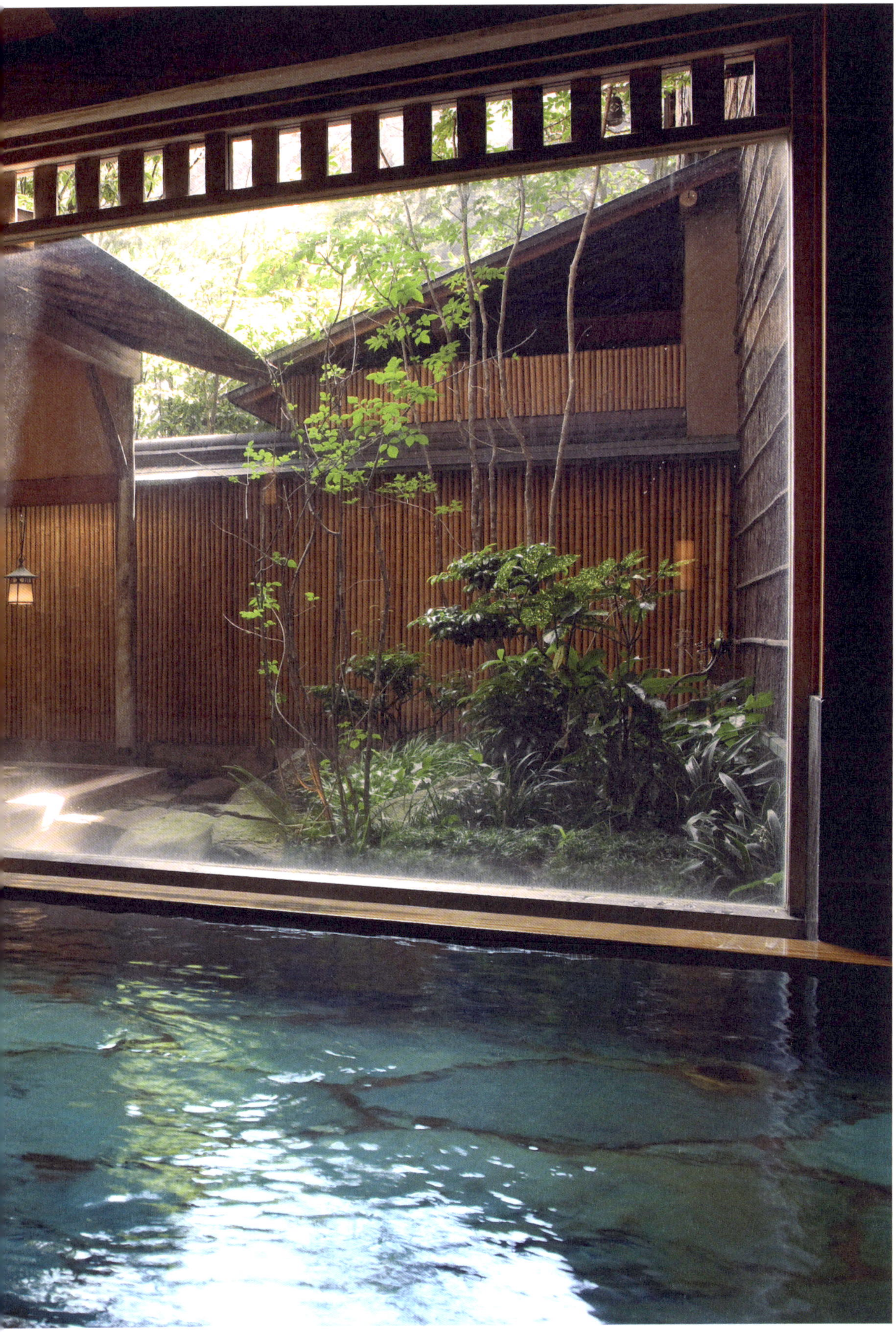

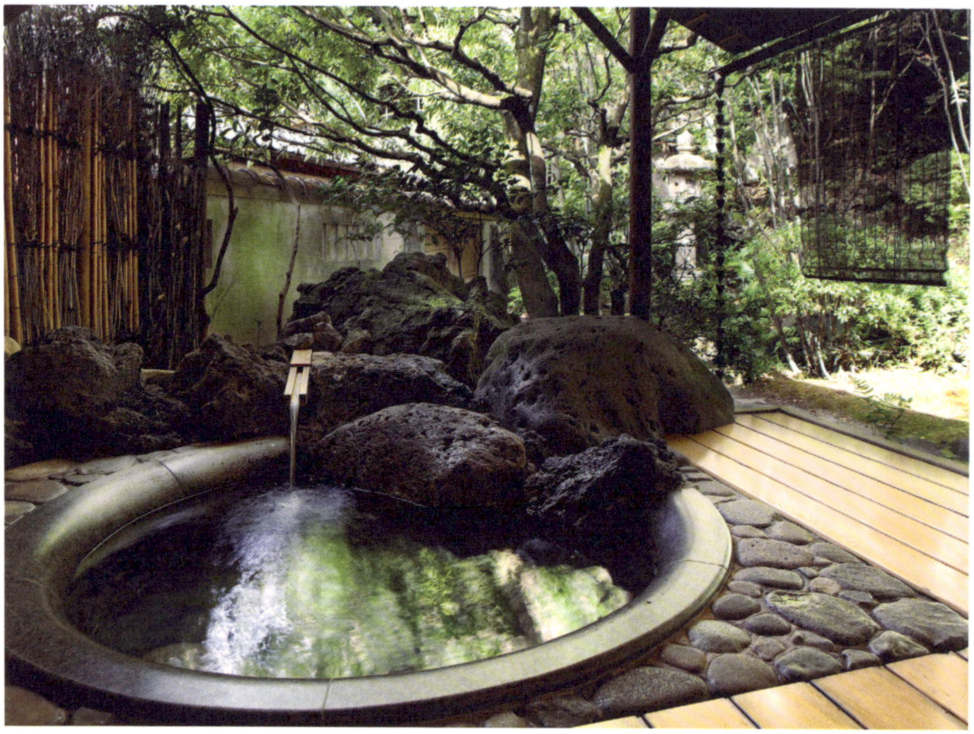

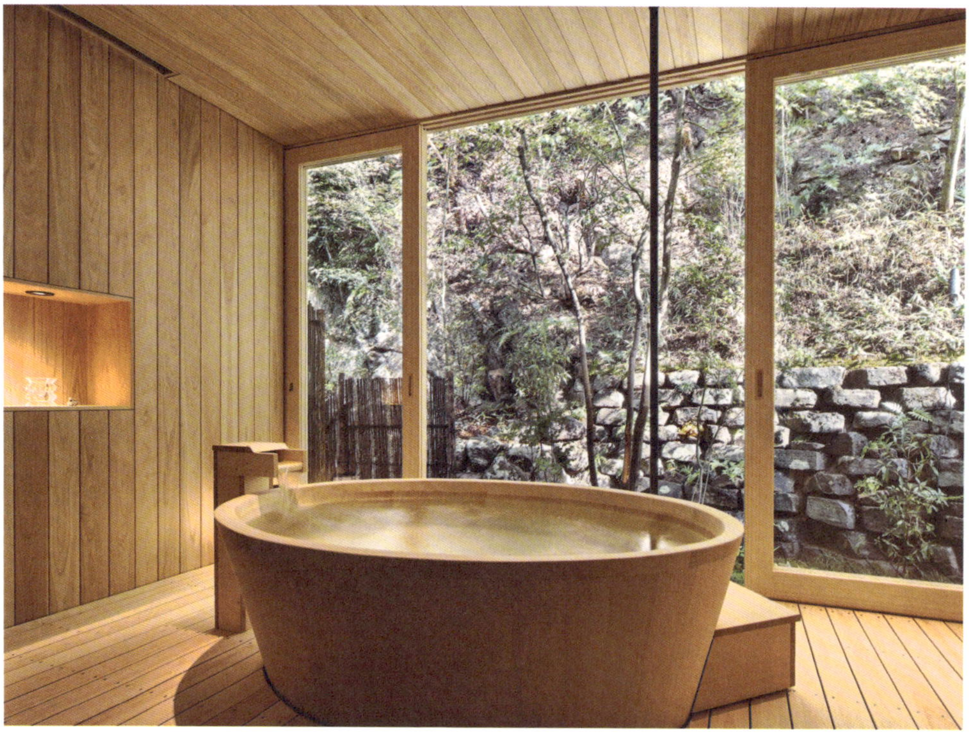

ABOVE AND TOP Private Shigaraki and hinoki baths feature in several rooms.

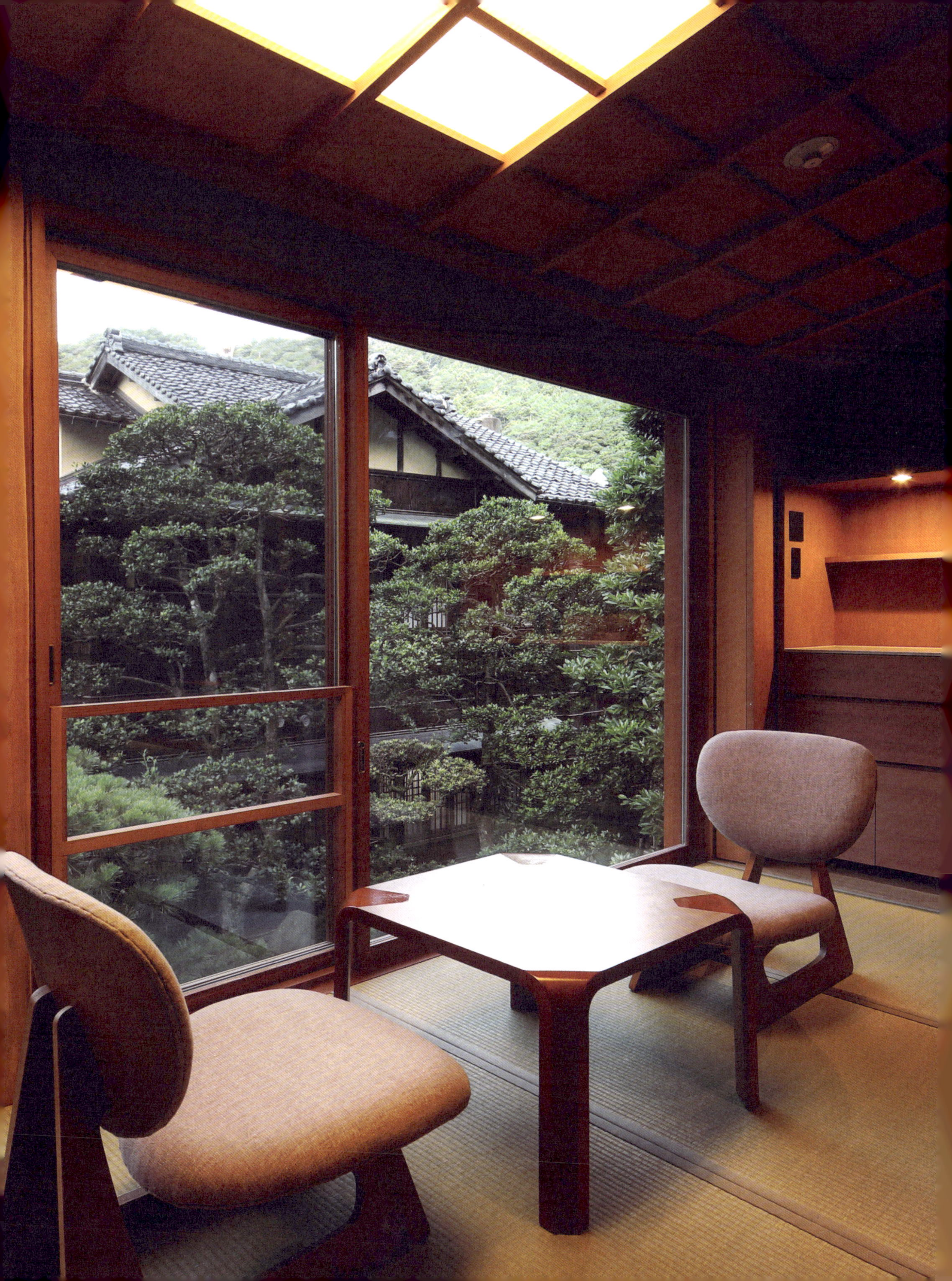

Kamenoi Besso
Yufu • Oita Prefecture

UNWIND AT THE FORMER PRIVATE HAVEN OF A KEY FIGURE IN JAPANESE TOURISM

Detailed luxury, refined sophistication, and timeless elegance await guests at this onsen ryokan in one of Japan's most beautiful onsen towns.

With a rich history dating back over 100 years, Kamenoi Besso within Yufuin Onsen has a special origin story. First opening its doors in 1921, it began life as a private villa for the VIP guests of Kumahachi Aburaya, an important figure in Oita Prefecture history. Known as the founding father of tourism for neighboring Beppu Onsen, it was Kumahachi-san who, after returning to Japan at age 49 from the United States, was inspired to implement his vision of sharing the distinct charms of Kyushu with the Japanese people and the world. It was Kumahachi-san who dreamt up the idea of the now-famous Beppu "hells" tour, which would be imitated across Japan's other Hell Valleys, such as Noboribetsu and Unzen.

Today, Kumahachi-san's private villa has grown to encompass 11 individual cottages and six Western-style rooms spread across a vast forest and garden whose grounds border the shores of the picturesque Lake Kinrin. Both the cottages and rooms are the epitome of luxury, with spacious areas filled with interior elements that fuse Japanese and European design principles. Exquisite Danish design furniture is paired with traditional artisanal pieces, creating a splendid, welcoming, peaceful refuge for guests. Kamenoi Besso's accommodations feature separate areas within the main structure, from comfortable bedrooms to spaces for lounging, relaxing, and sometimes dining. The Japanese-style rooms in the cottages are especially magnificent, as guests will be transported back to a time of old-world luxury, with cozy alcoves, warm tatami floors, sliding shoji doors, and other refined touches.

Whether cottage or room, each accommodation contains its own private indoor or outdoor onsen bath, crafted from Japan's beloved hinoki or hiba wood. Kamenoi Besso's onsen water, which flows into the private onsen baths and the site's grand onsen, streams from beneath the mountains.

Although leaving the luxurious comfort of one's room might prove arduous, guests will certainly want to devote a few hours to Kamenoi Besso's grand bath. Here, they can soak away in the impressive indoor rock bath with sliding doors that open to the outside air, or two outdoor onsen baths—one circular and made of hinoki, the other rectangular. However they choose to spend their stay, guests will likely leave Kamenoi Besso deeply refreshed and rejuvenated in body and soul.

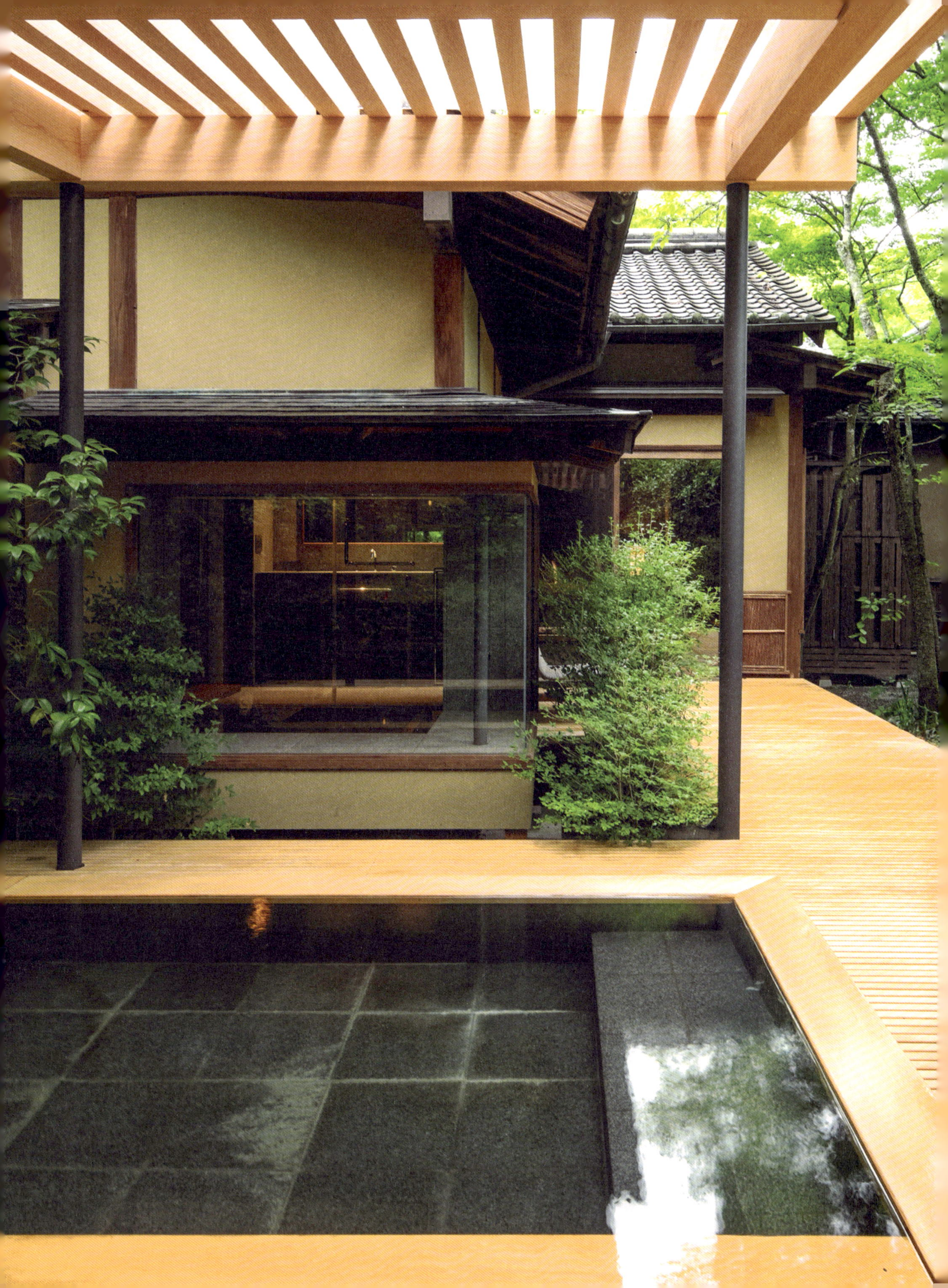

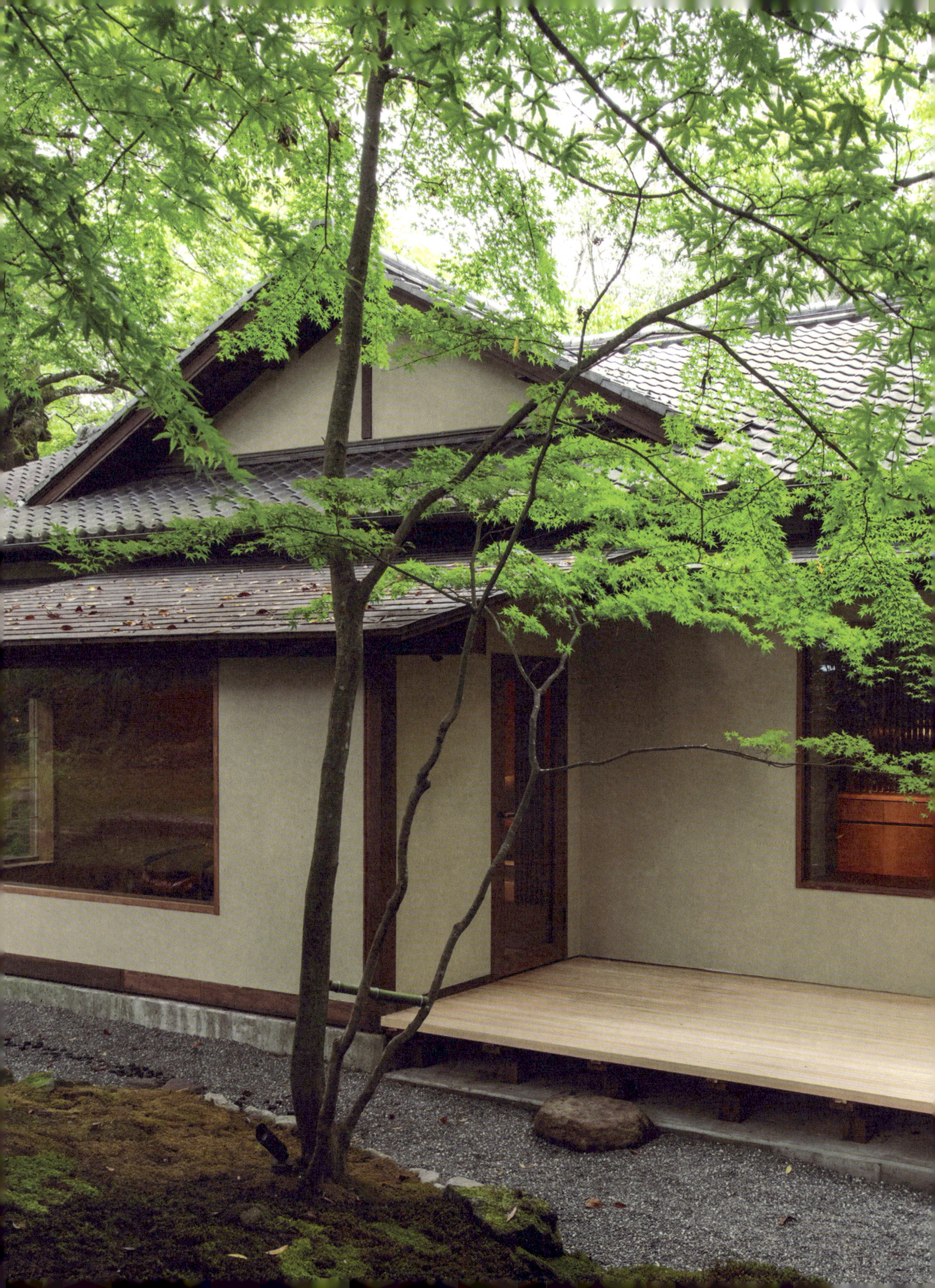

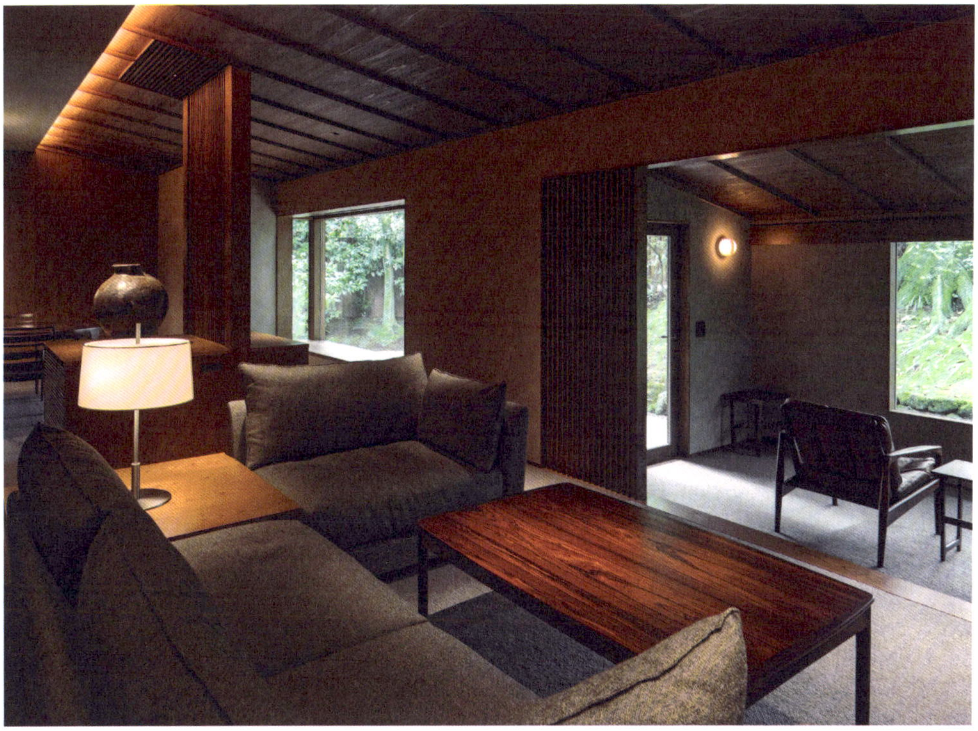

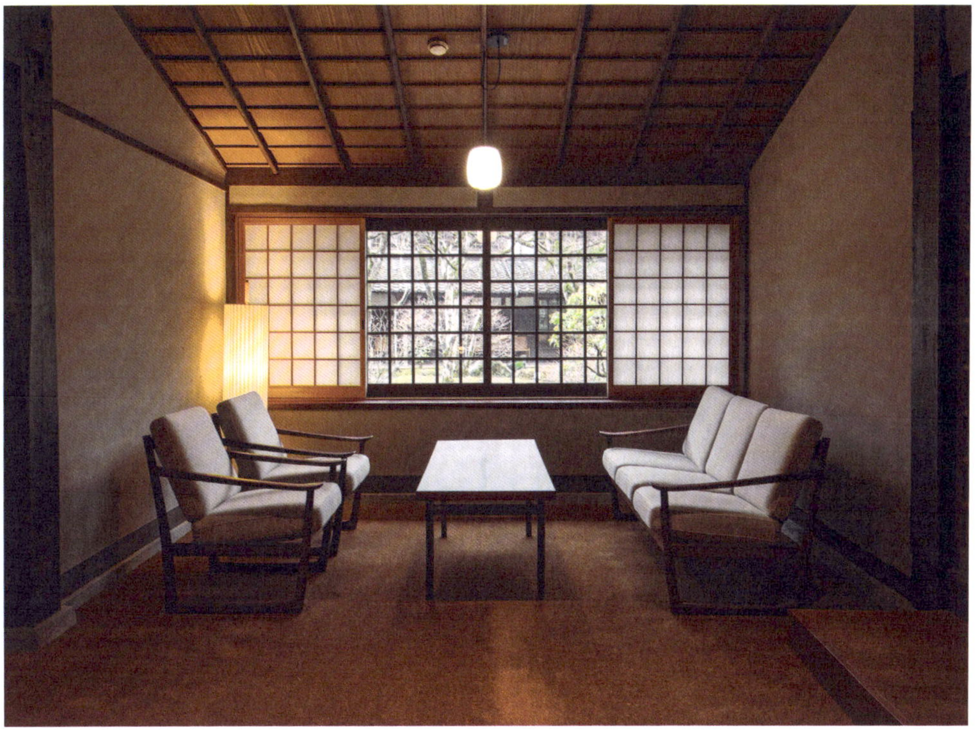

ABOVE AND TOP Elegant, comfortable lounges make guests feel at home.

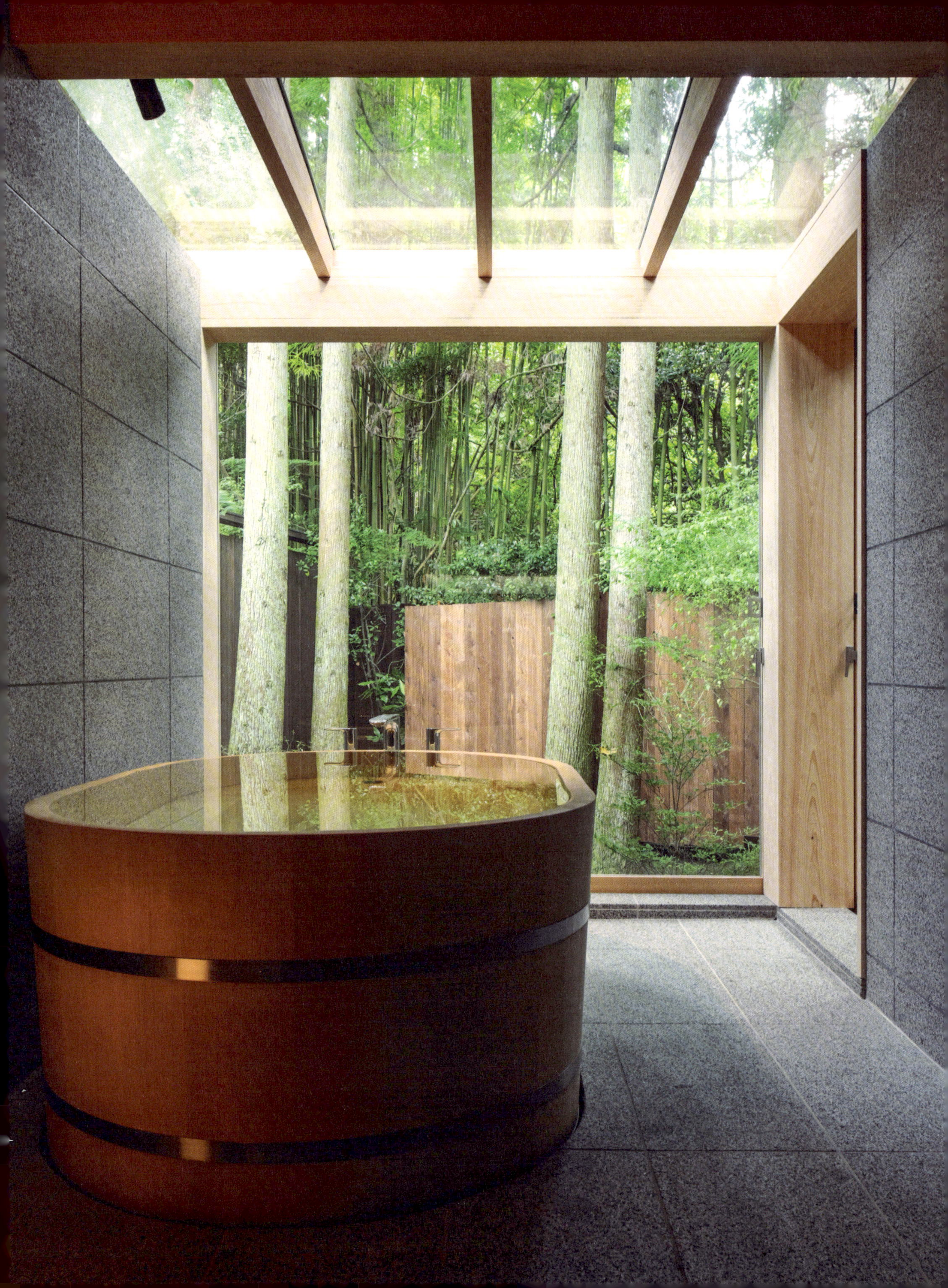

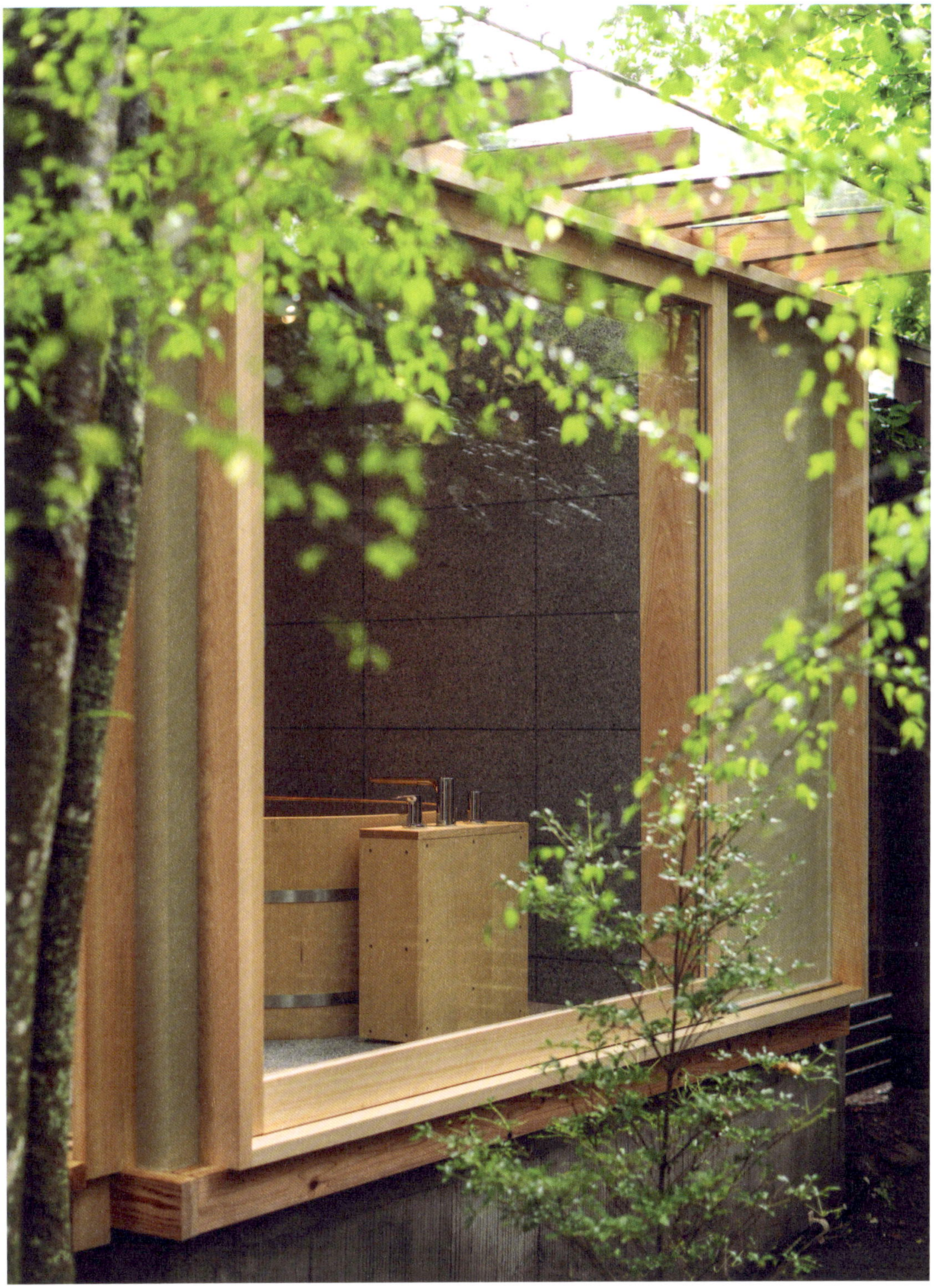

ABOVE AND LEFT Set before wide windows, these spacious hinoki baths create a peaceful ambiance.

Sekizenkan
Nakanojo • Gunma Prefecture

QUIETLY WHILE AWAY THE DAYS IN THIS HISTORIC ONSEN RYOKAN

Believed to have inspired memorable scenes in the acclaimed film *Spirited Away* (*Sen to Chihiro no Kamikakushi*), the iconic red bridge of this ryokan is not to be missed.

In the mountains of Gunma Prefecture lies one of the oldest onsen towns: Shima Onsen. With a history dating back to 989 and designated as the country's first national hot spring resort, Shima Onsen is acclaimed as one of the three best onsen in Gunma and also ranks as one of the top three for healing gastrointestinal diseases.

Shima's name represents the number 40,000, and it is said that its onsen waters can heal some 40,000 diseases. The town's origins are reflected in two legends: the first tells that the onsen was discovered when, during the reign of Emperor Kanmu, Sakanoue no Tamuramaro bathed in its waters when he came to conquer Ezo. The second tells that during the Enryaku era, a vassal named Usui Hyuga no Kami Sadamitsu was reading sutras at night when a child appeared and announced that it was the divine spirit of the mountain and revealed the location of the onsen source.

The town still retains a quaint, nostalgic Showa ambiance, with its roughly 35 onsen ryokan scattered across the land, and none of which are more iconic than Sekizenkan. With a history dating back some 300 years, Sekizenkan is one of Shima's oldest ryokan, spread over three buildings that each showcase distinct eras of Japanese historic architecture and design. Currently managed by its 19th-generation family head, the ryokan has been owned by a family that traces its roots back to samurai Sato, whose descendant Sato Higonokami Kiyotada was given the surname Seki by the shogun Minamoto no Yoritomo.

Built in 1691, Honkan, the main building, is one of the oldest existing forms of Japanese *yuyado* architecture and, along with its vivid red bridge, is thought to be an inspiration for Yubaba's bathhouse in Miyazaki Hayao's *Spirited Away.* A stay at Honkan, where simple tatami rooms invite guests to lay out their own futons and dine on seasonal *kaiseki* meals, allows one to experience the old onsen *toji* ways. The ryokan's indoor onsen, Genroku no Yu, is evocative of the luxurious Taisho Roman architectural style popular at the time.

Beyond Honkan lies Sanso, a romantic mountain lodge built in the gorgeous Momoyama era architectural style, where guests can appreciate the lavish and intricate skills of Japanese carving and craftsmanship. Both Honkan and Sanso are designated cultural heritage properties.

Further luxury can be found in the third building, Kashotei, which unites the beauty of both traditional and modern Japanese aesthetics. Kashotei is where guests can also find the superb open-air onsen Mori no Yu, surrounded by gorgeous greenery. Both Sanso and Kashotei have reservable private onsen, and several rooms even contain their own onsen baths.

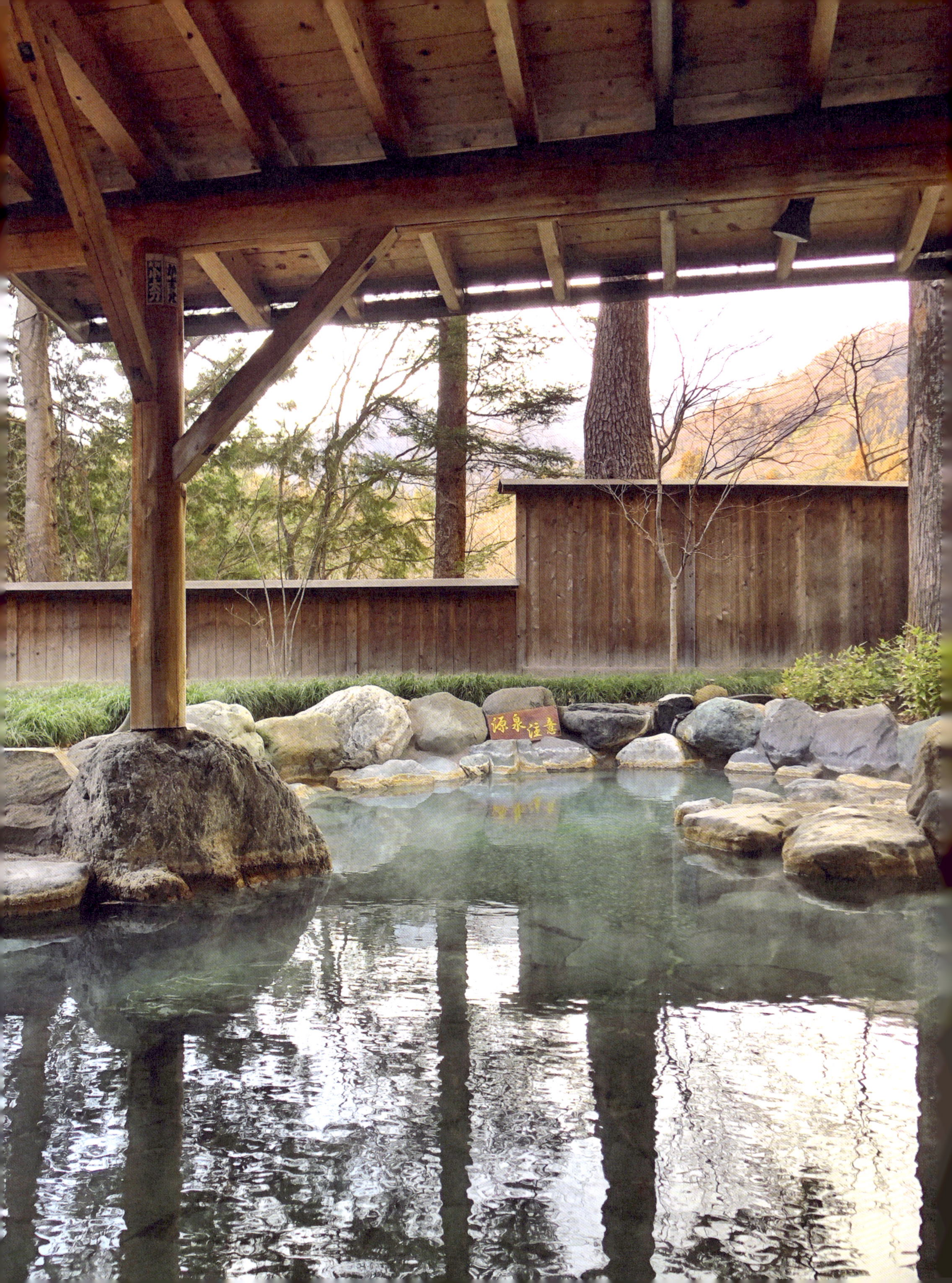
源泉注意

Fukiya Ryokan
Yugawara • Kanagawa Prefecture

A STYLISH, TASTEFUL DESTINATION FOR A WEEKEND GETAWAY

Treat yourself at this beautiful, family-run onsen ryokan not far from Tokyo, which offers spacious, luxurious rooms and superb onsen.

A short train ride from Shinjuku or Tokyo deposits one at the doorstep of Yugawara Onsen. Lying roughly midway between the popular onsen towns of Hakone and Atami, the quaint Yugawara provides a more tranquil, peaceful atmosphere devoid of crowds. Yugawara Onsen's history dates back to the Nara period when the town was mentioned as a place of healing in the *Man'yōshū*, Japan's oldest surviving anthology of *waka* poetry. Yugawara Onsen's beloved waters are known as Yakushi no Yu (medicine bath), and, over the years, the town has been host to countless onsen lovers, notable writers, and artists all seeking the onsen's healing properties.

Multiple ryokan are found throughout the onsen town, which follows the Chitose River and is especially beautiful in spring when the sakura bloom along its riverbanks. One of Yugawara's classiest, most beautiful onsen ryokan is undoubtedly Fukiya Ryokan. Founded in 1935, this elegant ryokan is perched on a gentle hillside and features 18 guest rooms, each reflecting one of seven distinct architectural or design styles. Currently helmed by the third-generation family head (*sandaime*) Okami Yamamoto-san, Fukiya Ryokan is named after the area's resilient *fuki* (butterbur) leaves.

A stay at Fukiya is an utterly serene, peaceful experience. Providing a retreat from the hustle and bustle of the city, the spacious tatami rooms have been tastefully designed utilizing techniques of Sukiya-zukuri architecture. Traditional touches honoring Japan's rich past include sliding shoji doors, cozy *tokonomas*, and intricate wooden patterns, all paired with modern comforts. Many of the rooms also feature their own indoor hinoki baths with onsen-sourced water.

Guests can also enjoy a mini onsen *meguri* within Fukiya Ryokan. There are three private, open-air onsen located on the ryokan's rooftop, that guests are free to reserve. The rooftop also offers an open terrace area with comfortable lounge seats from which bathers can dip their feet into onsen footbaths. The third open-air onsen is a charming, ovular wooden tub facing the landscaped garden and towering mountains that can be reserved once during one's stay for 40 minutes. More gorgeous seasonal scenes can be savored at the ryokan's public onsen: both feature an indoor bath with wide windows and an outdoor rock *rotenburo* bordered by lush nature. In spring, the larger *rotenburo* acts as a gorgeous *sakuramiburo*, or sakura-viewing bath.

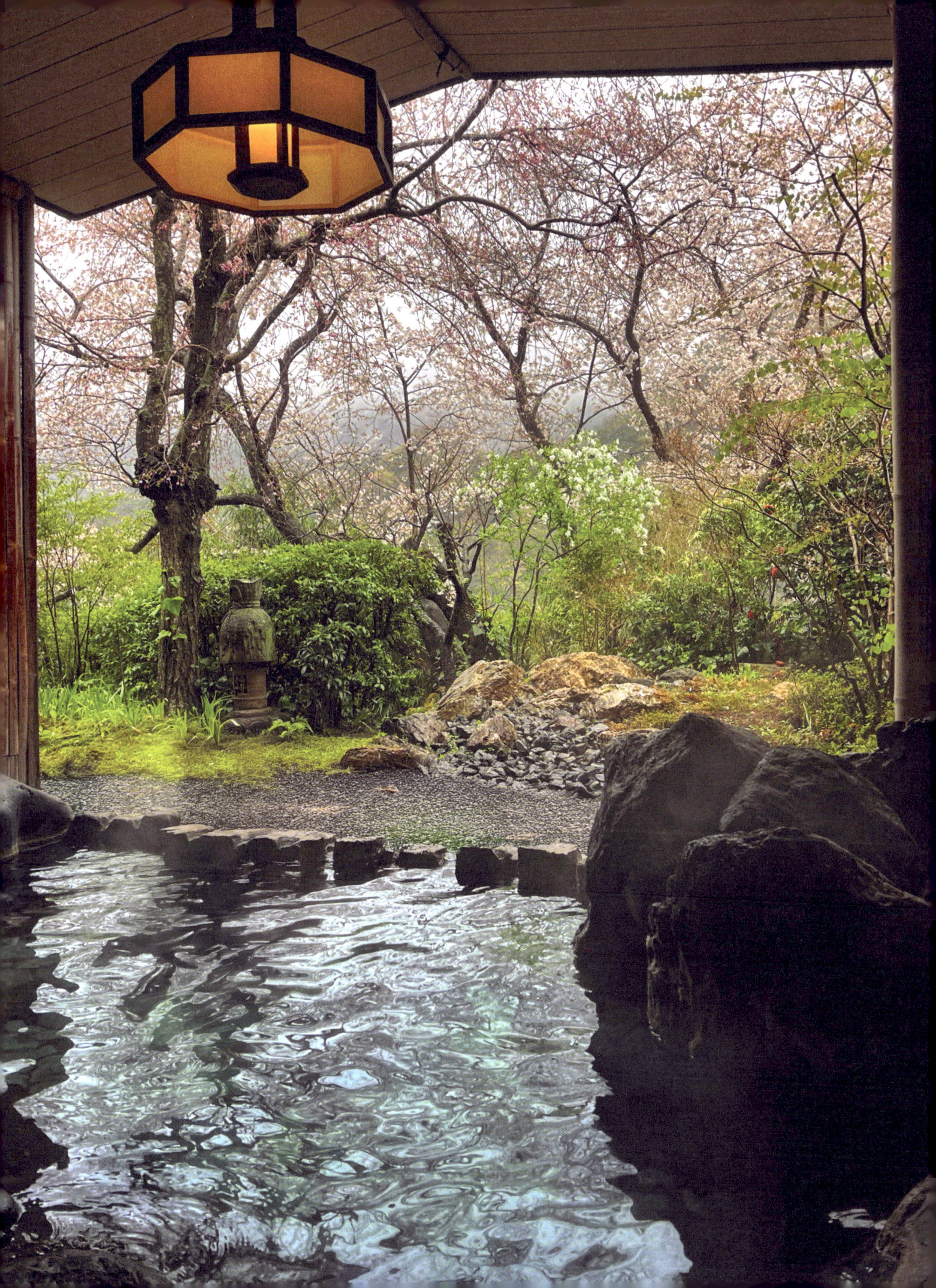

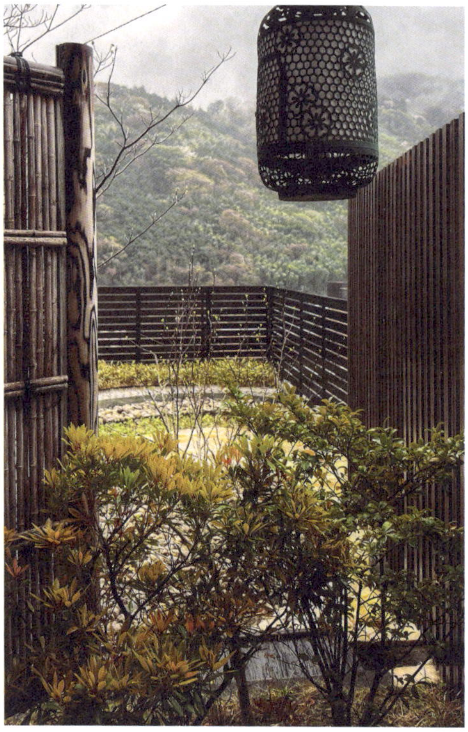

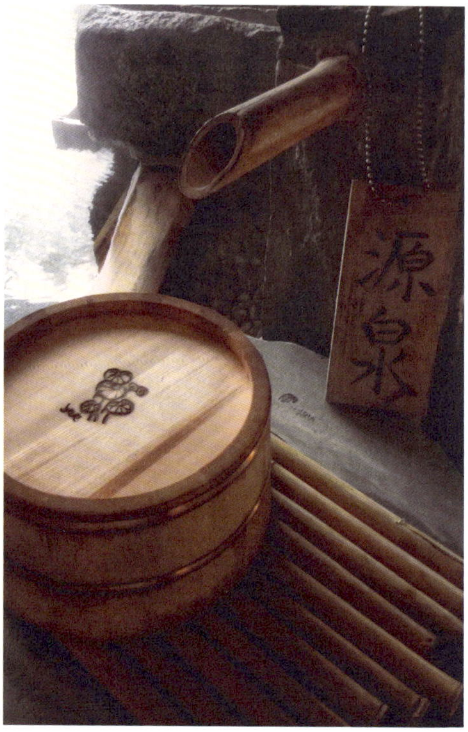

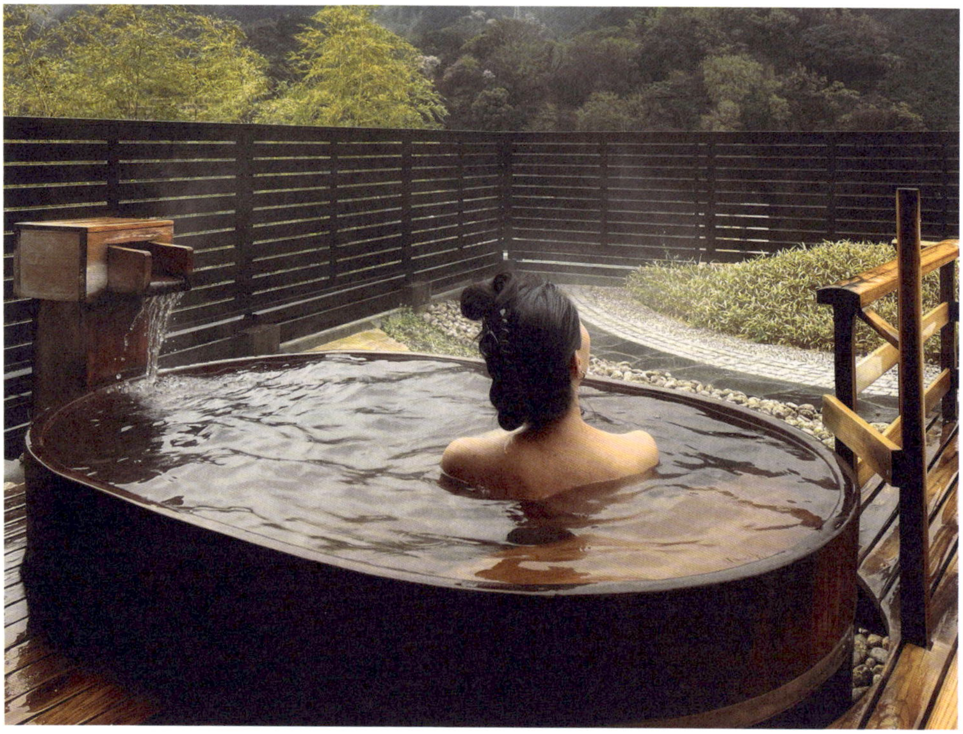

RIGHT The pretty grounds of Fukusenji, a nearby temple, offer the perfect place for a stroll.

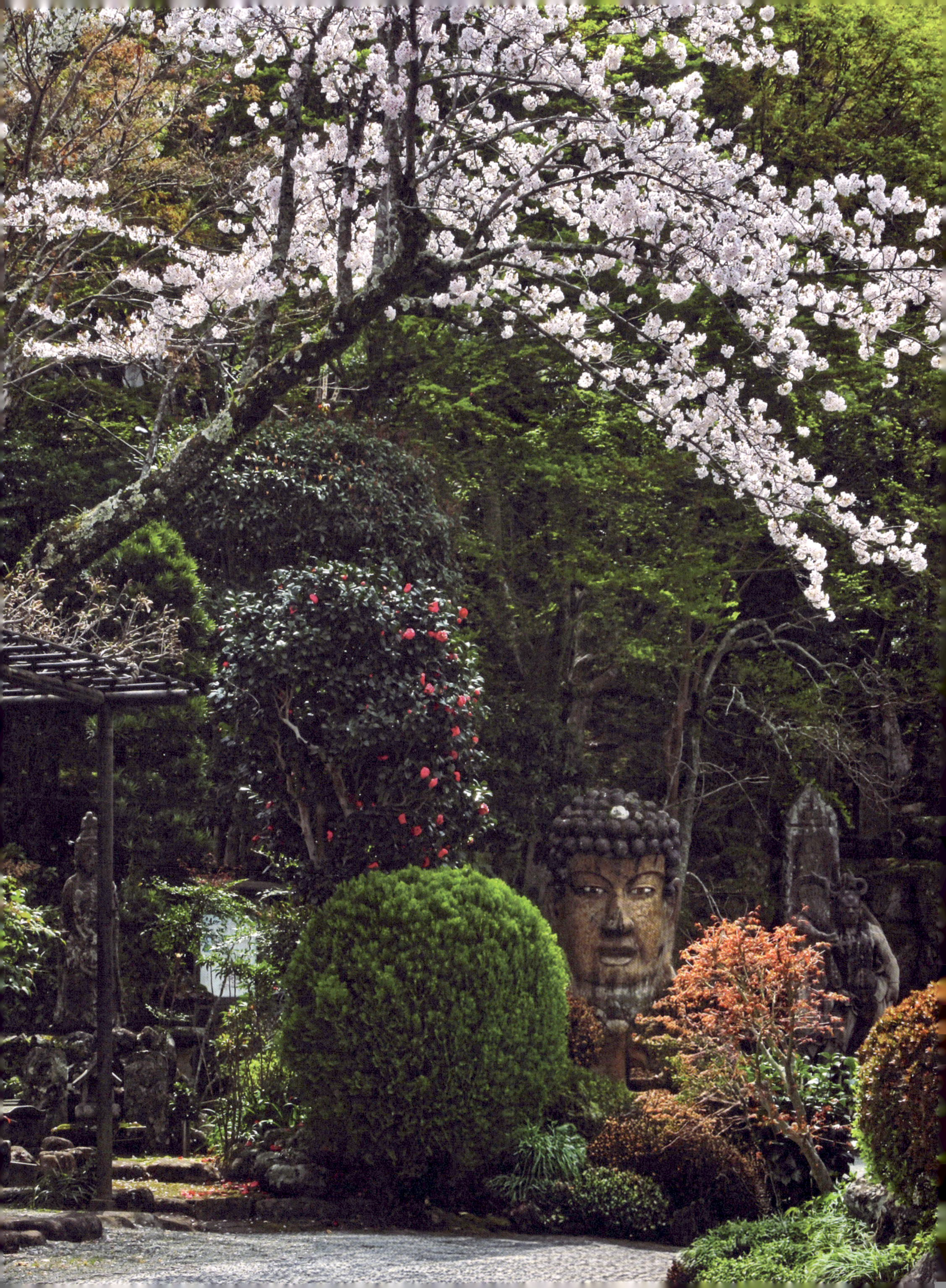

Nagato Yumoto Onsen
Nagato Yumoto • Yamaguchi Prefecture

A PICTURESQUE SETTING ENLIVENED BY CHERRY BLOSSOMS

Meander along the promenade of the oldest onsen town in Yamaguchi, resplendent with natural beauty and charming river stepping stones.

Local folklore tells the tale of the sea god Sumiyoshi Daimyojin, who revealed himself to the high priest Joan Shuzen (of nearby Taineiji Temple) in the guise of an elderly man. Sumiyoshi foretold that south of Taineiji, the high priest would come across a wondrous onsen source that would spill forth miraculous healing water from the rock's natural surface. It is said that loud, roaring thunder reverberated through the skies when the onsen source was discovered, and that the great sea god vanished from the earth in the form of an extraordinary dragon.

Nagato Yumoto Onsen prospered throughout the ruling years of the Ouchi and Mori clans, and in the subsequent Edo, Meiji, and Showa periods, it became a favorite onsen destination among travelers. A period of decline ensued during the Heisei period (1989–2019), as changes in travel and lifestyle led to the closing of the town's beloved public onsen, Onto, in 2017. Resolved to save his hometown, fifth-generation onsen ryokan owner Otani Kazuhiro revived Onto in 2020 with a new contemporary design, preserving the site's bathing traditions for future generations.

The Onto bathhouse is the beating heart of Nagato Yumoto and the town's central landmark. Built directly above the onsen source Moto-yu, Onto offers visitors a chance to experience the onsen flowing directly out of the bedrock. Its simple alkaline waters with a pH value of 9.62 distinguish the onsen as *bijin-no-yu*. Within the bathhouse, guests can also view the *shimenawa* (holy straw rope), which separates the onsen from the bedrock and lies in front of the enshrined stone statue of Sumiyoshi Daimyojin.

One of Japan's most attractive, yet lesser-known onsen towns, Onto awaits visitors at the end of a path that leads them down steps and through a swaying bamboo forest. Days can be spent by the riverside, relaxing on one of the many Kawadoko River terraces, soaking one's feet in the town's outdoor onsen footbaths, or strolling down the wide walking promenades bordered by weeping willows, overhanging sakura trees, and playful river stepping stones.

Many travelers will include a visit to neighboring Tawarayama Onsen, beloved for its retro Showa atmosphere, quaint traditional ryokan, rich onsen *toji* history, drinkable onsen waters, and the famed therapeutic onsen, Machi no Yu.

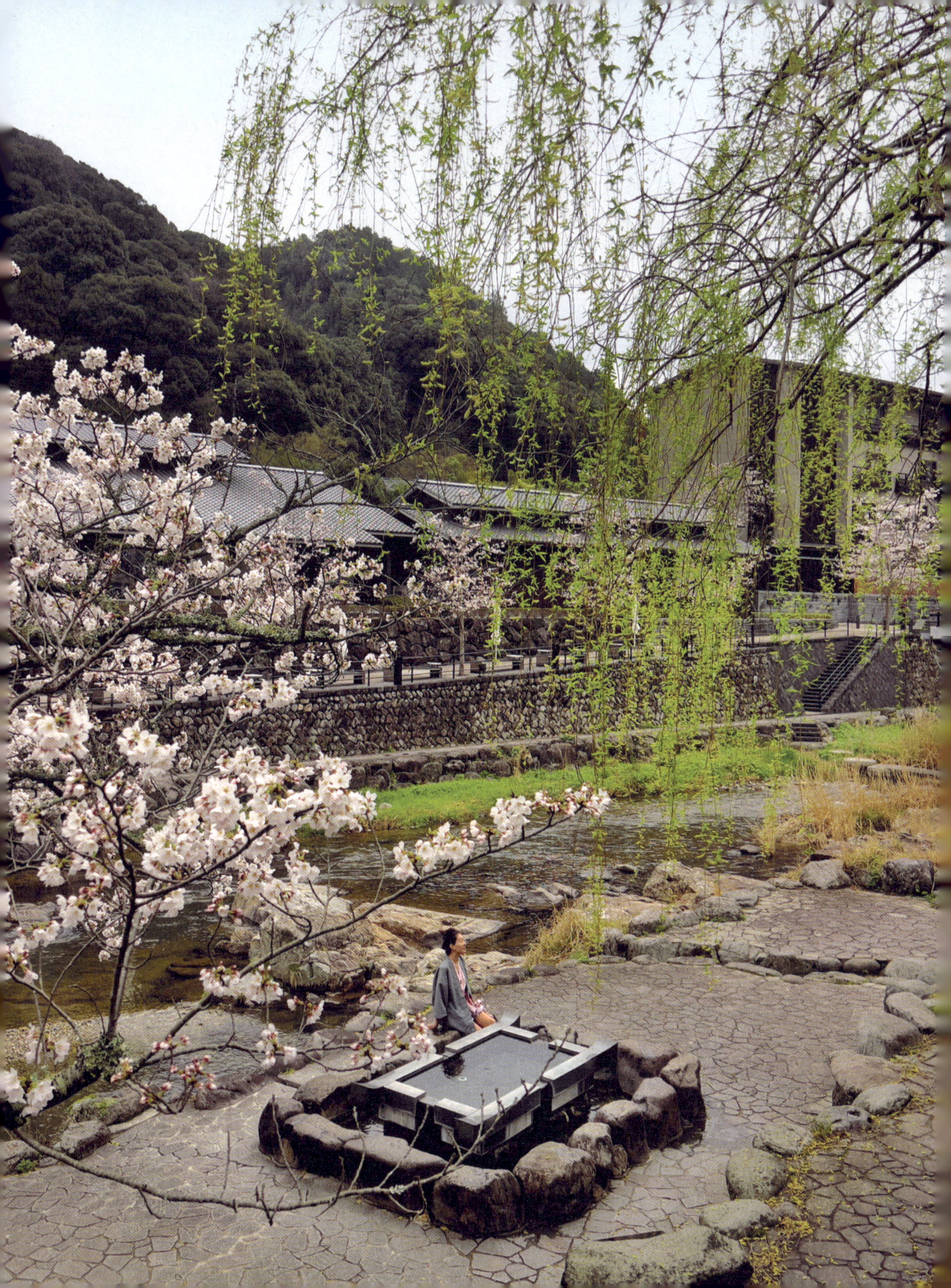

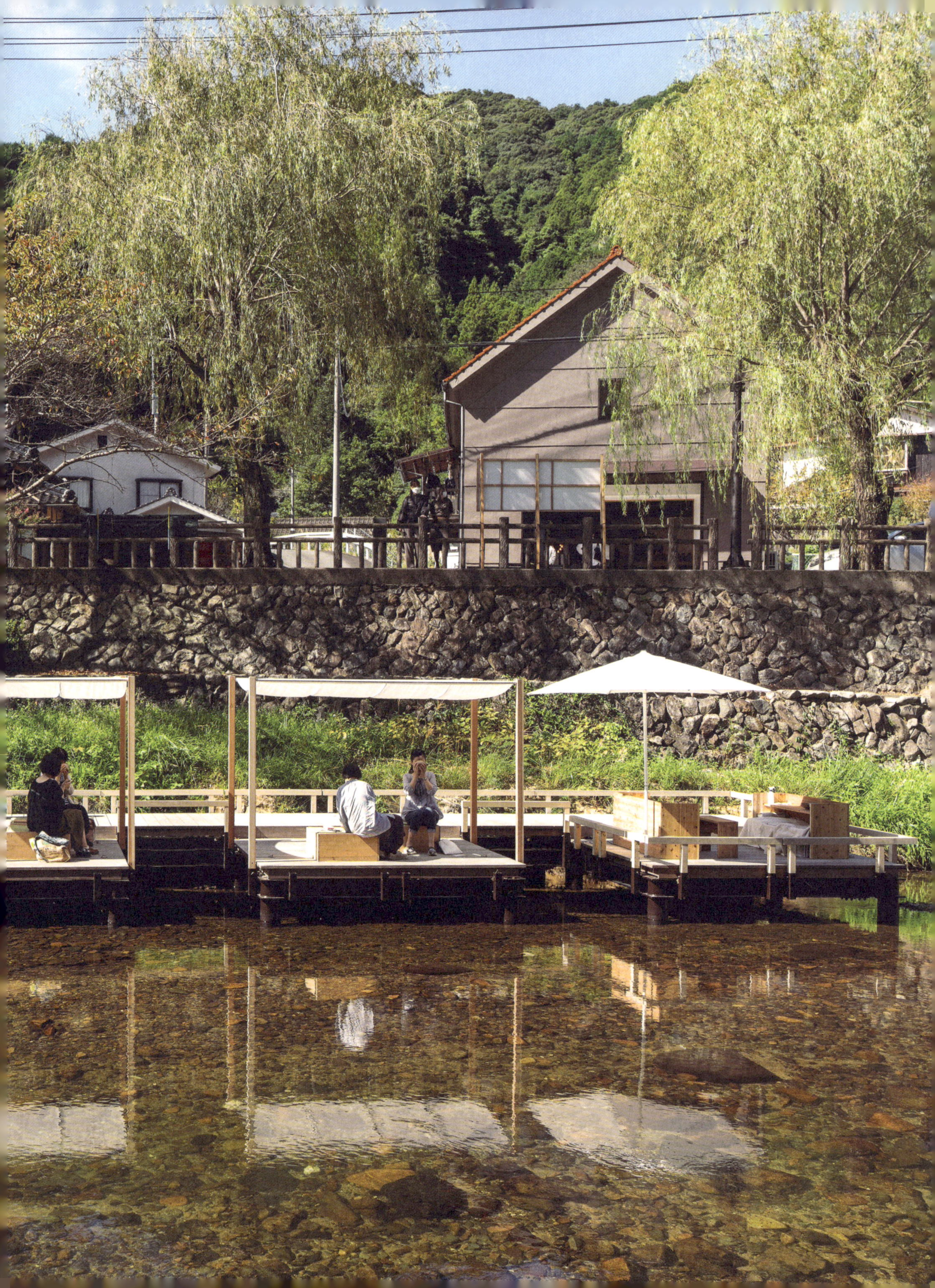

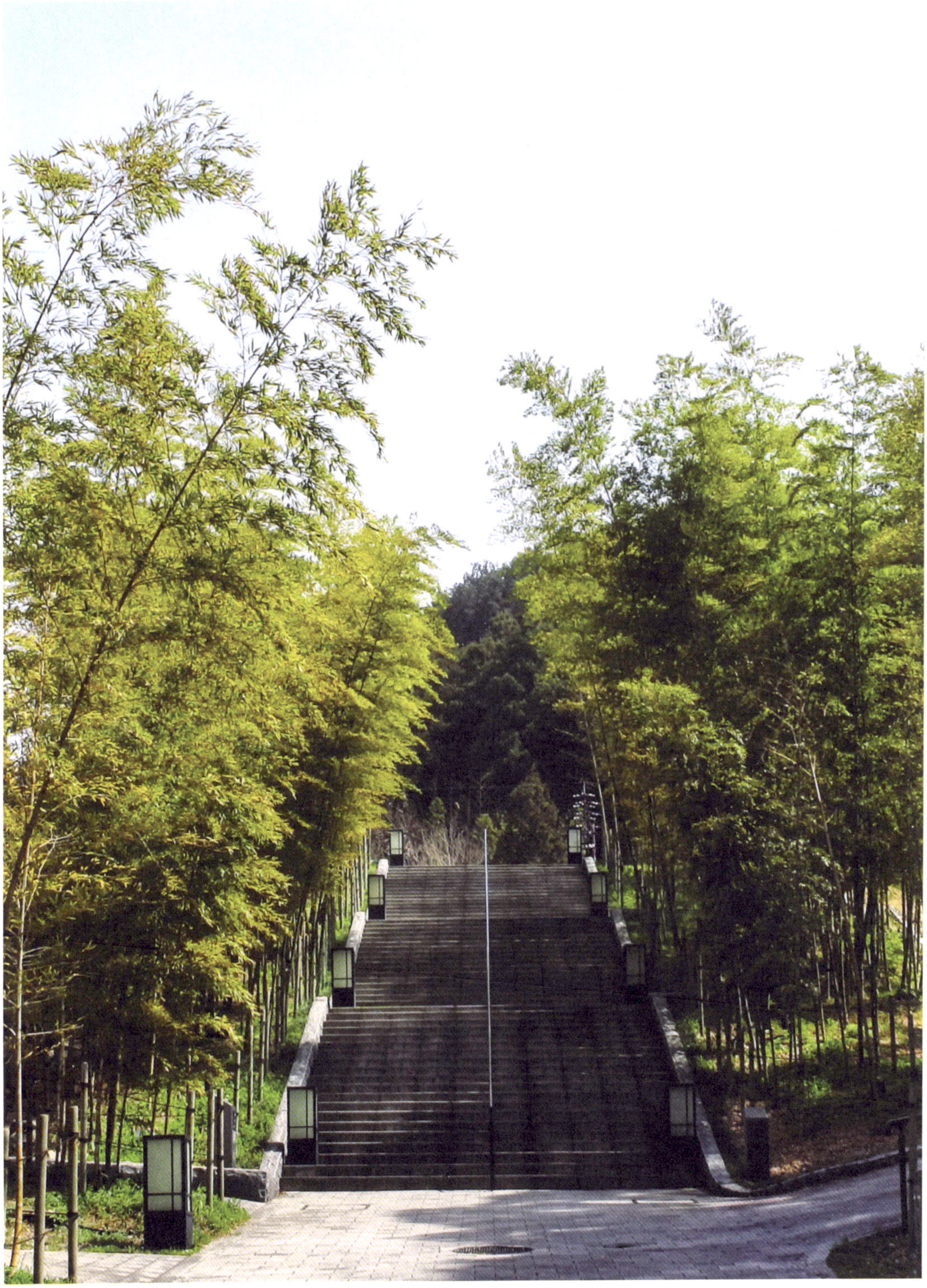

LEFT Relax on one of the many "Kawadoko" terraces lining the Otozure River.

Kinosaki Onsen
Toyooka ● Hyogo Prefecture

JAPAN'S MOST TATTOO-FRIENDLY ONSEN TOWN

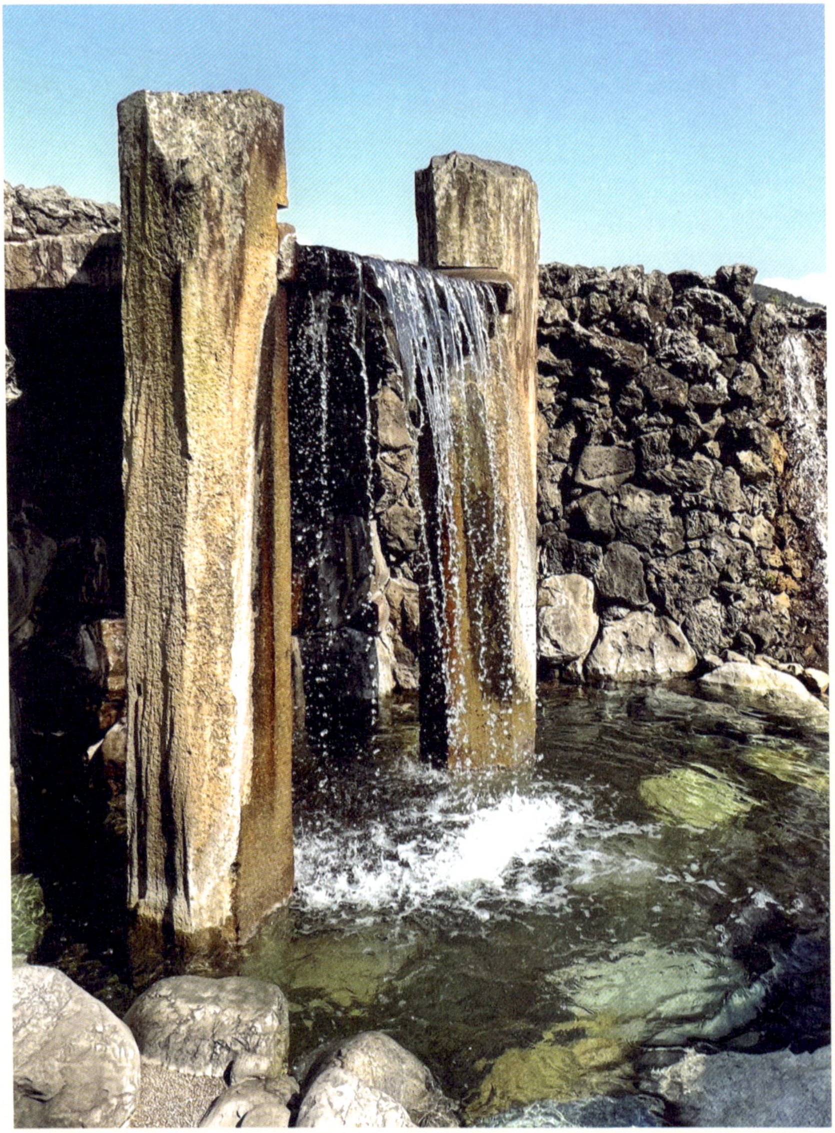

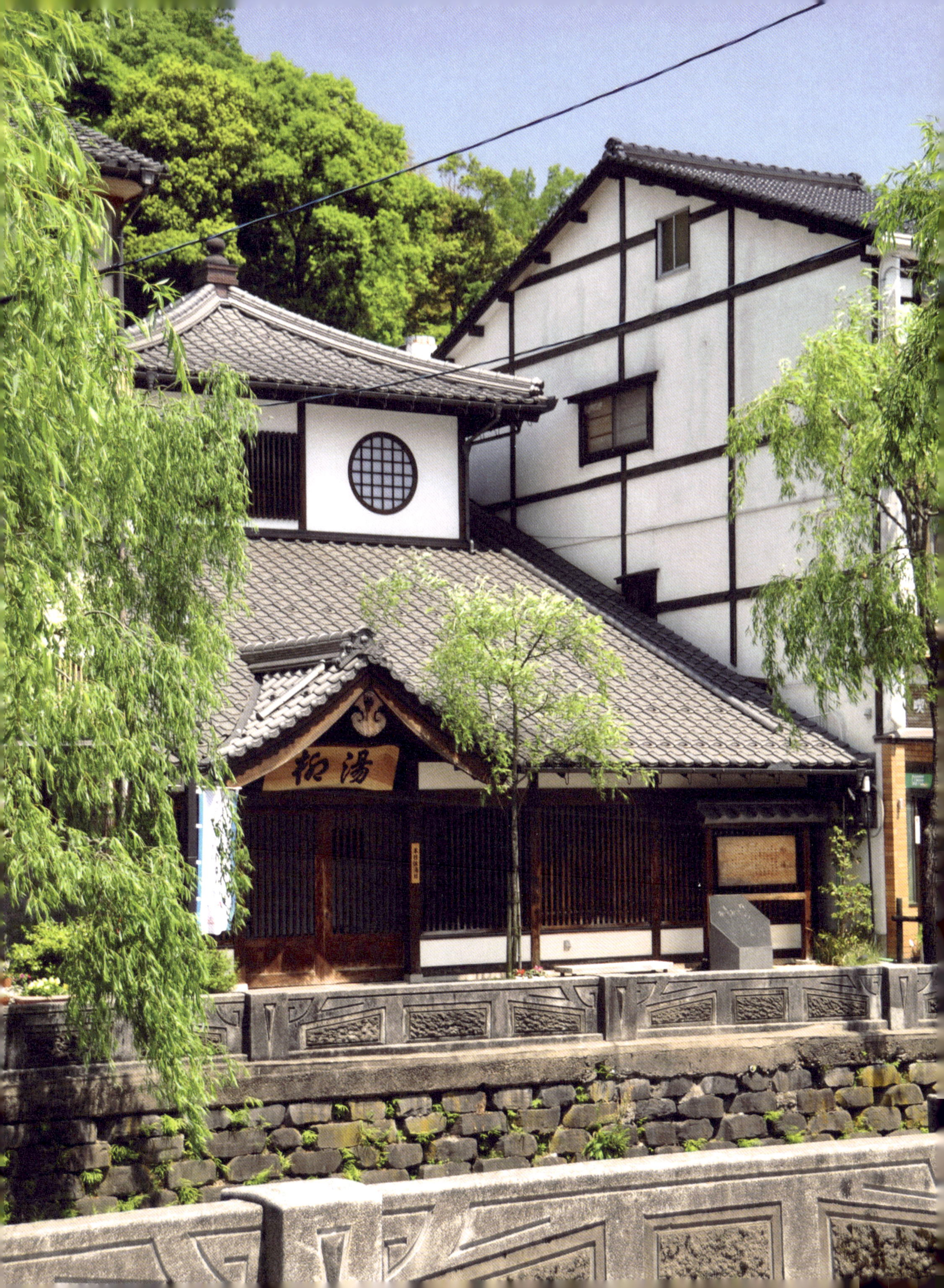
柳湯

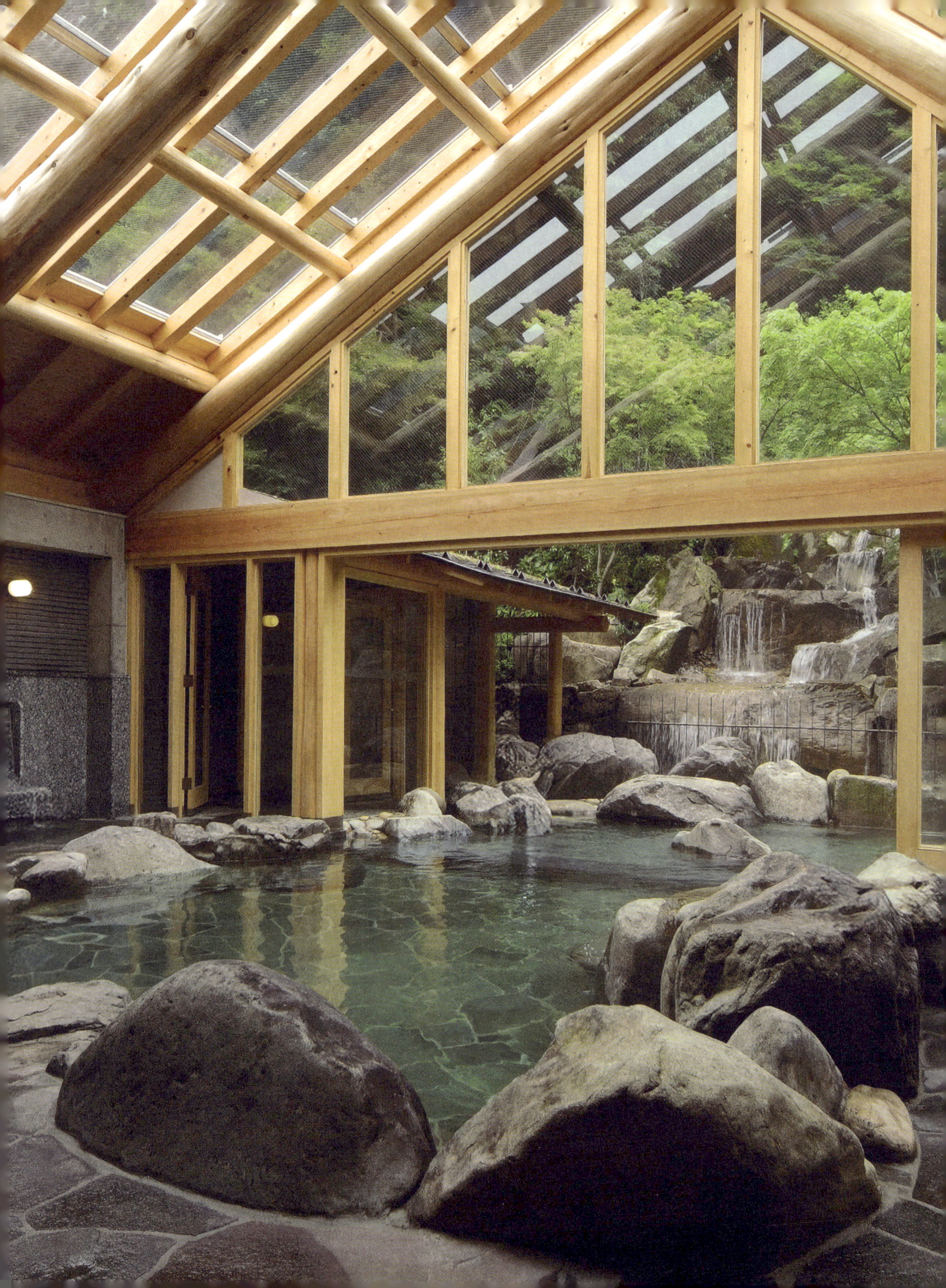

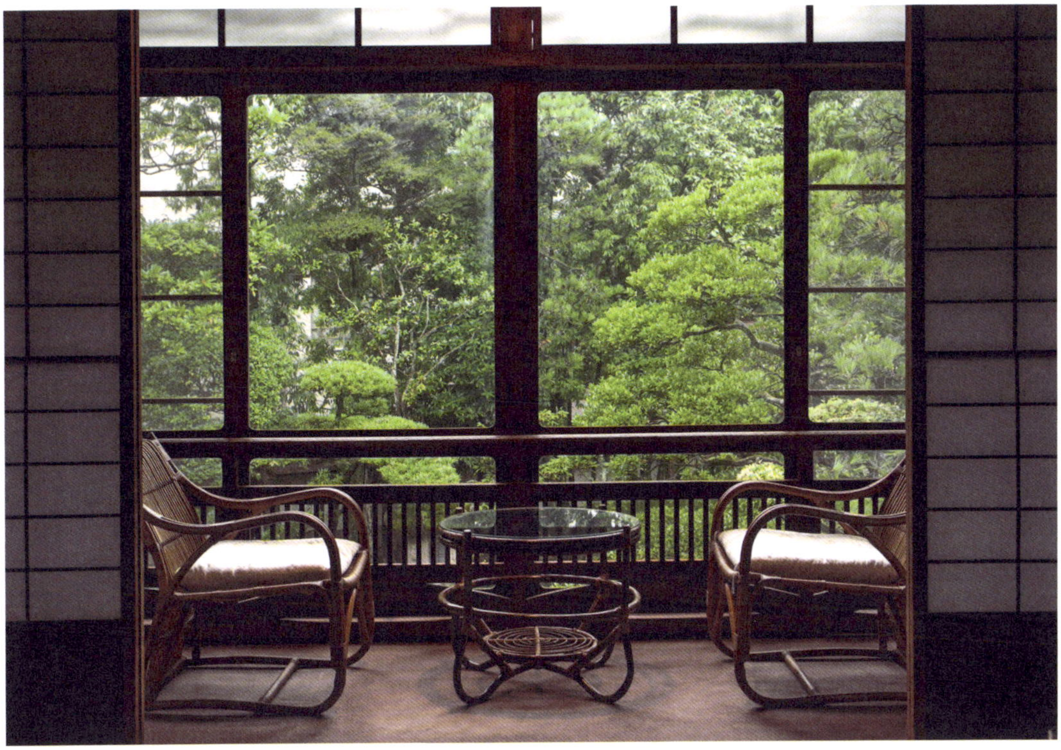

LEFT The impressive outdoor *rotenburo* at Gosho no Yu (Water of Beauty), one of Kinosaki's seven mystic onsen.

Seven superb, public baths form the backbone of this picturesque onsen town, which is easily accessible to travelers from Kyoto, Osaka, and Kobe.

Home to roughly 3,500 people and with a founding date of 720 BCE, Kinosaki is one of the oldest towns in Japan and, as such, is wonderfully picturesque, with its stone bridges, weeping willow trees, and decorative lanterns. The town is famous throughout Japan for its multiple, spiritually important hot springs as well as its literary significance—a number of notable writers were inspired by their trips to Kinosaki, including Shiga Naoya, the acclaimed and beloved novelist whose 1917 novella *At Kinosaki* depicted his stay.

Local lore states that when the Buddhist priest Dochi Shonin was traveling around the country in search of ways to heal the sick, he received a vision from an oracle who instructed him to chant a Buddhist sutra for 1,000 consecutive days. On the 1,000th day, it is said that onsen water erupted from the ground in the area that became Kinosaki Onsen. Today, the site of this onsen water source can be found at Mandara-yu, one of the seven public onsen of Kinosaki. Mandara-yu, meaning "the enlightened mind," is traditionally the starting point for one's onsen *meguri*, or bathing pilgrimage through the town.

Historically, the onsen of Kinosaki were considered *shinyu*, a blessing from the divine, and were thus sacred; in earlier times, visitors were required to hike up Mt. Daishi to reach Onsenji Temple, where they would offer prayers to the guardian of the onsen in hopes of being granted permission to enter the sacred waters and partake in their legendary healing benefits. In return, one would receive a *yu-shaku* (wooden ladle) that would act as proof of visiting the temple and as a ticket to enter all of the bathhouses.

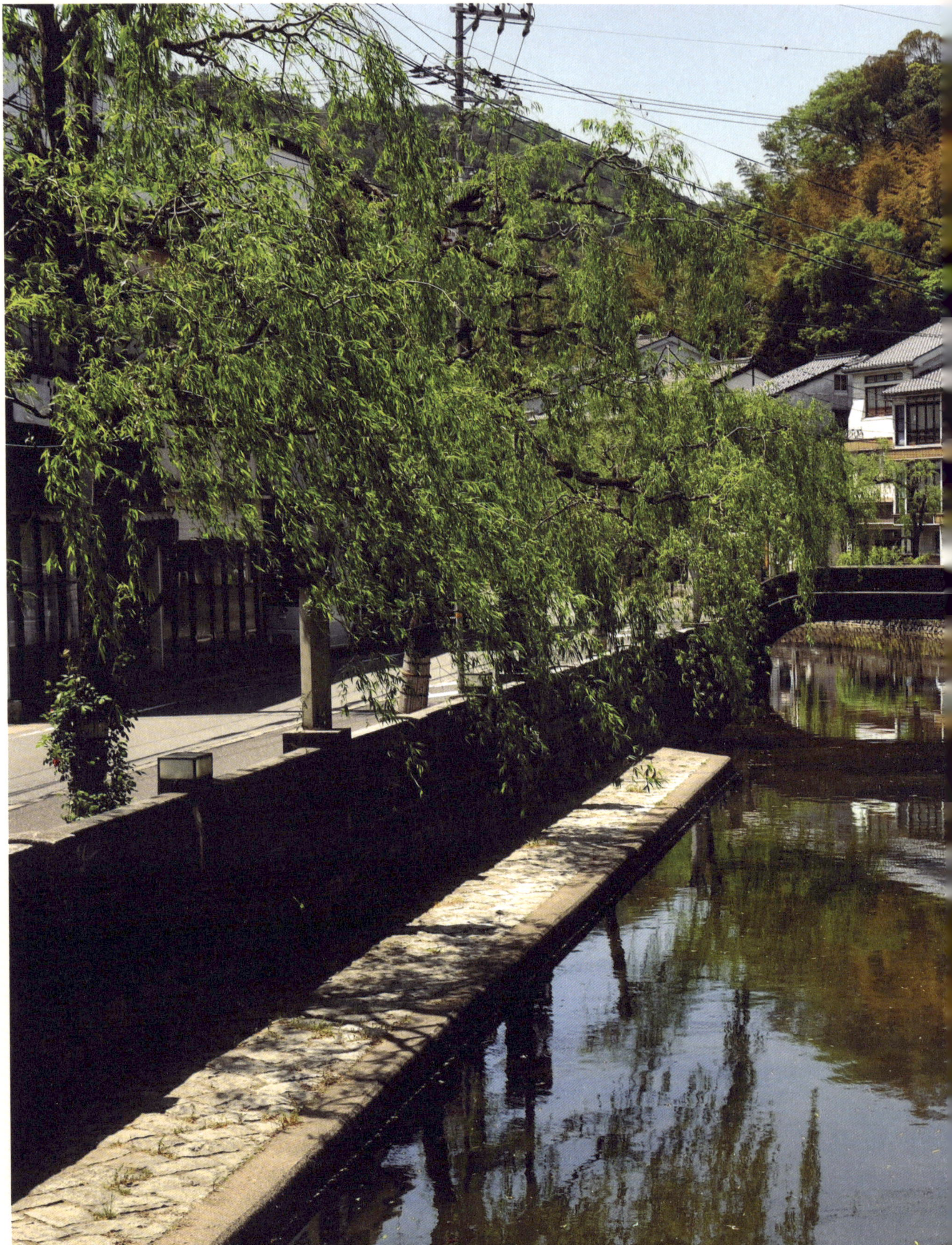

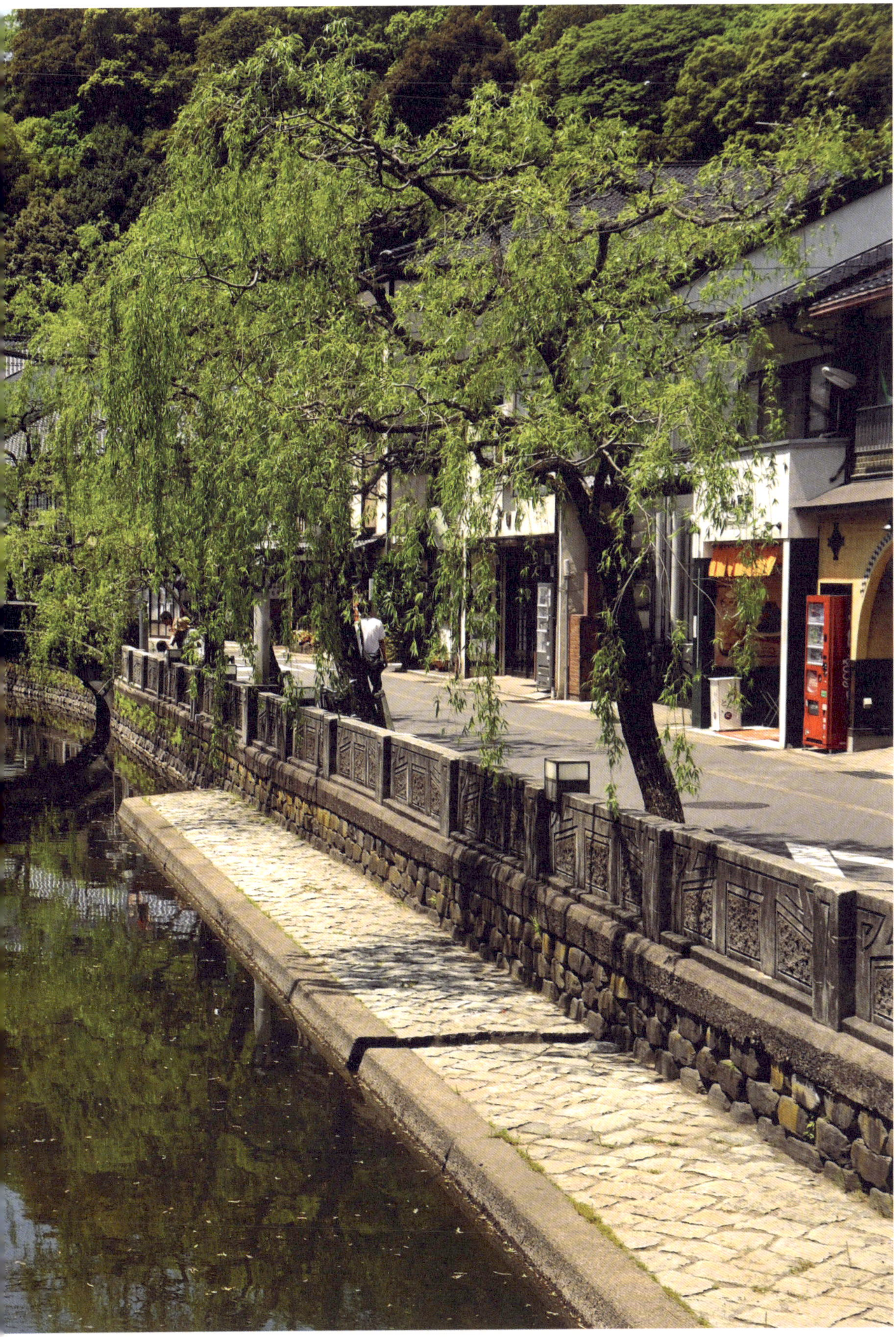

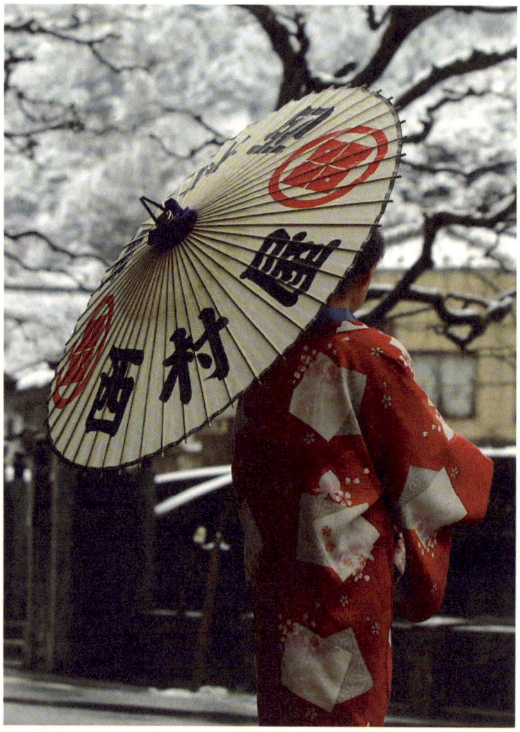

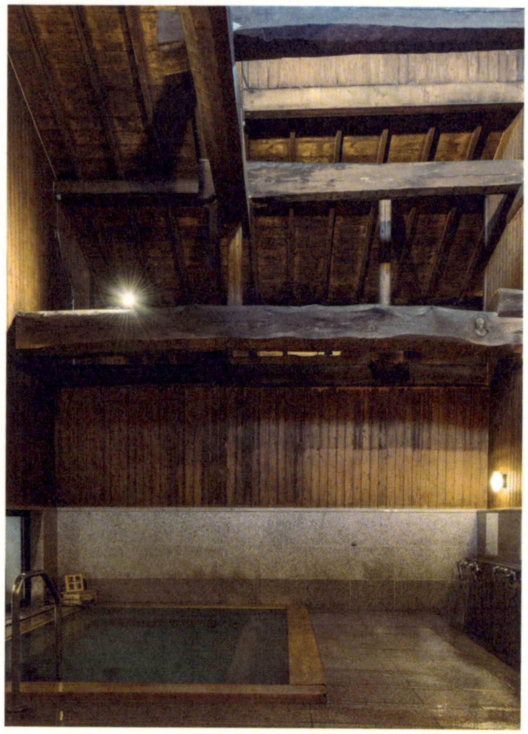

RIGHT Kinosaki's beloved cherry blossoms glowing by lantern light.

Entry would be denied if one did not possess this ladle. Today, however, visitors can simply pay an entrance fee to each of the public onsen.

The philosophy of "one town and one ryokan" stemmed from the tragedy of May 25th, 1925, when the North Tajima fire and earthquake devastated the region, and countless wooden homes, businesses, and lives were destroyed. From this horrific tragedy, the people of Kinosaki found strength in their community and rebuilt their homes according to this principle, in which all citizens and their businesses would coexist and prosper together. To remember the lives lost during the earthquake, the Toronagashi Festival is held every summer, during which residents and visitors send decorated paper lanterns with wishes for a good life down the river.

This vision of the town as one large ryokan is particularly striking. Under this philosophy, locals view Kinosaki Train Station as the actual entrance to the ryokan, while the streets are seen as its hallways, each ryokan is a single room, and the seven, tattoo-friendly public onsen are the baths.

In the 1950s, it was decided that preference would be given to these seven public bathhouses rather than individual onsen belonging to the ryokan, thereby fostering interaction, communication, and a love of bathing in both locals and visitors alike. Subsequently, all the onsen ryokan in Kinosaki that have a private, open-air, or indoor bath as part of their rooms do not use onsen water. Certain ryokan are allowed to have their own onsen, depending on the size of their premises and the number of guests that stay—they are either public or private via reservation. This was a conscious decision to conserve onsen water and cause minimal disruption to the earth due to the complicated construction of laying onsen pipes underground.

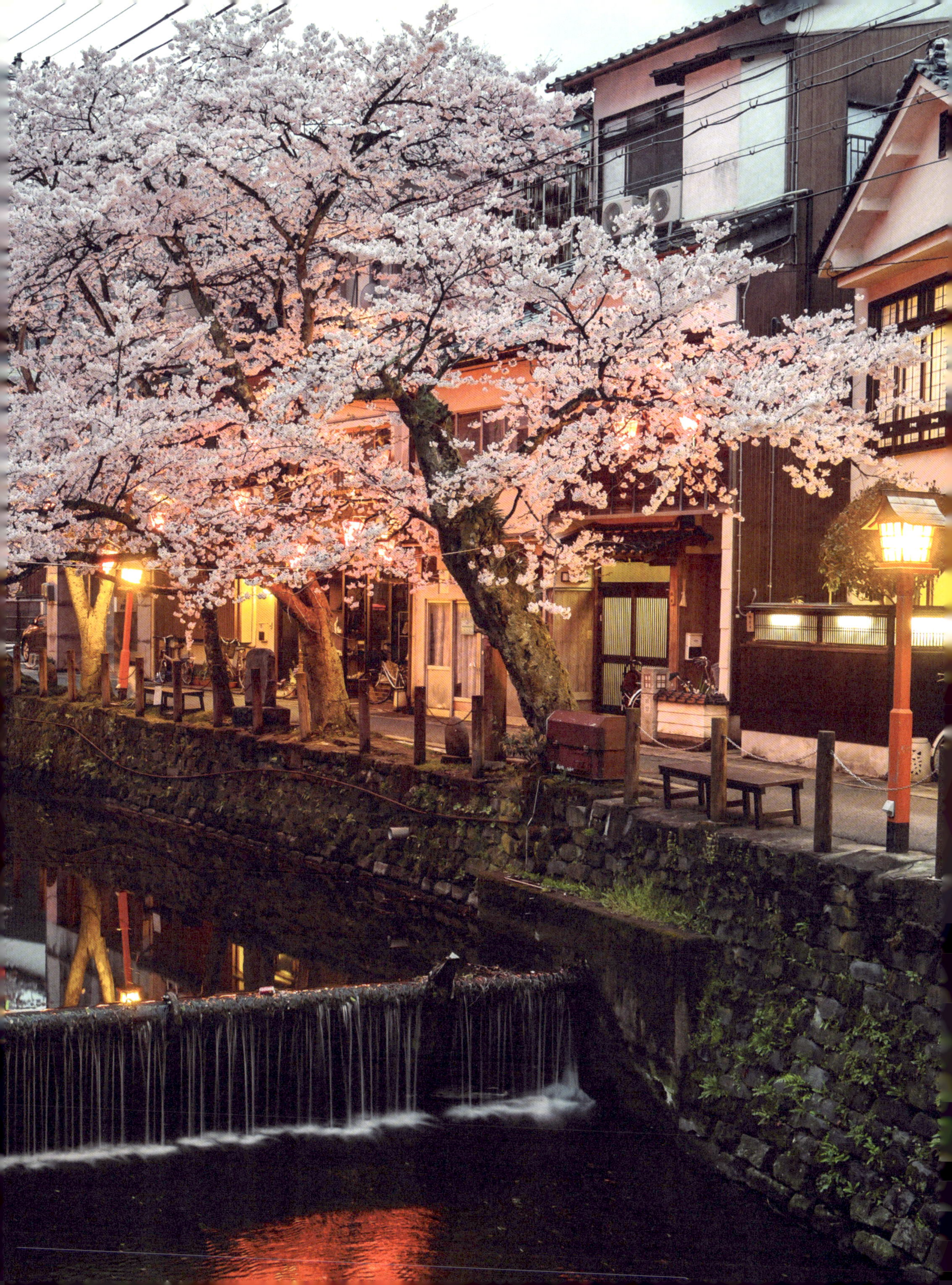

Hana No Omotenashi Nanraku
Minamiizu • Shizuoka Prefecture

SOAK AWAY IN AN INTIMATE ONSEN *MEGURI*

Beyond an expansive border of cherry blossom trees and vivid yellow canola blooms lies an onsen ryokan with an impressive array of baths.

The popular Shizuoka Prefecture, which lies on the Pacific coast of Honshu, makes for an easy weekend getaway from Tokyo. At its southern tip one finds the Izu Peninsula, where the quiet town of Minamiizu is often overlooked in favor of the more easily accessible Kawazu. However, the time it takes to reach Minamiizu is worthwhile, especially during the enlivening months of early spring.

The town is a delightful destination not only for its onsen, but for the annual Minamiizu Sakura and Nanohana Festival, when approximately 800 sakura trees lining both sides of the Aono River are in full bloom and compliment the swaying *sasa* grasses. Nearby, Hino Nanohana Field is a vivid carpet of sunshine-yellow *nanohana* blossoms. The vibrant pink and yellow hues contrast beautifully with the imposing mountains in the distance and the rising clouds of onsen steam.

Many visitors are unaware that the area also features the unassuming Shimogamo Onsen. Although this onsen houses several ryokan, none are more impressive than Hana no Omotenashi Nanraku. Commonly known as simply Nanraku, one of the ryokan's entrances is delightfully hidden by rows of sakura trees.

Step through the fluttering *noren* curtains marking the main entrance and you will feel transported to a countryside environment, where furnishings of rich wood, a traditional *irori,* Japanese antiques, sweet local crafts, and cozy alcoves effortlessly complement one other. Built in the traditional Sukiya-zukuri style, Nanraku is a timeless ryokan escape, ensconced in its own small bamboo forest. Both the Nonohana-tei and Shimogamo-tei rooms are spacious and built in the same Sukiya-zukuri style, while the latter features a private *irori* and jar-shaped open-air onsen.

Nanraku's 22 baths, where guests are invited to embark on a remarkable onsen *meguri* tour, are the pride of the place. The site features over 10 different bathing locations and 17 different types of baths and guests can easily move between the two large, communal onsen set in natural surroundings or relax in peaceful seclusion in one of Nanraku's many private onsen baths. The private onsen are spacious and roomy, making them perfect for not only for shy individuals but couples and families as well. Half the fun is choosing which onsen to try: indoor or outdoor, or baths made from hinoki, stone, or pottery.

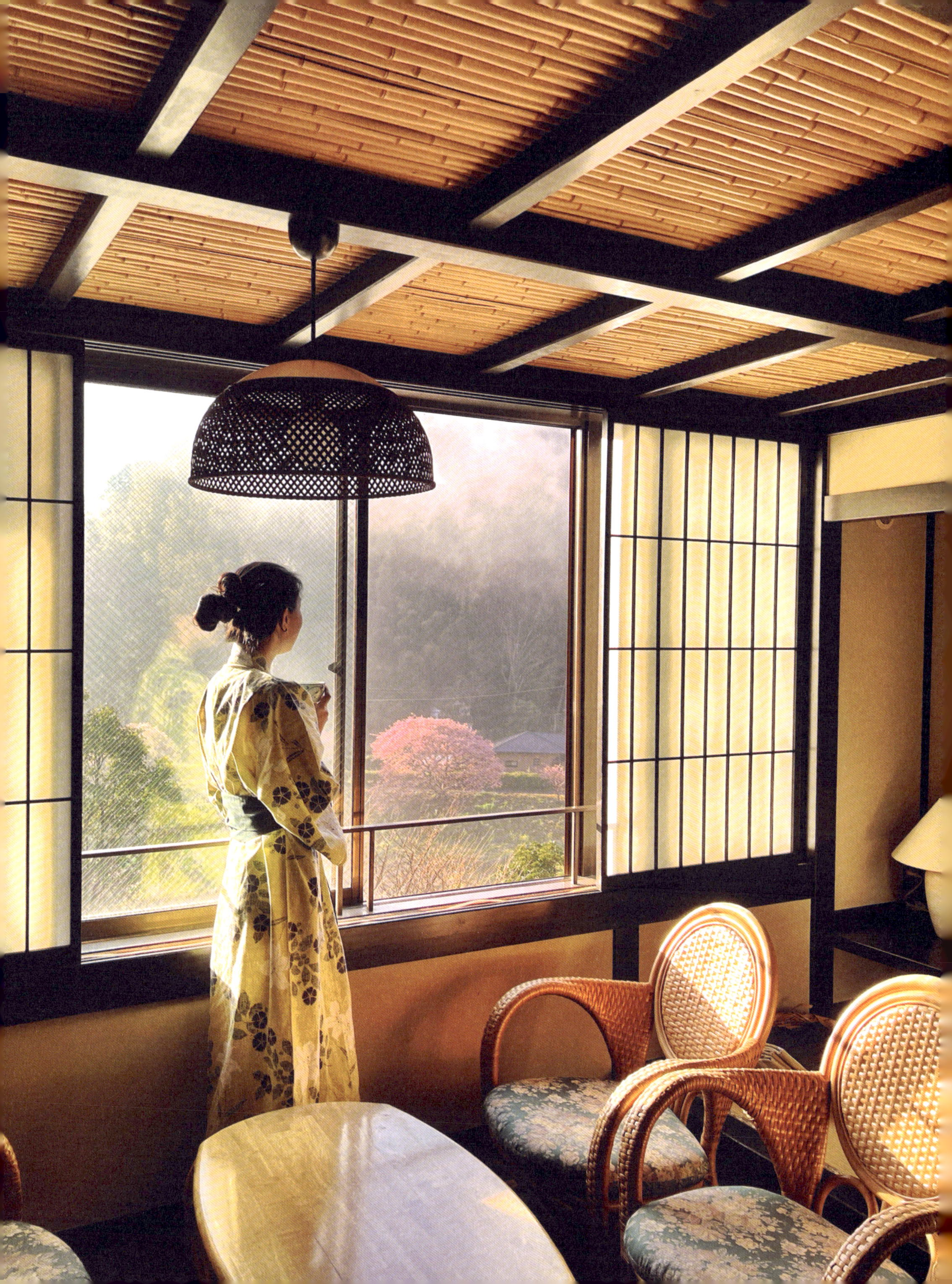

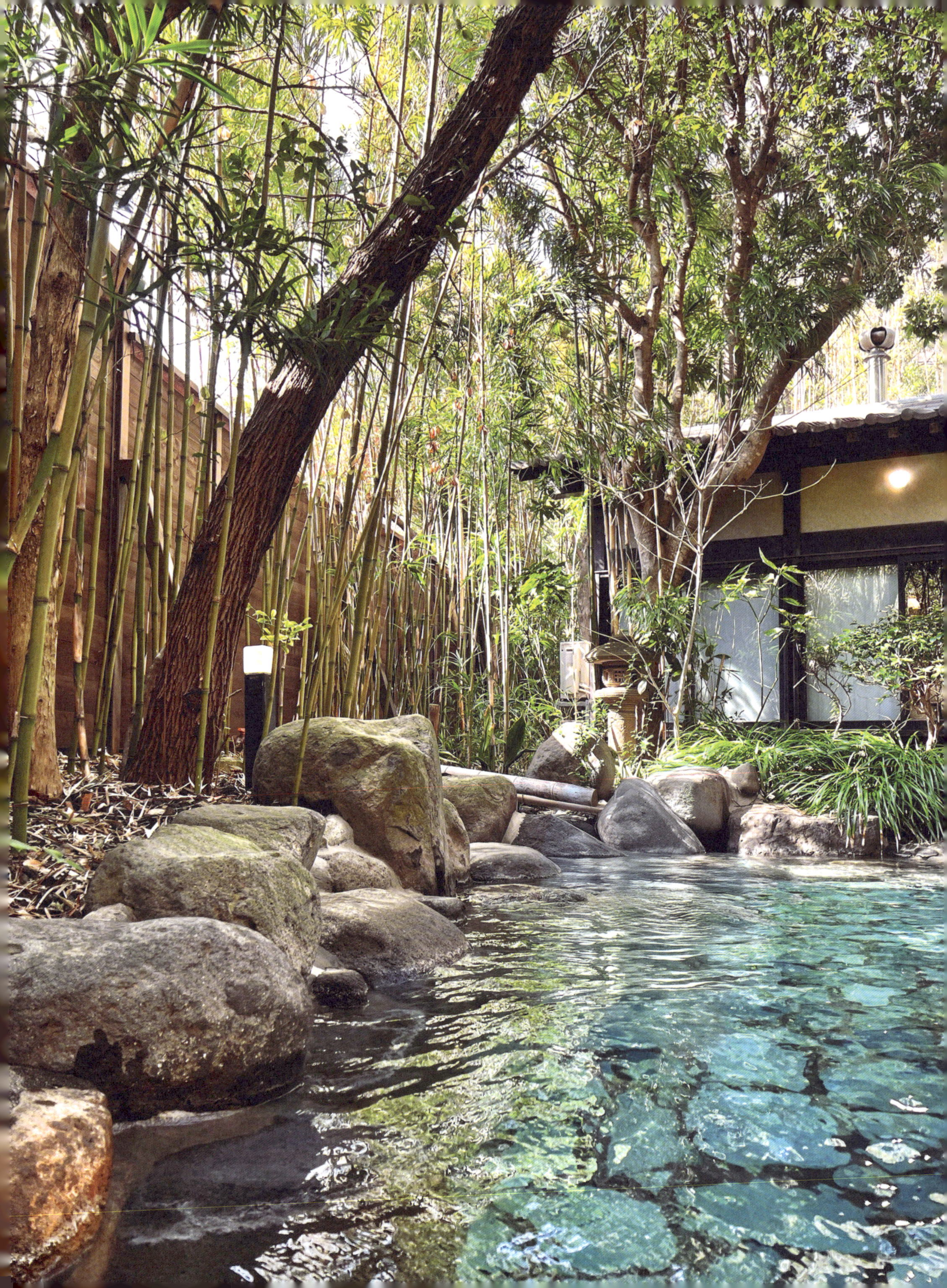

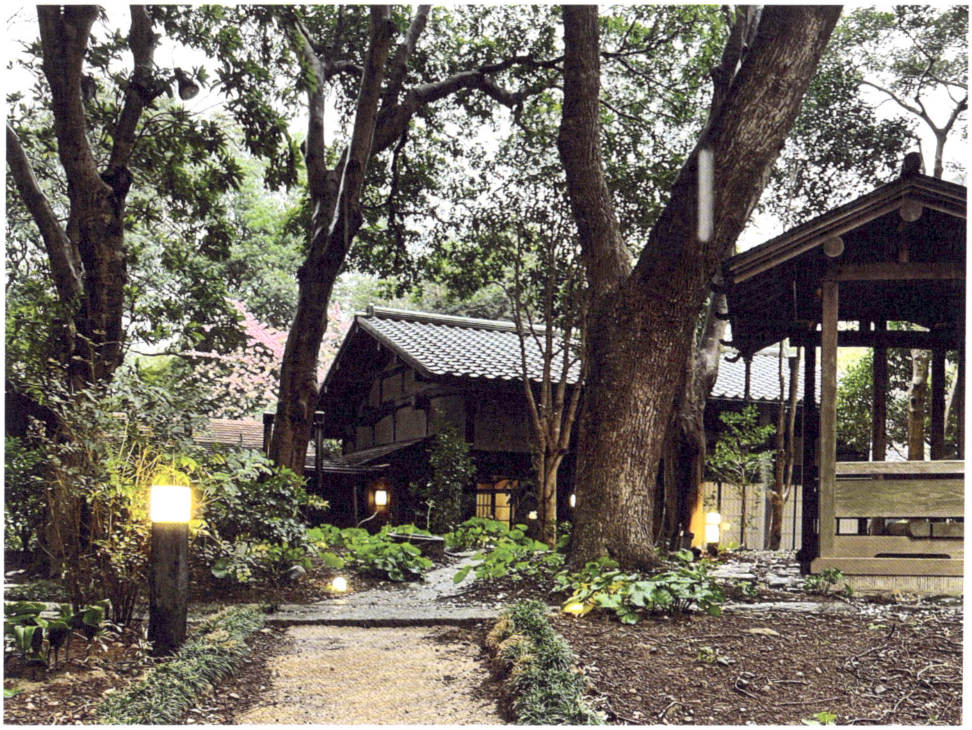

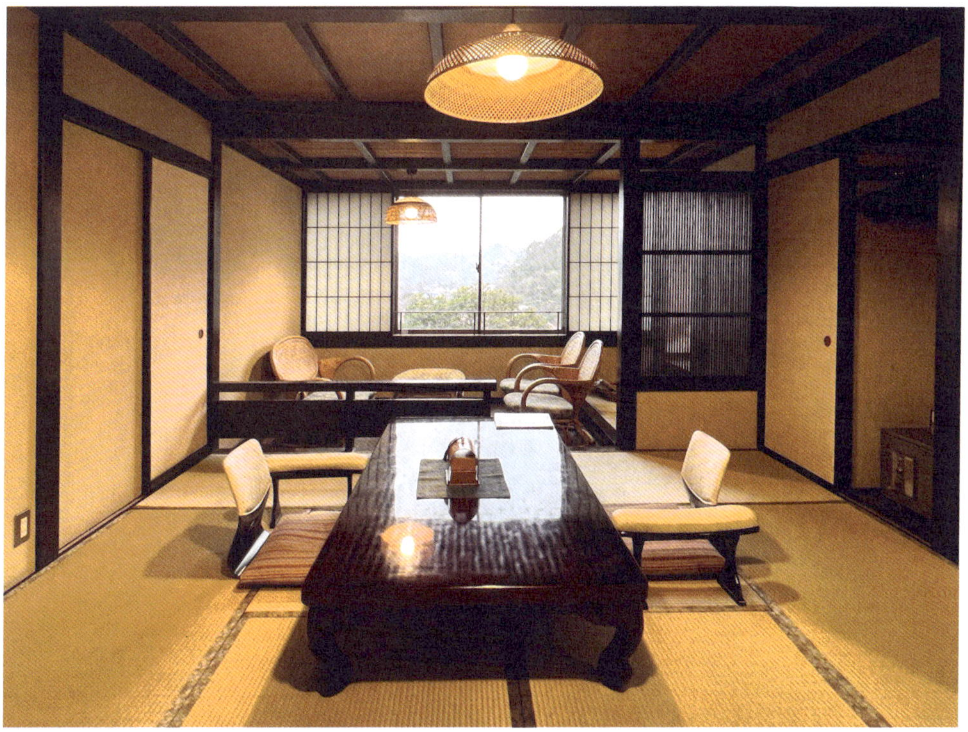

ABOVE Spacious Sukiya-zukuri-style rooms offer views of the beautiful Minamiizu area.

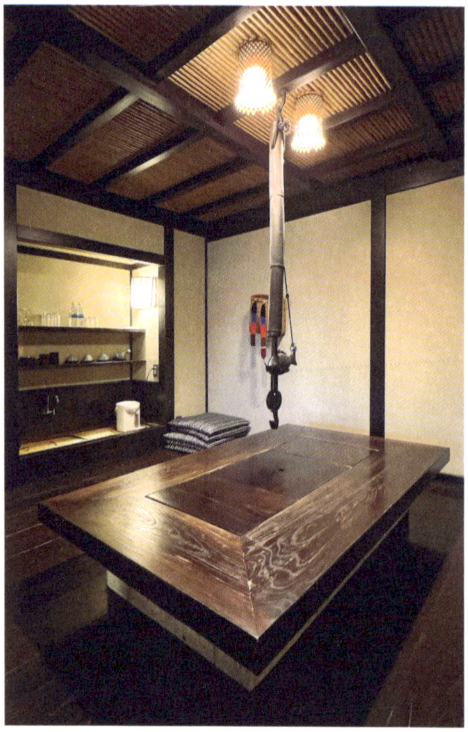

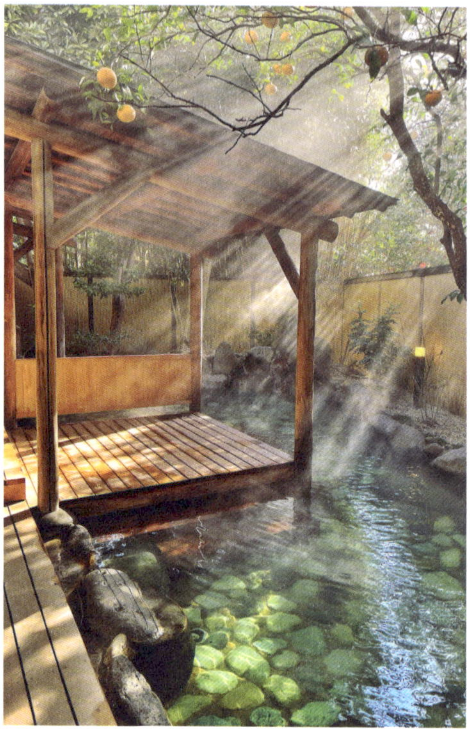

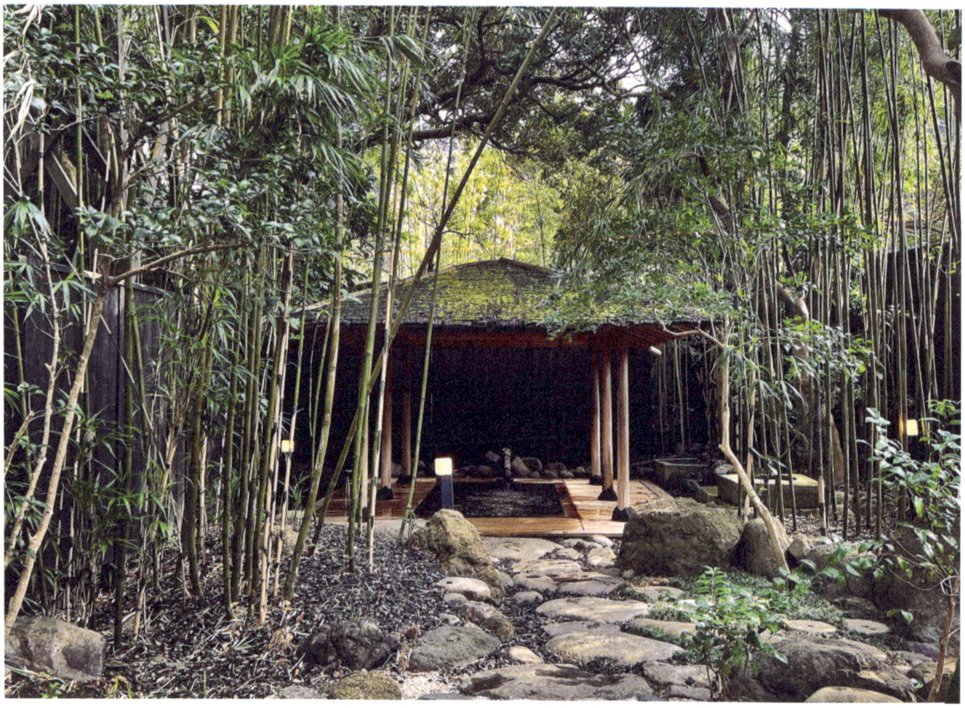

RIGHT Cherry blossoms in peak bloom during the Minamiizu Sakura and Nanohana Festival, which runs from late February to early March.

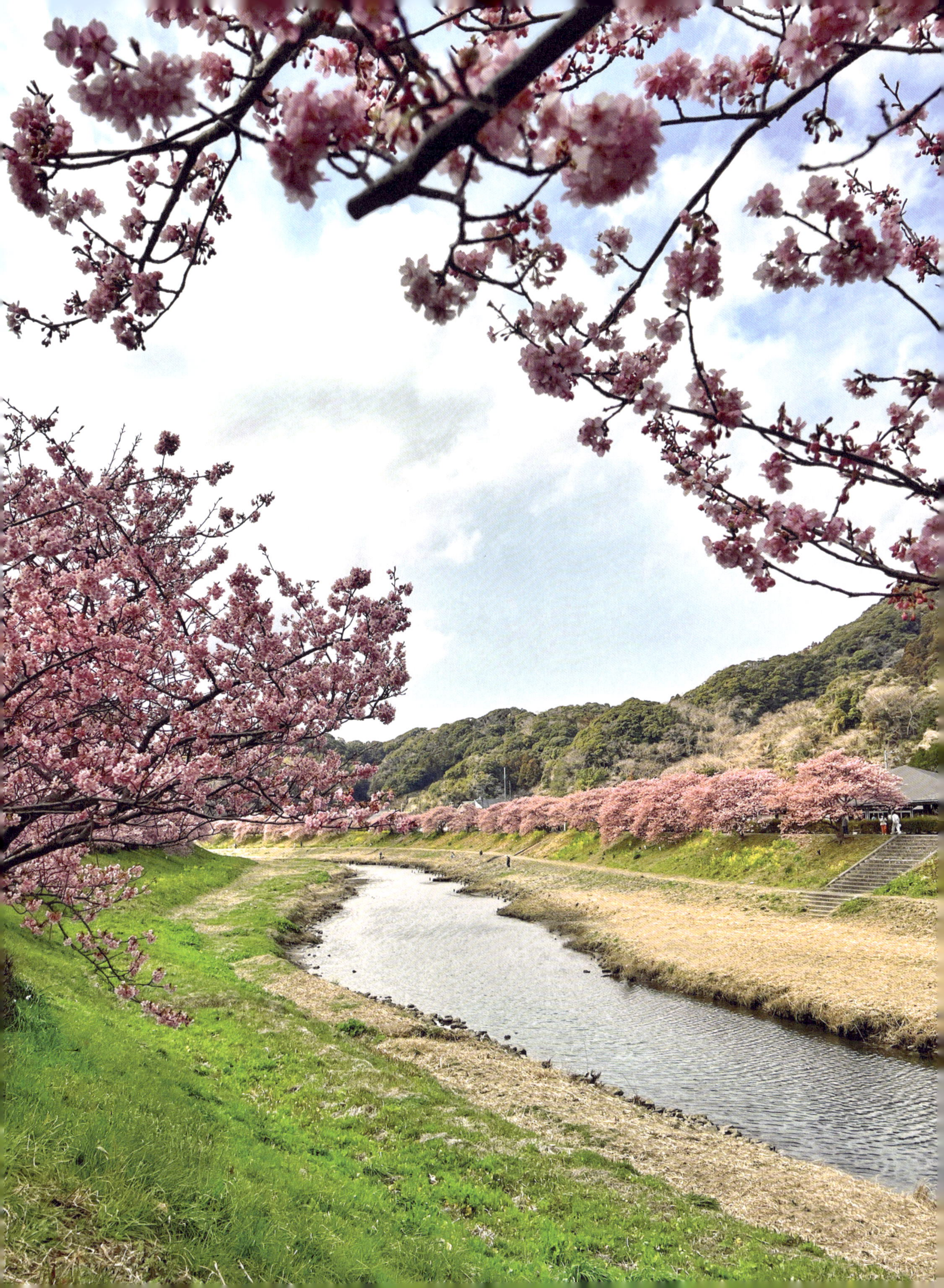

Fukuchi-in
Koyasan • Wakayama Prefecture

HAVE A PEACEFUL, SPIRITUAL STAY AT A TRADITIONAL *SHUKUBO*

While exploring the Kumano Kodō pilgrimage route and the sacred Koyasan, travelers are invited to overnight in the region's many Buddhist temples.

Historically, numerous Kumano Kodō pilgrims elected to stay at one of the venerable *shukubo* subtemples encircling Kongobu-ji and spread out across the sacred Koyasan (Mt. Koya). Today, these *shukubo* temple stays range from the most basic, minimalist form of accommodation to those of refined luxury, with spacious rooms adorned with gilded, hand-painted screens, precious antiques, and private Zen gardens.

Fukuchi-in is one of the larger sub-temples open to overnight guests; it was founded over 800 years ago by Kakuin Ajari in homage to the Buddha Aizen Myo-o, whom it was believed could bestow good fortune and the fulfillment of one's wishes. Fukuchi-in is the only *shukubo* that has its own private, natural onsen source—the only onsen, in fact, on the entire mountain of Koyasan.

The temple features two primary onsen baths: Togendai, which includes a serene indoor stone onsen, a sauna, a calming outdoor hinoki onsen, and two sunken Shigaraki pottery onsen designed specifically for men's relaxation; and Ten'nyo, which boasts a slightly larger indoor stone onsen, a sauna, and a rock *rotenburo* framed with low-lying shrubbery. Excepting the cold winter months, Fukuchi-in's indoor, carbonated onsen baths Tansansen no Yu are also available to guests. For those hesitant about communal bathing, Fukuchi-in also offers a reservable, private indoor onsen. Experiencing a traditional temple *shukubo* stay after hiking the pilgrimage route and cleansing oneself in Fukuchi-in's healing onsen waters offers visitors an extraordinary reminder of the sacred ties between the physical and spiritual worlds.

Within Fukuchi-in, travelers can admire a collection of antique art and treasures dating as far back as the Nara period, as well as the temple's three gardens: the Lotus Garden, created in the Horai style and featuring 15 rock formations; the Aizen Garden, which pays tribute to the temple's principle deity; and the Tosen Garden, inspired by Ryumon Falls (Dragon Gate Falls). Several room styles are available to guests: basic-yet-spacious, simple tatami rooms with shared bathrooms; larger rooms with garden views; and slightly more ornate quarters with their own private ensuite. During their stay, guests can also freely participate in the temple's early morning prayer.

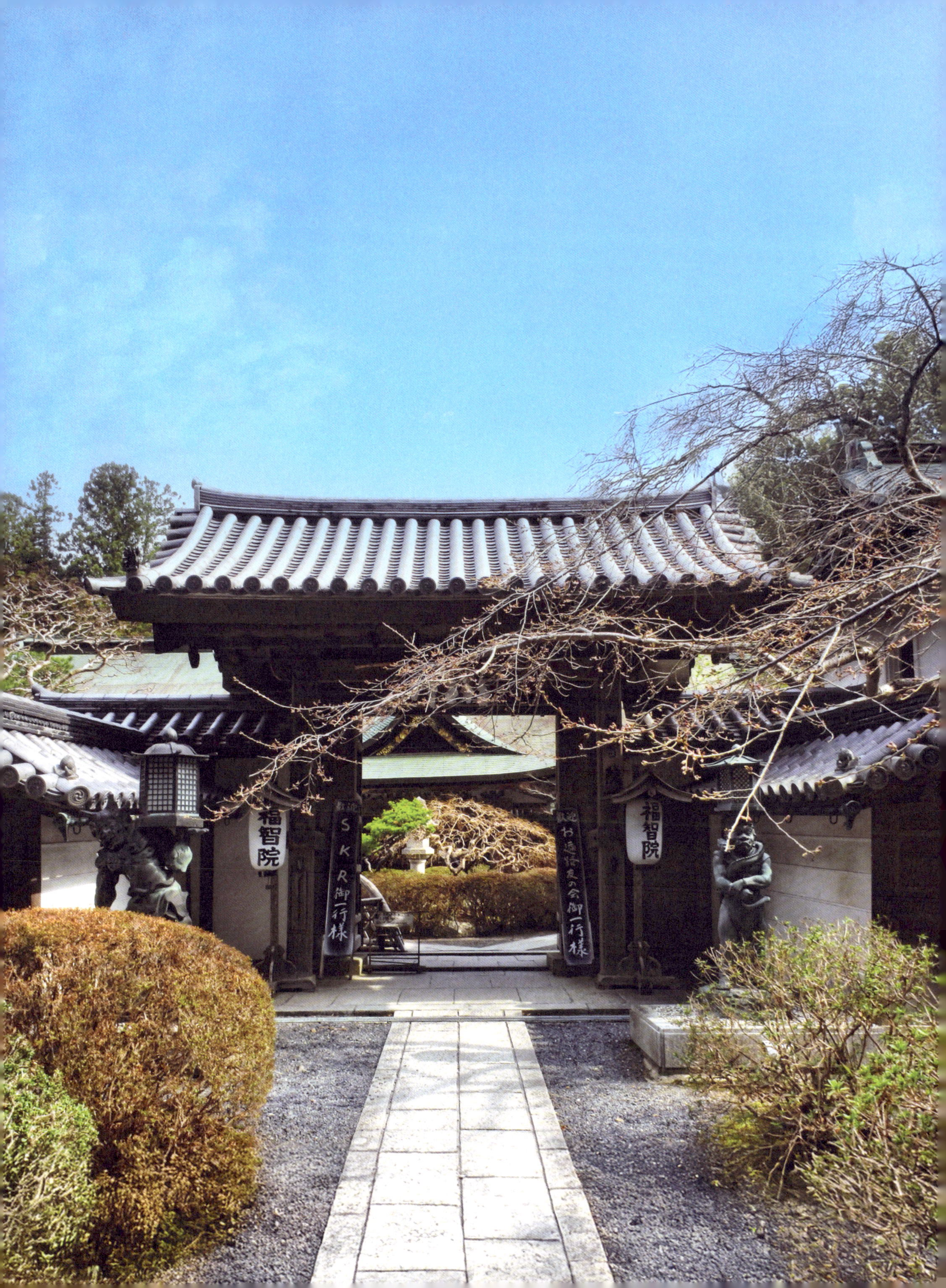
福智院
SKR御一行様
お遍路友の会御一行様
福智院

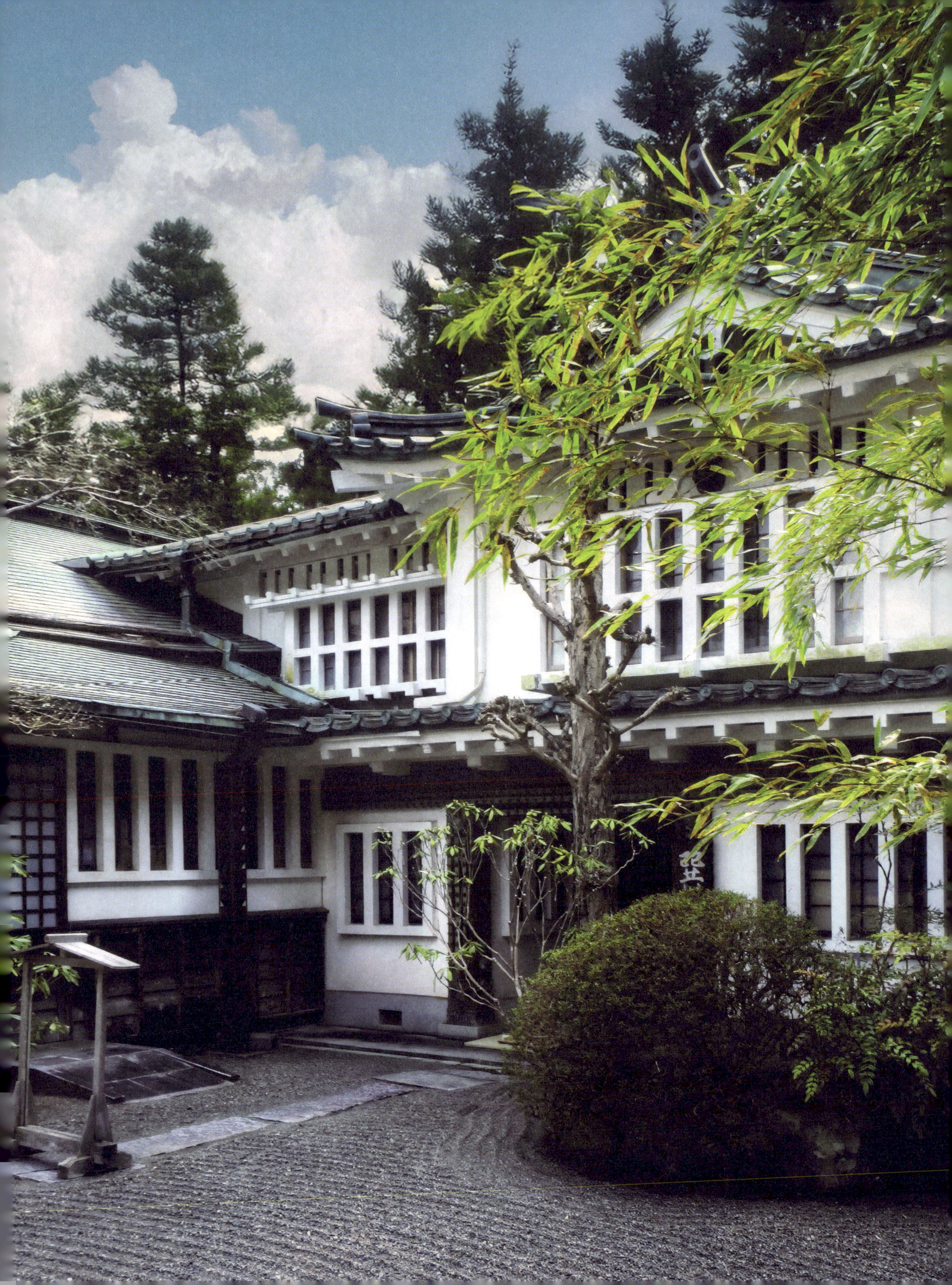

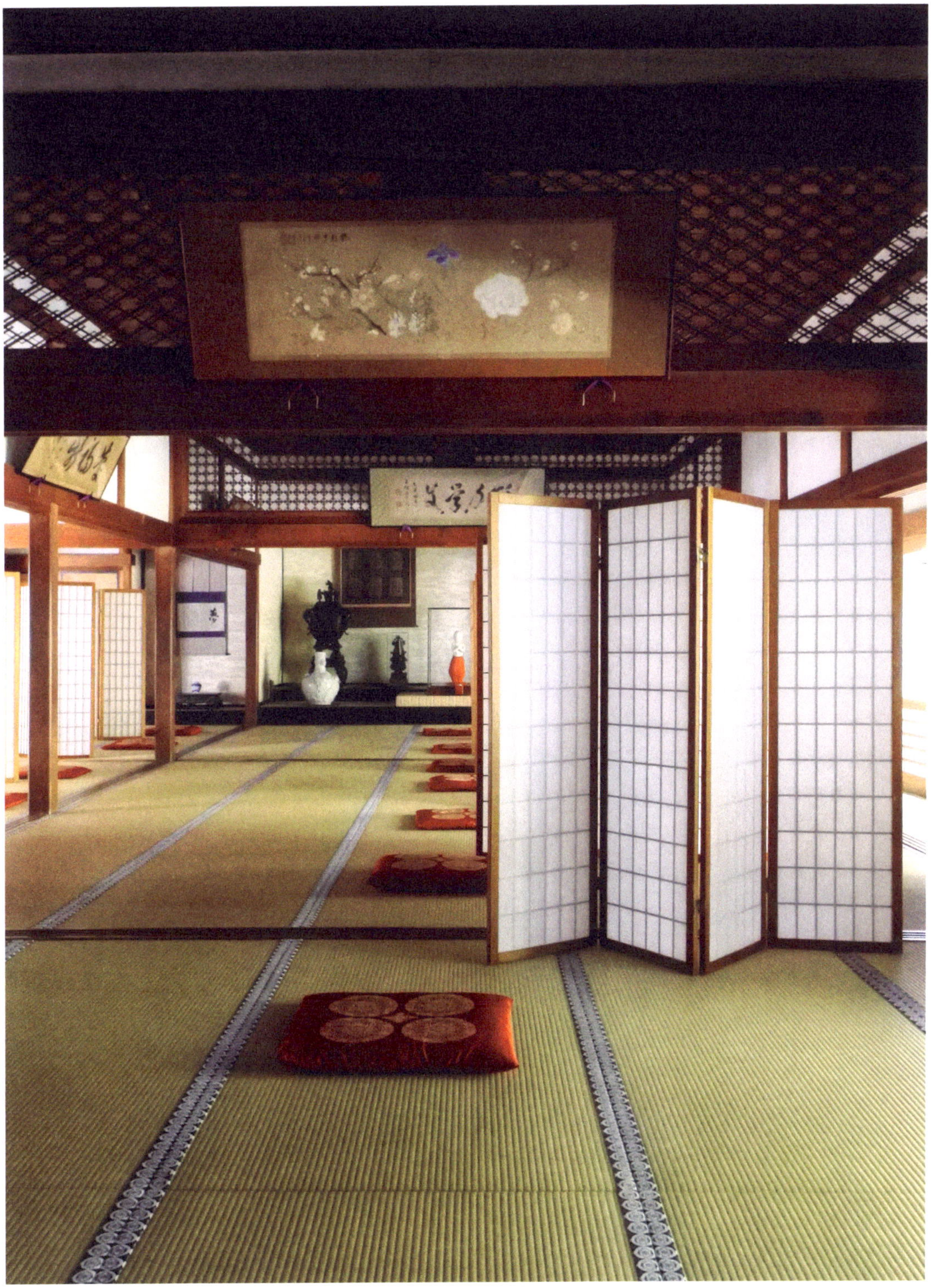

ABOVE Simple, seasonal *shojin-ryori* (Buddhist cuisine) meals are taken in communal dining halls during stays at Fukuchi-in.

KAI Ito

Ito ● Shizuoka Prefecture

ESCAPE TO AN ONSEN GETAWAY EASILY ACCESSIBLE FROM TOKYO

Experience the beauty of Japan's changing seasons, from blooming *sakura* blossoms to the delicious taste of fresh, regional delicacies.

A favorite of Tokyo dwellers looking to escape the hustle and bustle of the city, Ito Onsen along Shizuoka's Izu Peninsula has been a popular destination for hundreds of years. Famed for its abundance of onsen water, Ito Onsen lays claim to more than 700 onsen sources, making it the fourth-largest in the country, and one of Japan's top onsen towns.

Tracing its roots to Japan's ancient Jōmon period, Ito Onsen was officially discovered in the Heian era and saw significant development under the rule of the third shogun, Tokugawa Iemitsu. Tokugawa Iemitsu recognized the therapeutic benefits of Ito and officially designated it as a place of healing. The onsen gained further prominence as a healing retreat after many acclaimed novelists, artists, and notable cultural individuals, such as Yosano Akiko, Saishū Onoe, and Kawabata Yasunari found rest, inspiration, and creativity there.

Travelers are spoiled for choice in Ito Onsen, with accommodations ranging from budget-friendly to serious splurge, and from small, cozy boutique lodgings to impressive onsen resorts. For those in search of a modern luxury experience, a stay at KAI Ito will certainly not disappoint. Part of the Hoshino Resorts group, a family-run organization currently managed by its fourth-generation head, Hoshino Yoshiharu, the KAI properties are found throughout the country and dedicated to showcasing the rich beauty and culture of each onsen area; guests are invited to relax in sumptuous, contemporary rooms, and offered a range of cultural experiences to indulge in.

Each of KAI Ito's 30 spacious rooms offers a seamless blend of traditional Japanese aesthetics fused with modern design elements, celebrating artisanal crafts like Tsurushi-kazari, whereby auspicious handmade dolls are dangled on strings in odd numbers to attract long life, good health, and the prosperity of one's children. The rooms themselves are designed around Japan's *hanagoyomi* flower calendar, with lovely, artistic touches throughout showcasing the changing floral landscape of the seasons. Guests are also invited to participate in a camellia (*tsubaki*) oil workshop, honoring a native flower whose oil is beloved for its moisturizing, anti-aging, and anti-inflammatory properties.

Every room also draws its bathwater from one of KAI Ito's four onsen sources, whether it be an indoor hinoki bath or a private outdoor *rotenburo*. Its public onsen baths are truly spectacular, with large, indoor hinoki baths offering stunning views of the outdoor *rotenburo* enlivened by a gorgeous waterfall. The seasonal beauty of Japan's seasons present at KAI Ito will forever stay imprinted upon one's memories.

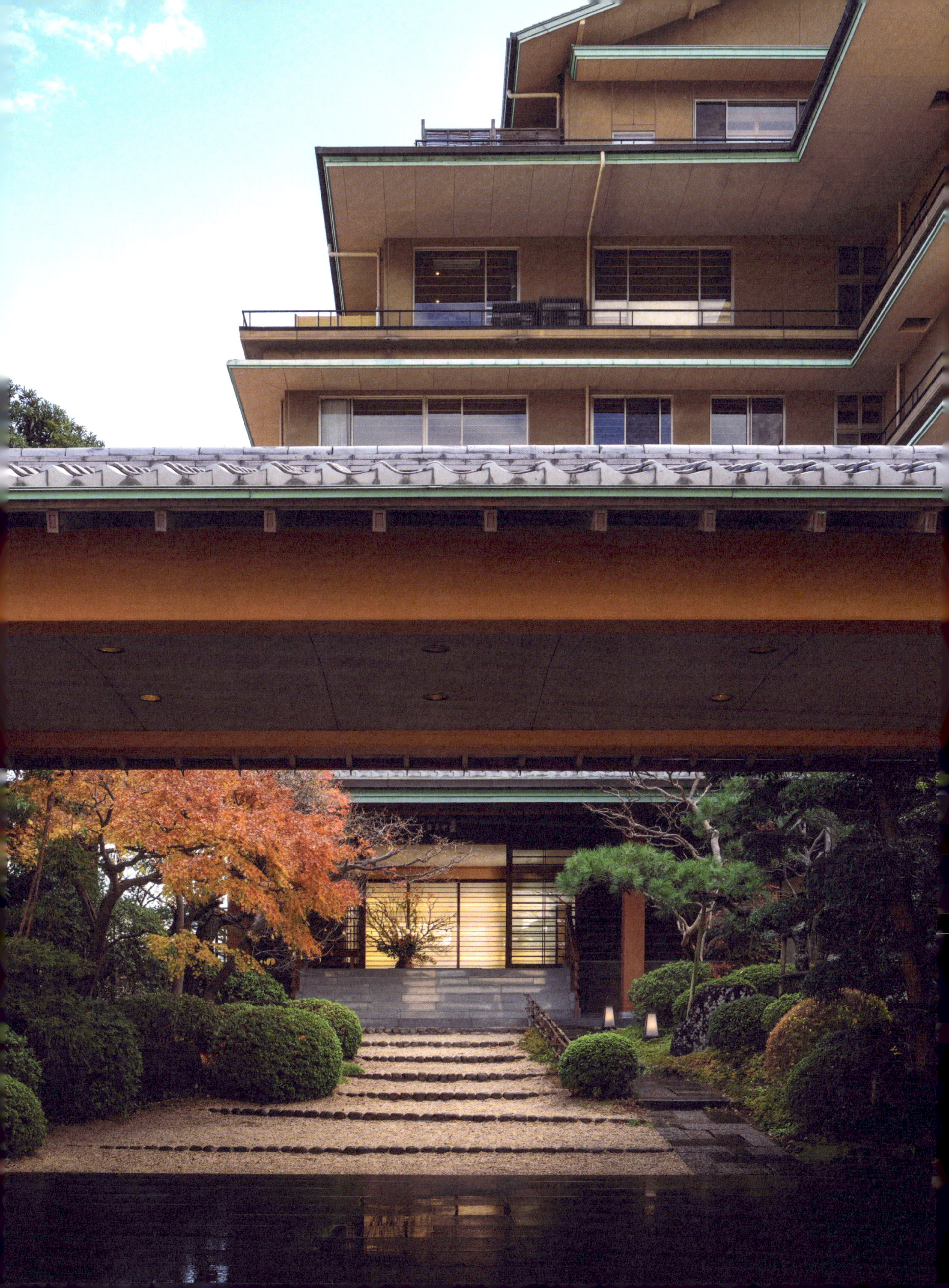

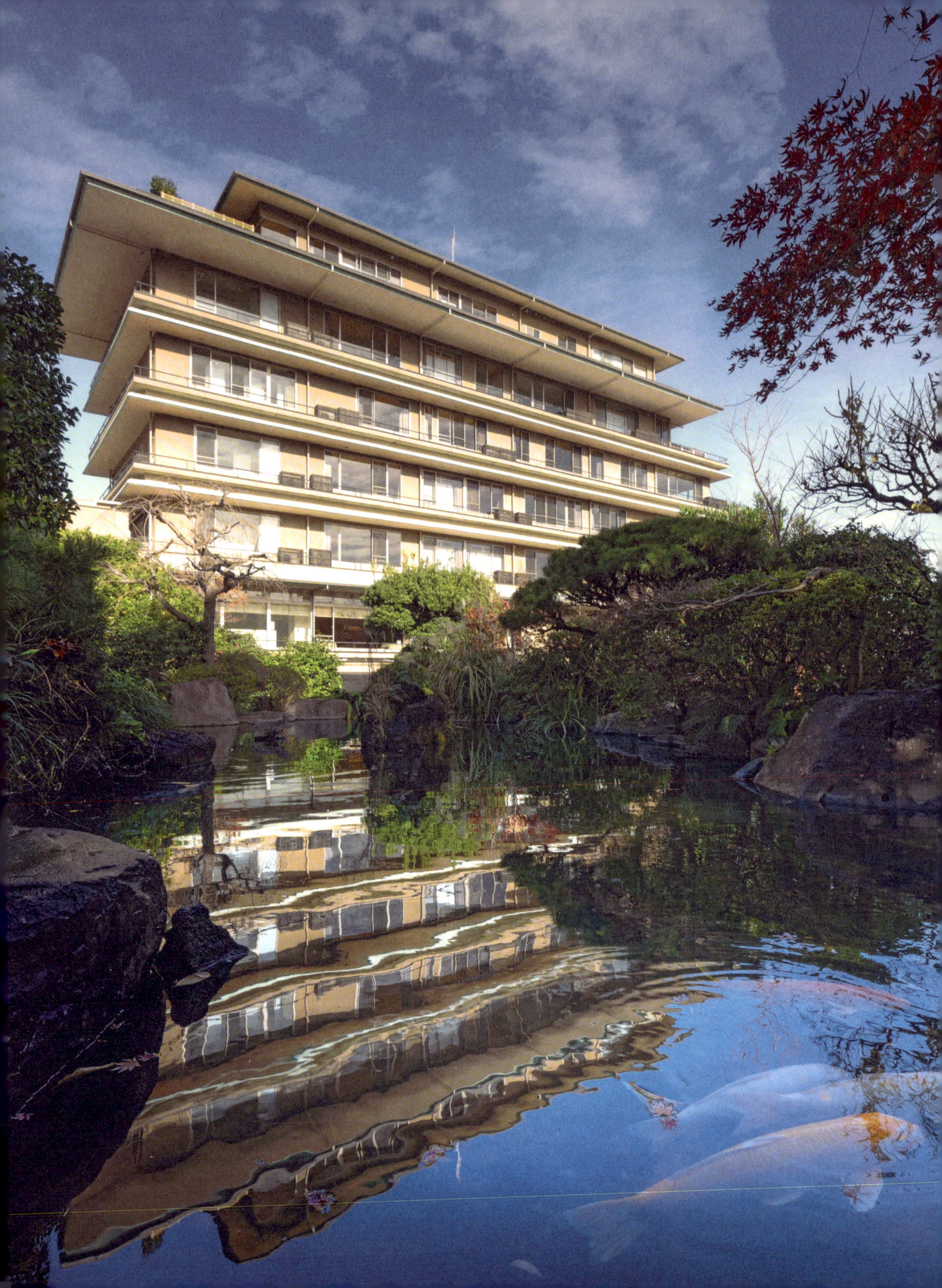

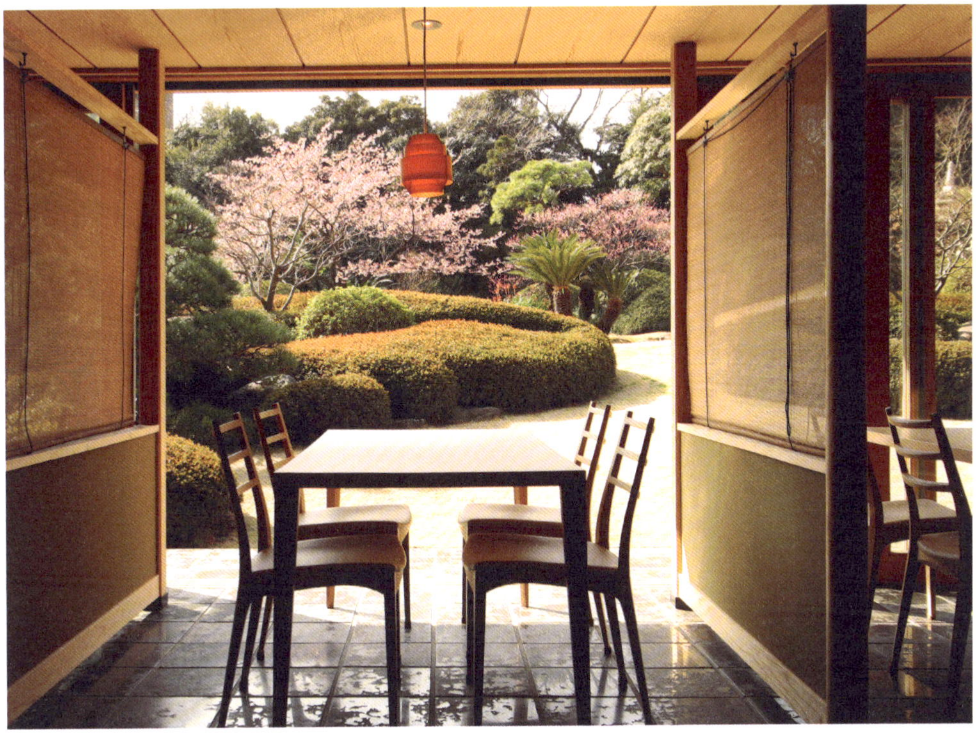

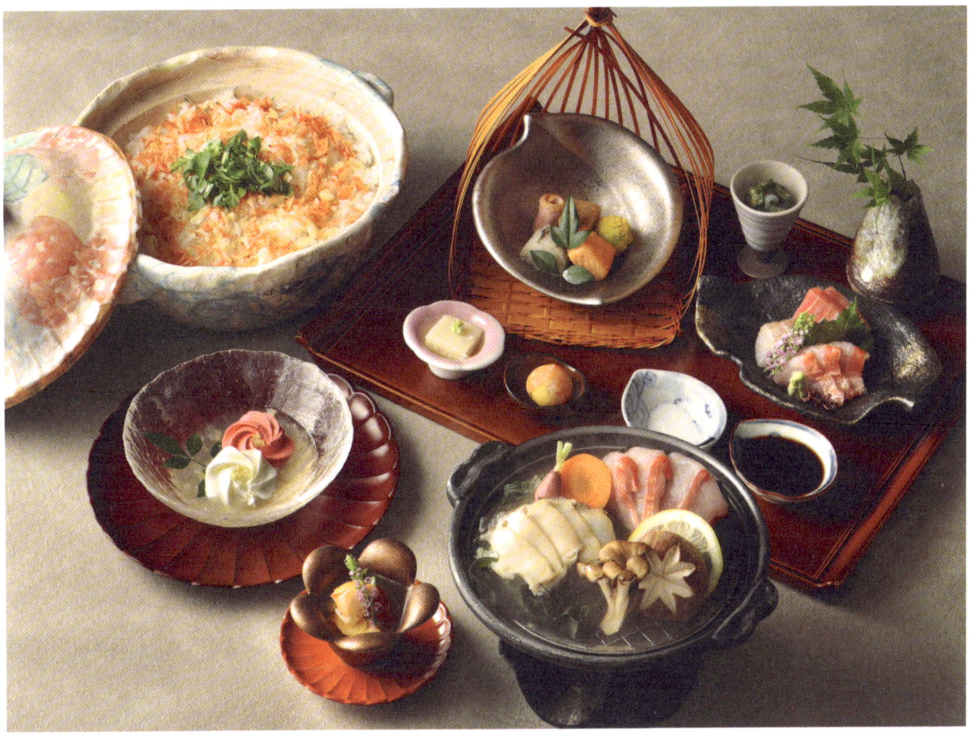

ABOVE AND TOP Feast on sumptuous *kaiseki* meals with scenic views of the garden.

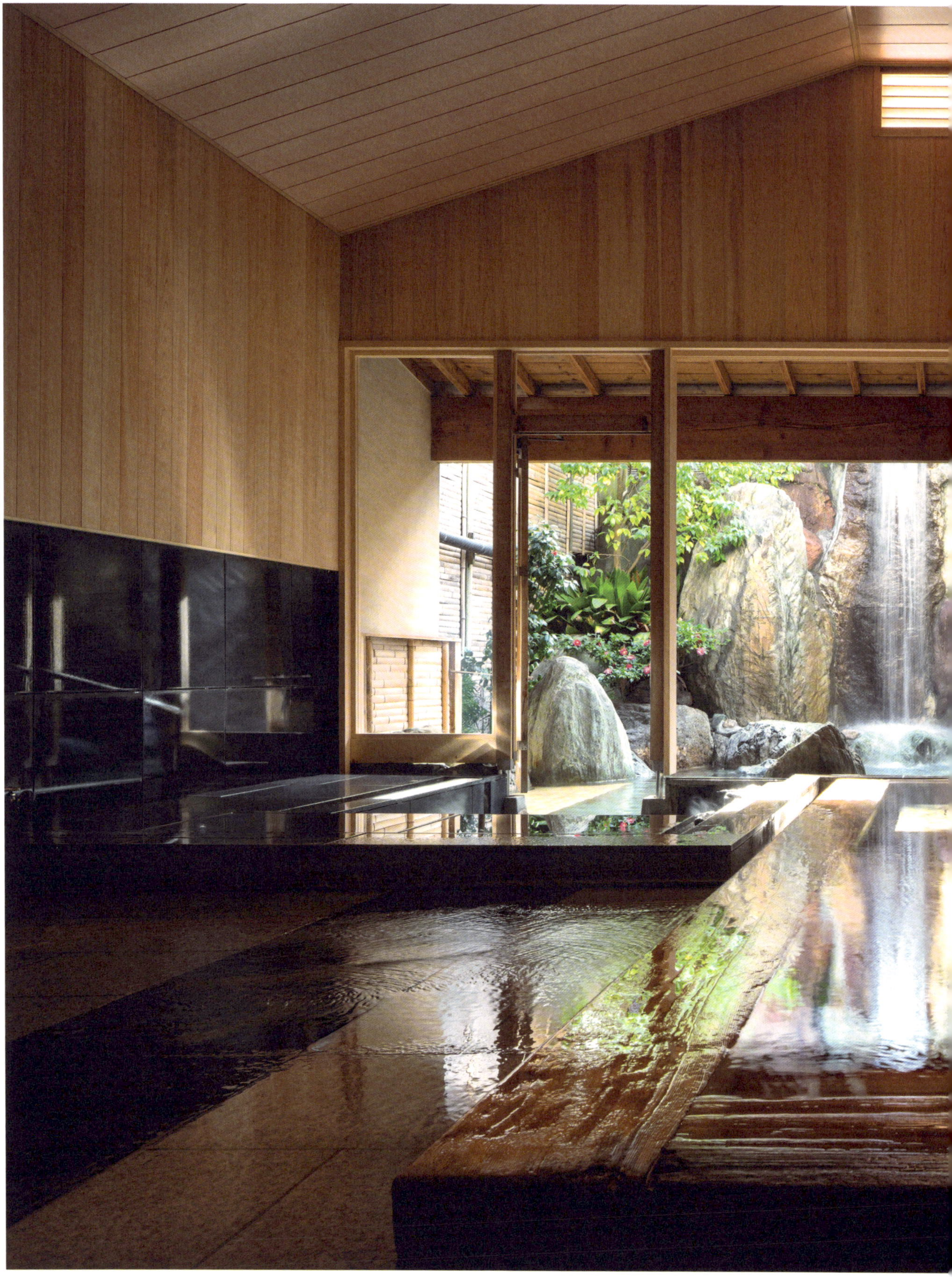

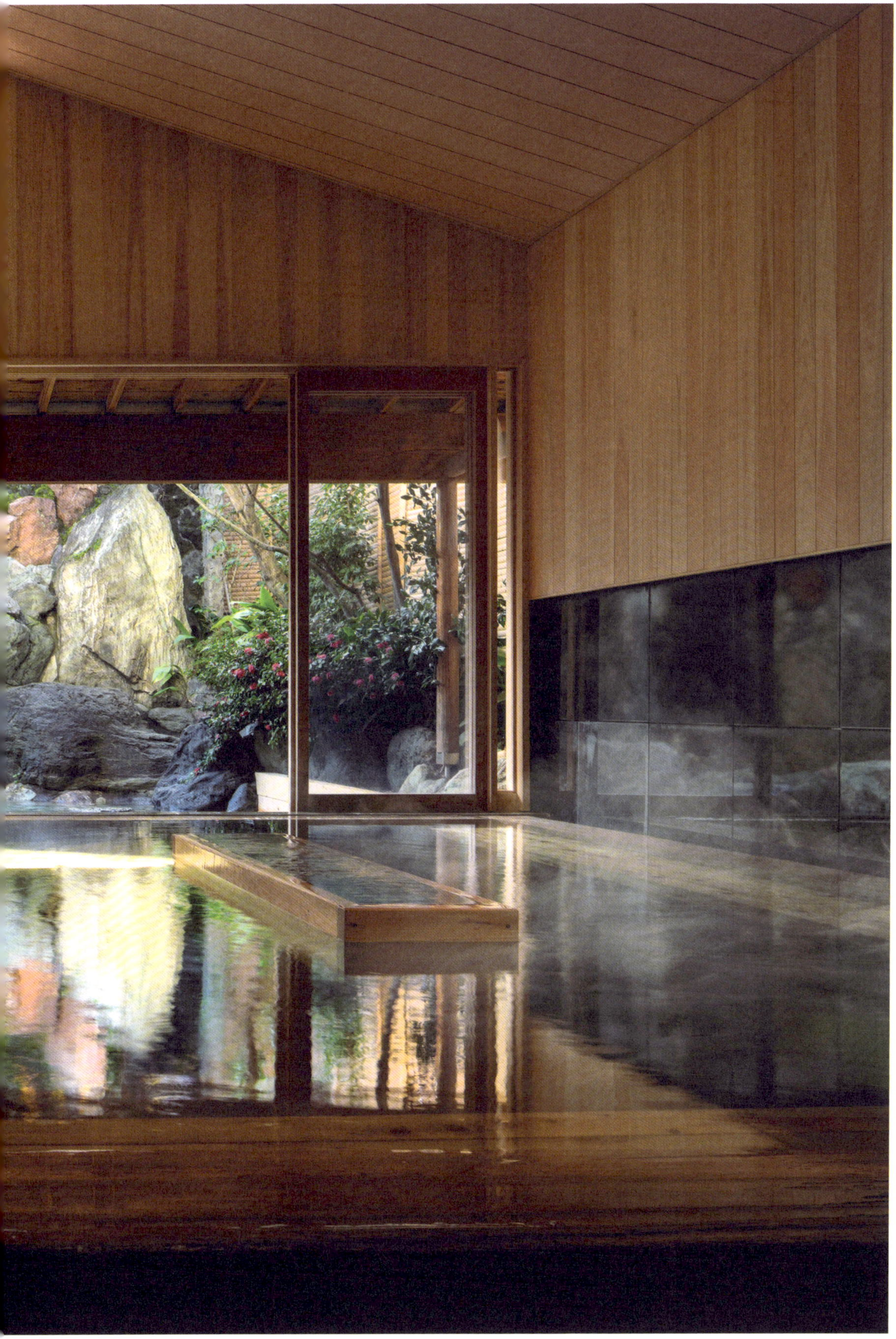

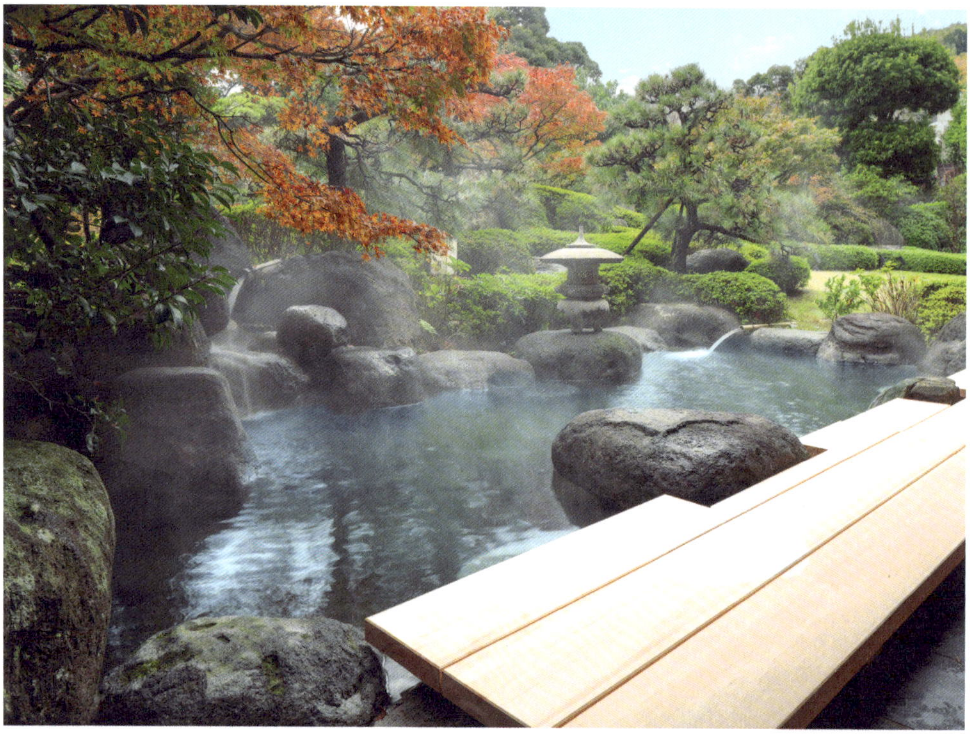

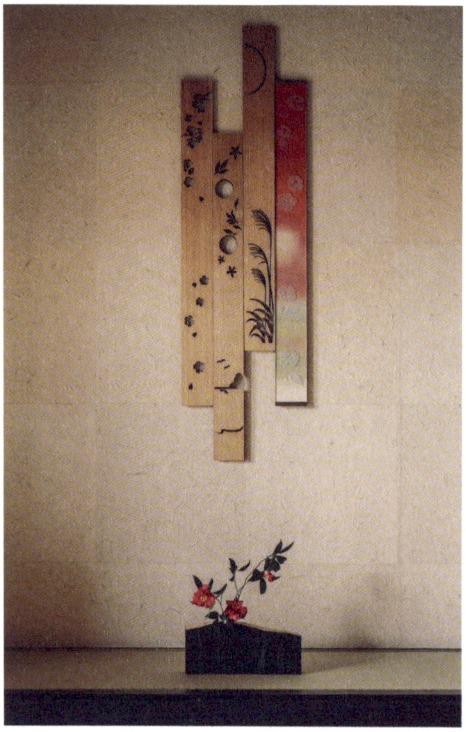

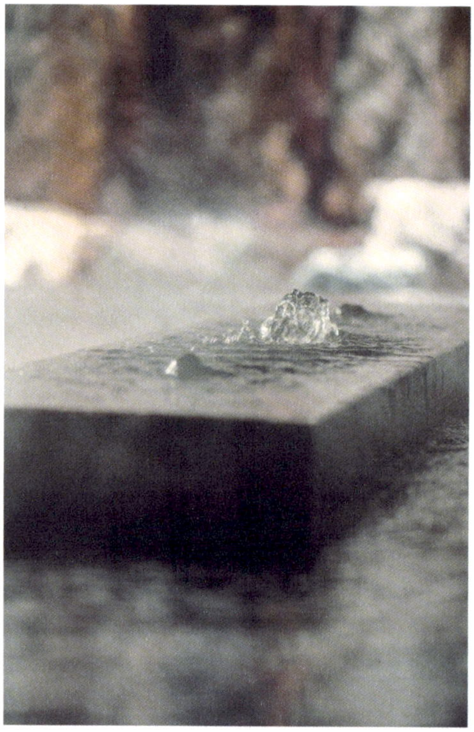

TOP One can enjoy peaceful moments while soaking one's feet in the garden's onsen footbath.

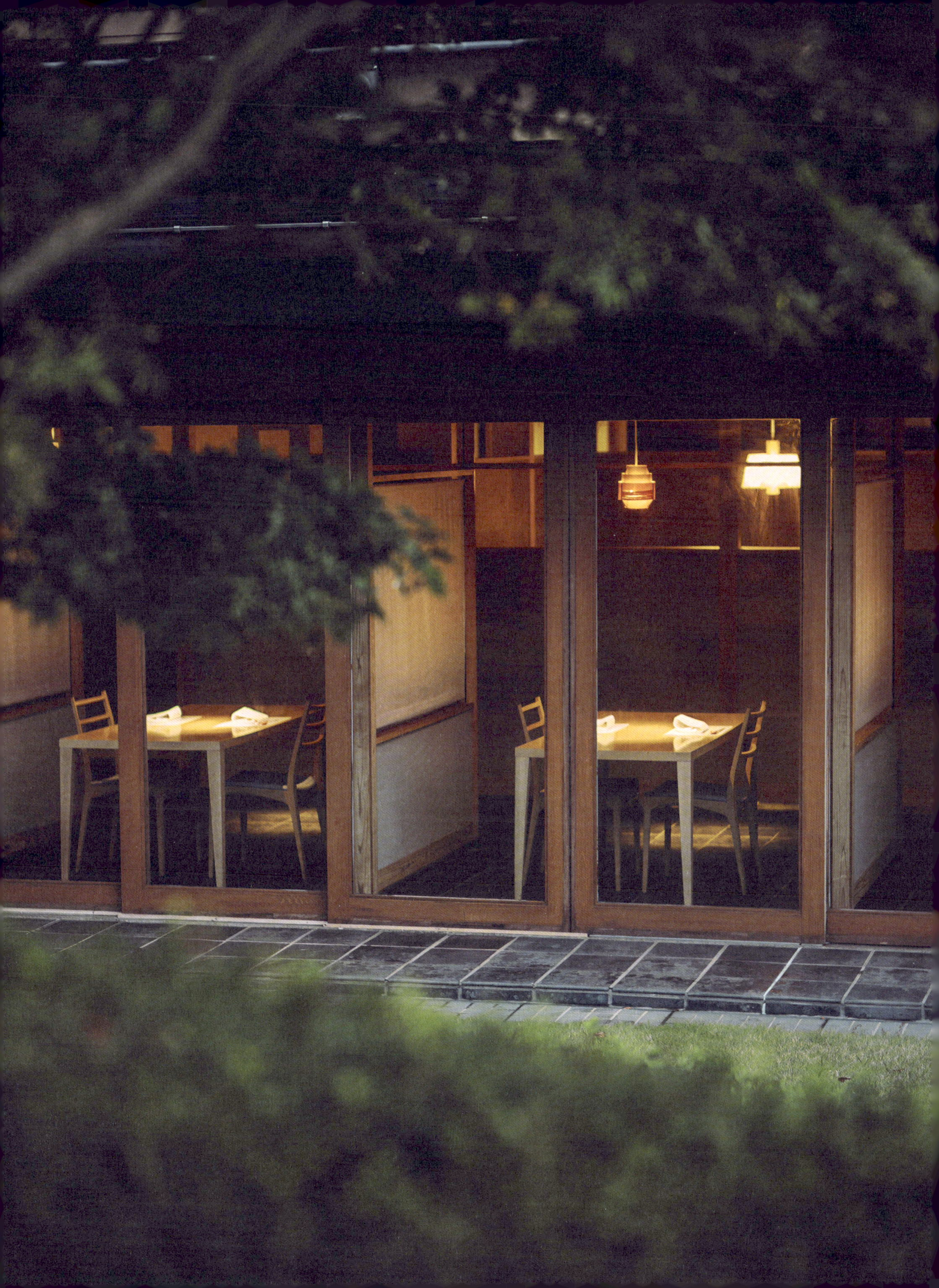

Bettei Otozure
Nagato • Yamaguchi Prefecture

PAMPER YOURSELF IN THIS ELEGANT, PRIVATE ONSEN RYOKAN

Behind secluded sliding doors lies a world of cozy luxury and refined intimacy, where both Japanese and Western aesthetics are celebrated.

Around the corner from Otani Sanso lies a sister property, the luxury onsen ryokan Bettei Otozure. A vision of Otani Kazuhiro's father, Bettei Otozure was created to provide travelers with a more intimate and exclusive experience of *omotenashi* in an onsen setting. With only 18 rooms available, a stay at this ryokan offers an opportunity to relax in the atmosphere of a traditional, opulent Japanese home, rich with cultural and historical touches.

The main entrance to Bettei Otozure is an unassuming traditional gate near the center of Nagato Yumoto onsen town. With no identifying external signage, a curving stone path leads up to the main building, where a subtle entrance door awaits, opening to reveal a courtyard water garden within. As guests stroll past the tranquil waters, which reflect the low buildings, the mountains, and the sky, they will happen upon several sliding doors, whereupon the entrance hall emerges—an open space with hanging lanterns and elegant patio chairs facing a traditional Japanese garden. After slipping off your shoes, the kimono-clad staff will guide you to a beautiful, garden-ensconced tea house, where local sweets and Japanese tea will be served in welcome.

Patter barefoot across the wooden floors and the rest of the premises, whether it be to the comfort of your room, down to the onsen, to the library for book browsing, or to Otozure's bar for a complimentary early evening drink.

The rooms of Bettei Otozure are quiet havens with a modern, cozy lodge ambiance; all contain their own private open-air onsen baths on their wide balconies, where one can take in peaceful views of the seasonal greenery. Some of the rooms are maisonettes split across two floors, while others are sprawling, single-story villas, replete with bedrooms, and separate areas for living, lounging, and even dining.

Guests at Bettei Otozure can wander over to Otani Sanso and use the public onsen there, but within the retreat's own grounds, one also finds a separate public onsen for men and women. Both baths have two indoor onsen to try, including a sleeping onsen, where one can fully recline, and an outdoor onsen set against a wall of trees. Regardless of how long one's trip is, a stay at Bettei Otozure offers a restful, healing sojourn.

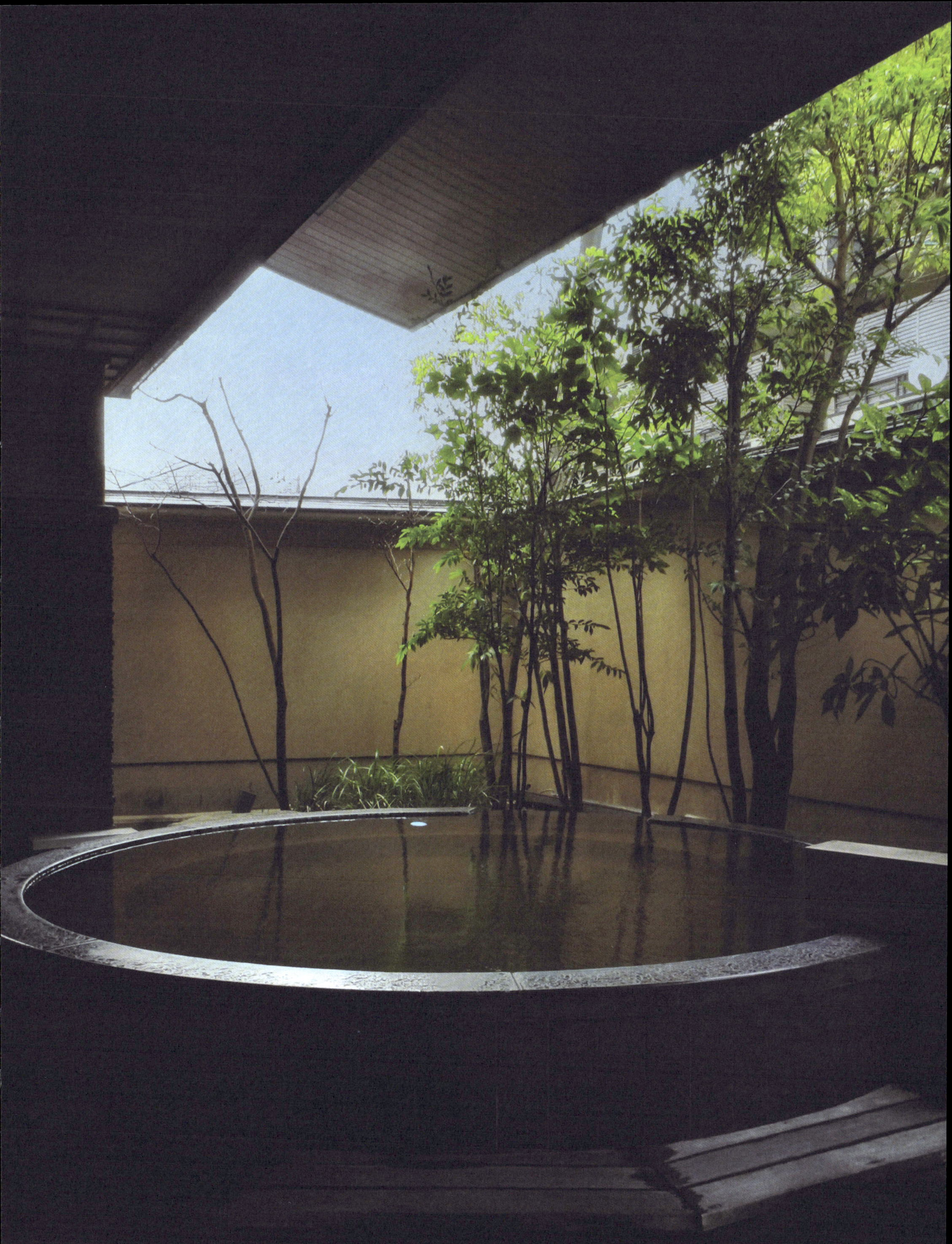

Kumano Kodō & Mt. Koya
Koyosan • Wakayama Prefecture

ONE OF THE WORLD'S OLDEST AND MOST BEAUTIFUL PILGRIMAGE ROUTES

Across the rugged Kii Peninsula stretch sacred roads that lead to stunning mountain temples.

Wakayama Prefecture is often regarded as Japan's deeply rooted spiritual heartland by many. For over 1,000 years, a series of ancient pilgrimage routes known as the Kumano Kodō have been used by pilgrims to visit the Kumano Sanzan (the Three Grand Shrines of Kumano): Kumano Hongu Taisha, Kumano Nachi Taisha, and Kumano Hayatama Taisha.

Historically, Shugendō monks would guide pilgrims to these Kumano holy sites. The Kumano faith, which predates all modern religions in Japan, incorporated elements later found in Shinto, Shugendō, mountain worship, and Buddhism. Kumano was open to all people, including women, who in the past were banned from other sacred sites in Japan.

Yatagarasu, the three-legged crow of Shinto myths, is the emblem of the Kumano region, and is worshipped as the servant of Susanoo-no-Mikoto, one of Japan's central deities. Legend tells that Yatagarasu's three legs are symbolic of heaven, the natural world, and humankind.

The Kodō (old way) routes see travelers traverse the well-trod, uneven stone steps and winding dirt paths through otherworldly mountain forests, where soft light filters through the canopy of towering trees. With a rich cultural history and deeply mystical natural environment, the sacred Kumano Kodō, Kumano Sanzan, and Koyasan became UNESCO World Heritage Sites in 2004.

Located higher along the Kii Peninsula, the holy mountain of Koyasan is considered the home of Shingon, a school of Buddhism founded 12 centuries ago by the priest Kukai (posthumously known as Kobo Daishi). Many beautiful temples surround the impressive central Kongobu-ji complex; however, another must-visit is Japan's largest cemetery, Okuno-in, where Kobo Daishi lies. Surrounded by a vast, verdant forest of massive cedars, the tranquil, expansive grounds are filled with moss-covered tombstones, torii gates, *jizo* statues, and dappled sunlight, producing a serene, spiritual atmosphere.

Throughout their journey in this revered region, many travelers will ease their aching and tired limbs by visiting some of its natural hot springs, including hidden onsen villages, a river onsen, a temple *shukubo,* and the only onsen in the world registered as a UNESCO World Heritage Site.

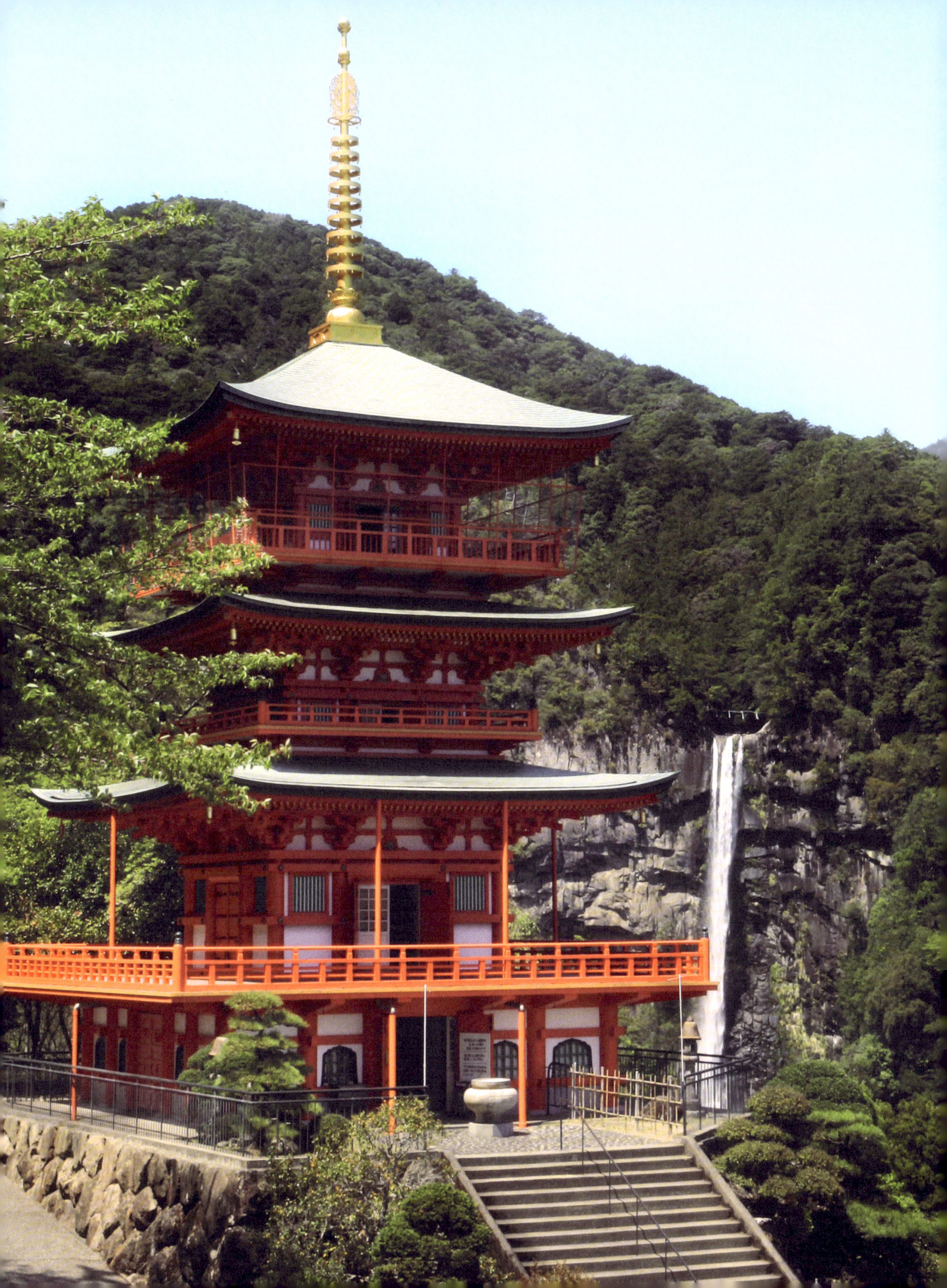

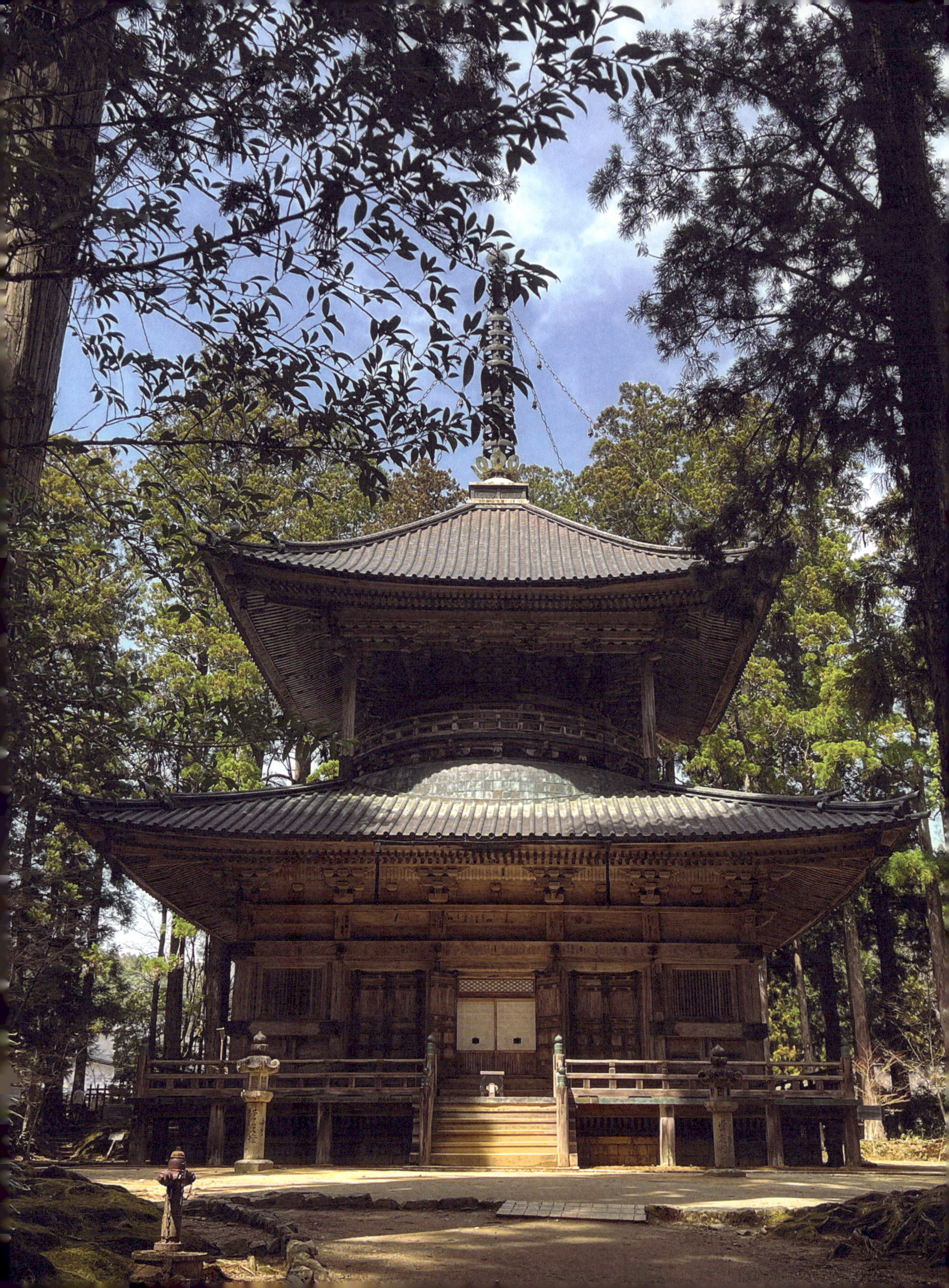

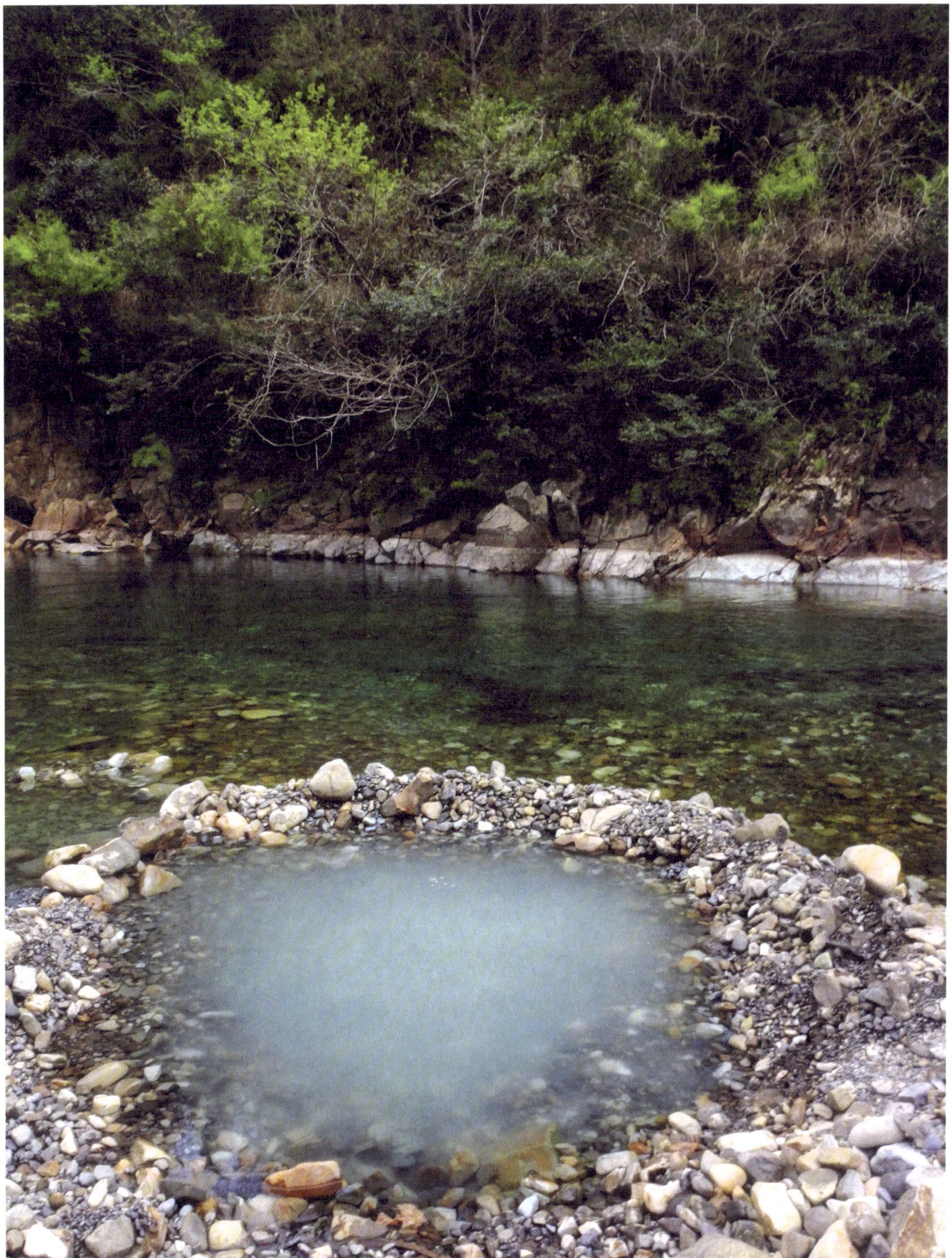

ABOVE A natural onsen source, the Kawayu River sees visitors and locals dig deep into the stones in the riverbed to create their own outdoor *rotenburo*.

Tsuru no Yu
Semboku • Akita Prefecture

BATHE AS ONE IN OLDEN, BYGONE TIMES

The cloudy onsen waters of this remote mountain destination have enchanted visitors for centuries.

Nestled within a beech forest at the foot of Mt. Nyuto lies Nyuto Onsen Village, part of Akita Prefecture's Towada Hachimantai National Park. Several secluded onsen ryokan are scattered around the village, with the oldest, and perhaps most legendary, being Tsuru no Yu.

Tsuru no Yu is another throwback to the slow onsen rituals of yesteryear. Built in the Tohoku region's architectural style, the buildings, with their engraved wooden pillars greeting you as you enter, retain a traditional mountain inn atmosphere. Tsuru no Yu's establishment traces back almost 400 years; however, the site's oldest remaining building, Honjin, was constructed around 1860. Originally known as Tazawa no Yu, the ryokan was later renamed, according to local lore, in honor of a crane (*tsuru* in Japanese) who was discovered healing its wounds in the onsen waters by a hunter called Kansuke.

Rooms are spread across five different buildings, ranging from the simplest tatami rooms in the original structures to those in the newer building, which contain *irori* hearths, *engawa* spaces, and private toilets. In keeping with the old *toji* experience, no rooms contain private bathrooms. Depending on one's accommodations, meals will either be served in-room or in one of two communal dining areas. The food is rustic, delicious, hearty Akita fare, with an abundance of mountain vegetables, a mountain yam *nabe* hotpot, and *ayu* (a sweet freshwater fish) that is slow-cooked over the *irori*.

Picturesque throughout all seasons, Tsuru no Yu is particularly beloved during the fall and winter: in autumn, rich, vibrant foliage in hues of red, orange, and yellow transforms the landscape, while deep winter sees gorgeous snowfalls blanketing the ground, the trees, and the building's roofs.

One's senses are especially heightened as one soaks away in Tsuru no Yu's four different onsen springs: Shiroyu, Kuroyu, Naka no Yu, and Taki no Yu, each with unique characteristics. The most famous onsen bath is the mixed *konyoku,* which lies just over a bridge. An open-air *rotenburo* with a small, simple wooden pagoda seating area, it has onsen waters that are a striking shade of bright pastel turquoise. Separate gender onsen baths can also be enjoyed, with the women's bath featuring a gorgeous open-air hinoki onsen with similar milky-blue waters. For shyer guests, Tsuru no Yu also offers a reservable, private onsen.

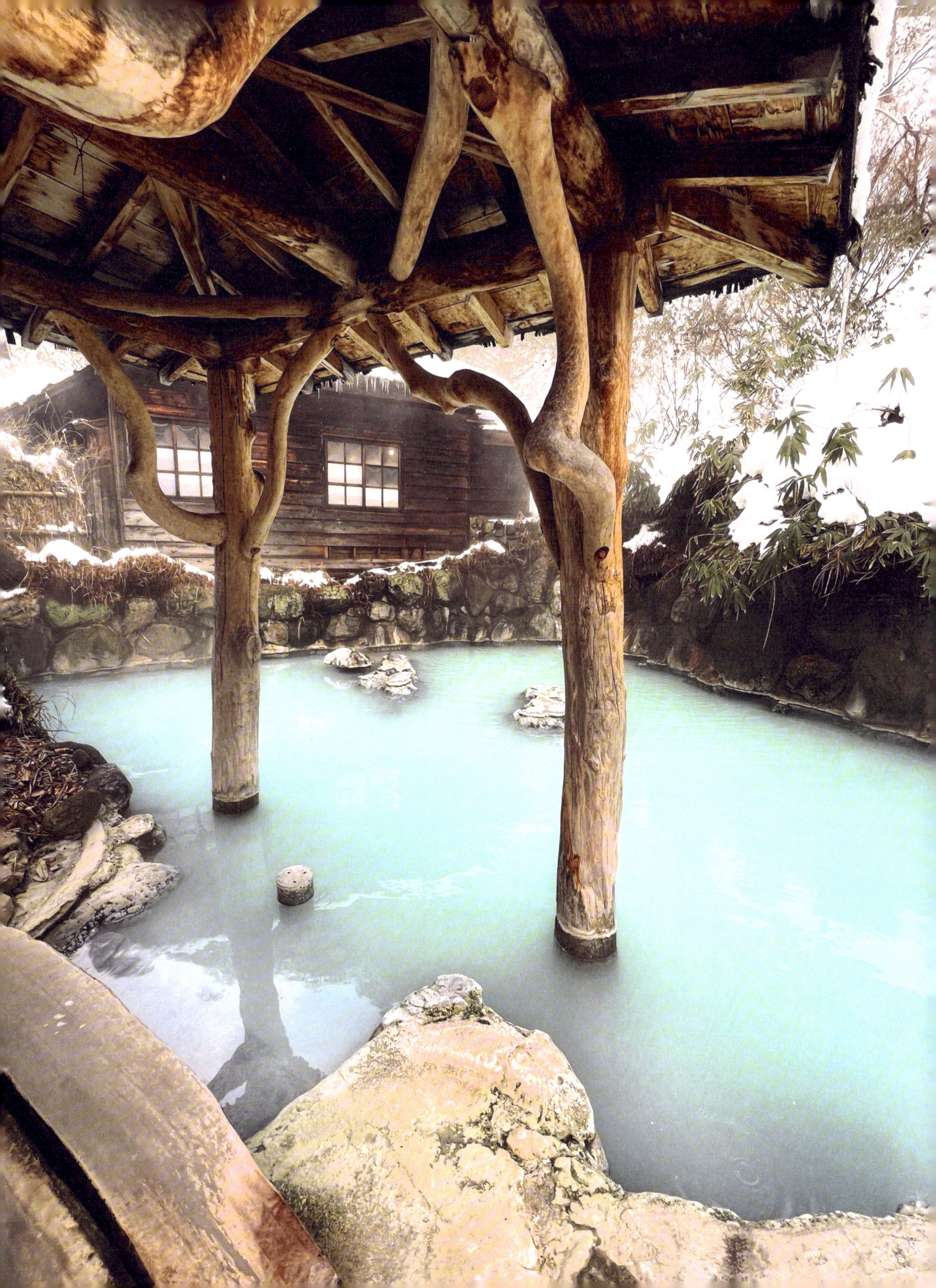

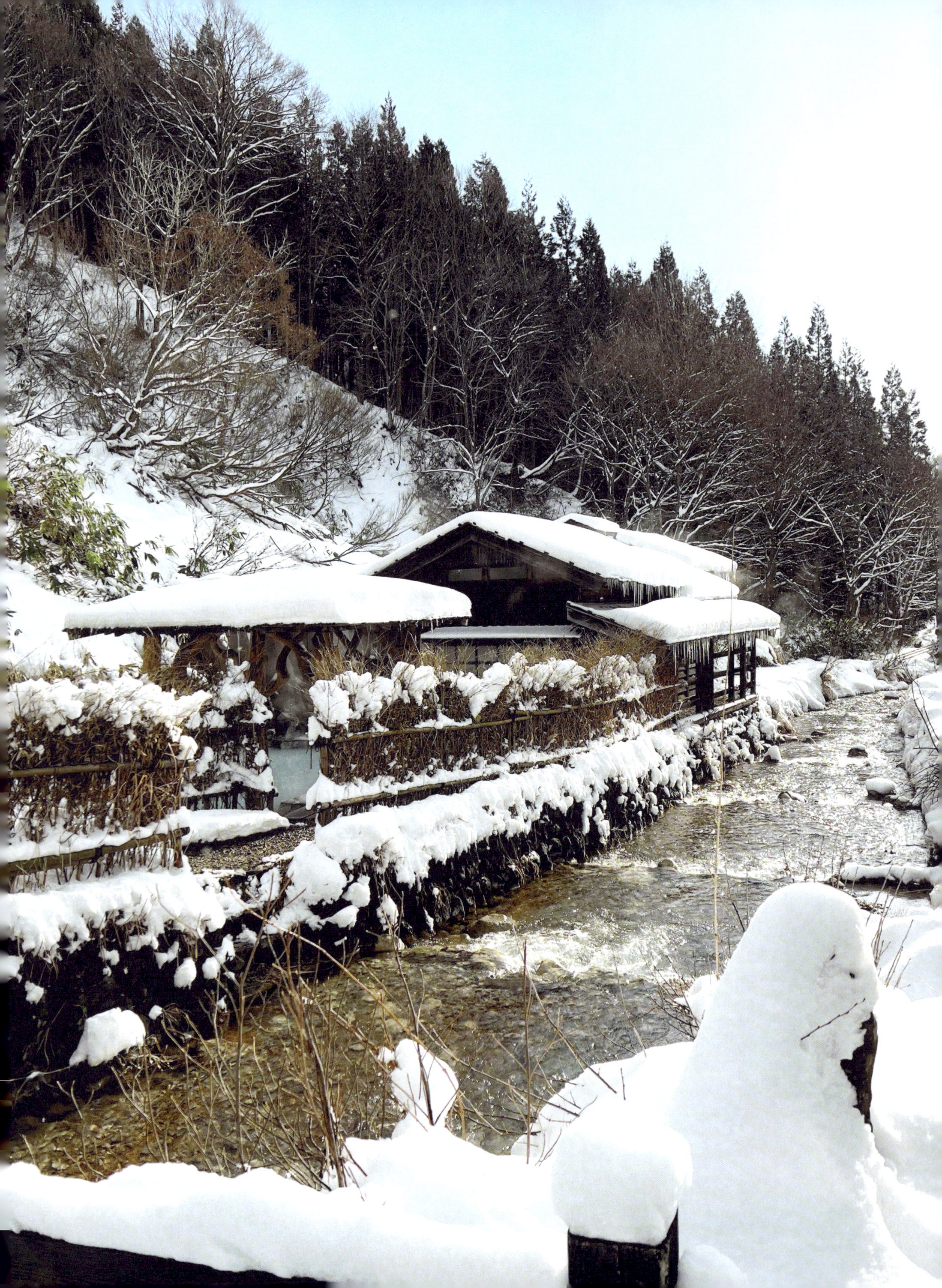

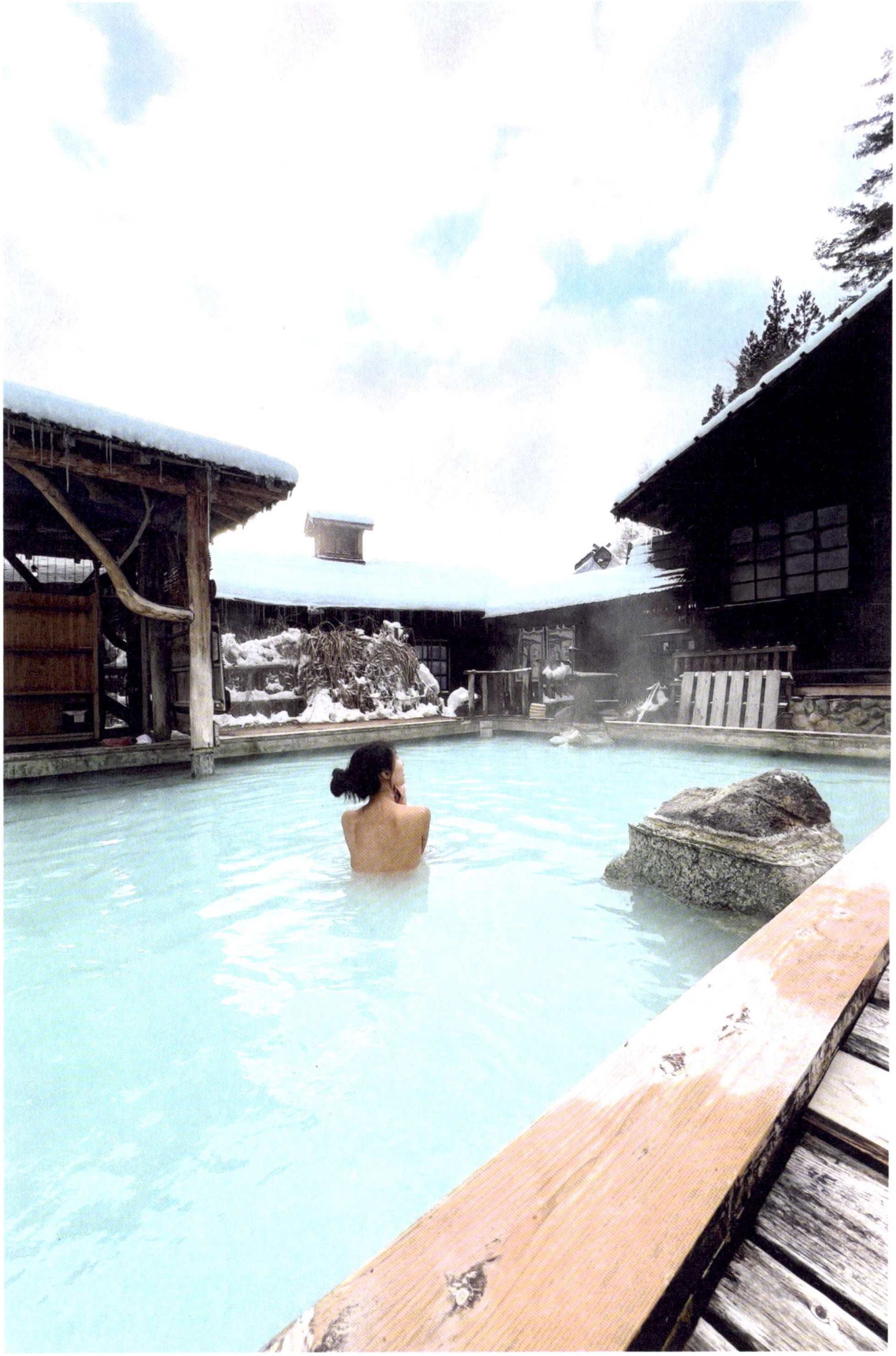

ABOVE At Tsuru no Yu, women can enjoy the same milky onsen waters found in the famed mixed onsen.

Iya Bijin
Miyoshi • Tokushima Prefecture

DISCOVER ONE OF JAPAN'S BEAUTIFULLY SCENIC, LESS-TRAVELED PREFECTURES

Even today, reaching this pristine mountain refuge takes time, but one's efforts are always rewarded.

Deep within Tokushima Prefecture's mountainous region and surrounded by visually imposing, craggy slopes, as well as the striking Oboke and Koboke gorges, lies the Iya Valley. Historically, this secluded domain was practically cut off from the outside world, and its remoteness served as a perfect refuge for the remnants of the Taira (Heike) clan who fled to the valley for safe cover after losing the Genpei War (1180–85). The Taira discovered the rich, flowing onsen waters enjoyed today, and their legacy is preserved in the two magnificent, unique vine bridges (known as Oku-Iya Kazurabashi) the clan constructed to safely cross the gorges through which the Yoshino River flows.

A foray into this wild landscape reveals a relatively untouched region, where wild deer, boar, and monkeys still roam. Though access has become easier since the 20th century, narrow, one-way mountain roads and limited public transport have helped maintain the area's quiet serenity. Only a handful of lodgings are available to travelers, and none are more charming than the tiny hidden inn, Iya Bijin.

Iya Bijin began life as a local soba restaurant and is still a popular choice for those seeking a taste of fresh, handmade soba noodles, as well as other local specialties. Dine indoors or on the outdoor terrace perched above the river, where a cheeky statue of a *tanuki* (raccoon dog) urinates off the cliff edge, an homage to the statue placed at the awe-inspiring Hinoji Valley which was placed there to honor the past time of local children eager to prove their courage.

Featuring a mere nine rooms, Iya Bijin offers a lovely, intimate experience. No public onsen exists on-site; instead, each room has its own open-air onsen, where visitors enjoy views of the gorgeous landscape and the valley's soothing sounds. Comforting, rustic tatami rooms, with fluffy futons and antique decor, provide a restful atmosphere, with several rooms alternating between Shigaraki pottery or cypress-wood onsen baths. Two of the rooms, perfect for families or larger groups, have multiple bathing areas and feature both a Shigaraki and hinoki onsen. Travelers can leisurely explore the surrounding area with ease, taking comfort in the knowledge that a peaceful abode—along with delicious home-cooked mountain fare grilled over a traditional *irori*—awaits.

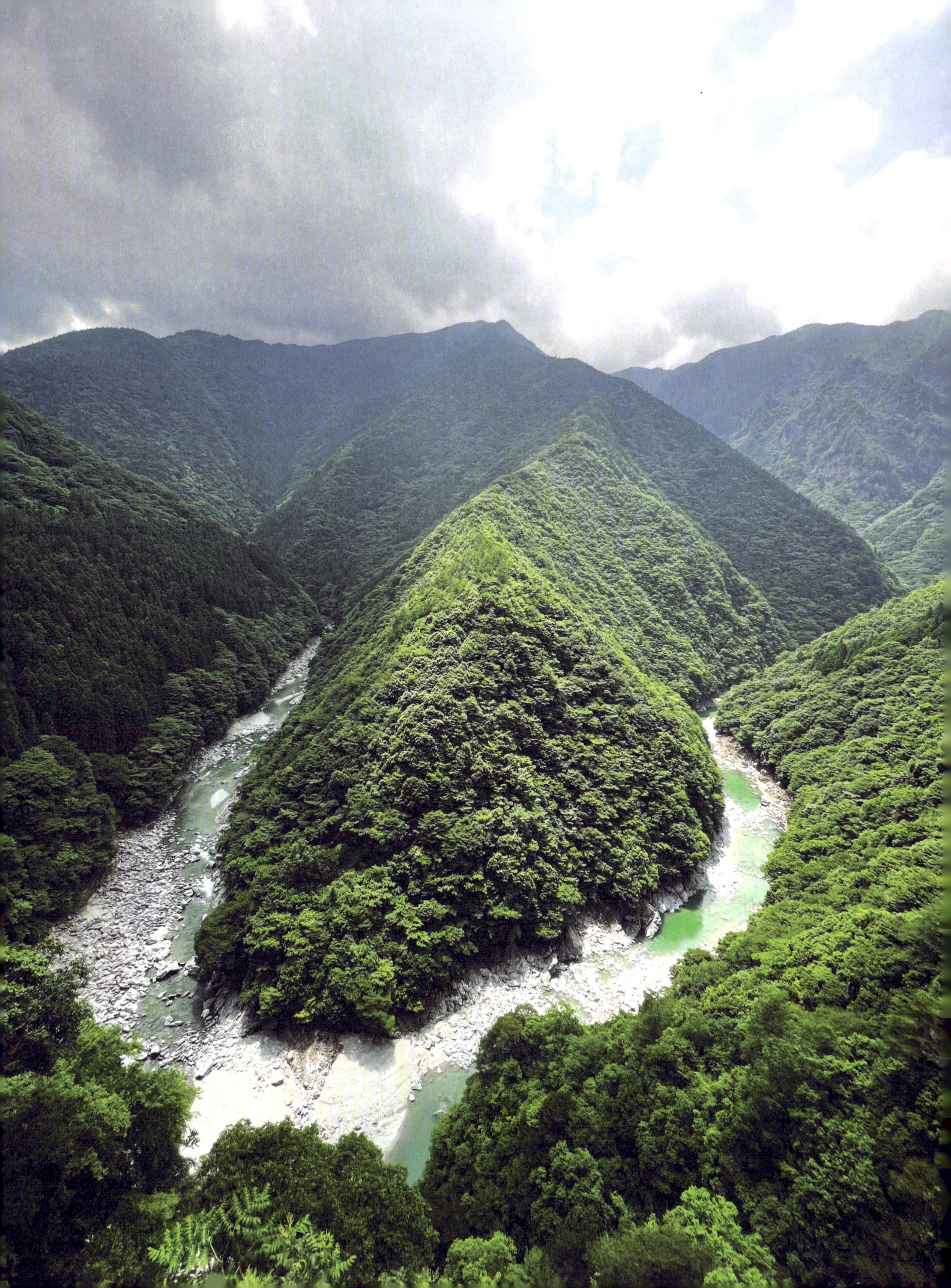

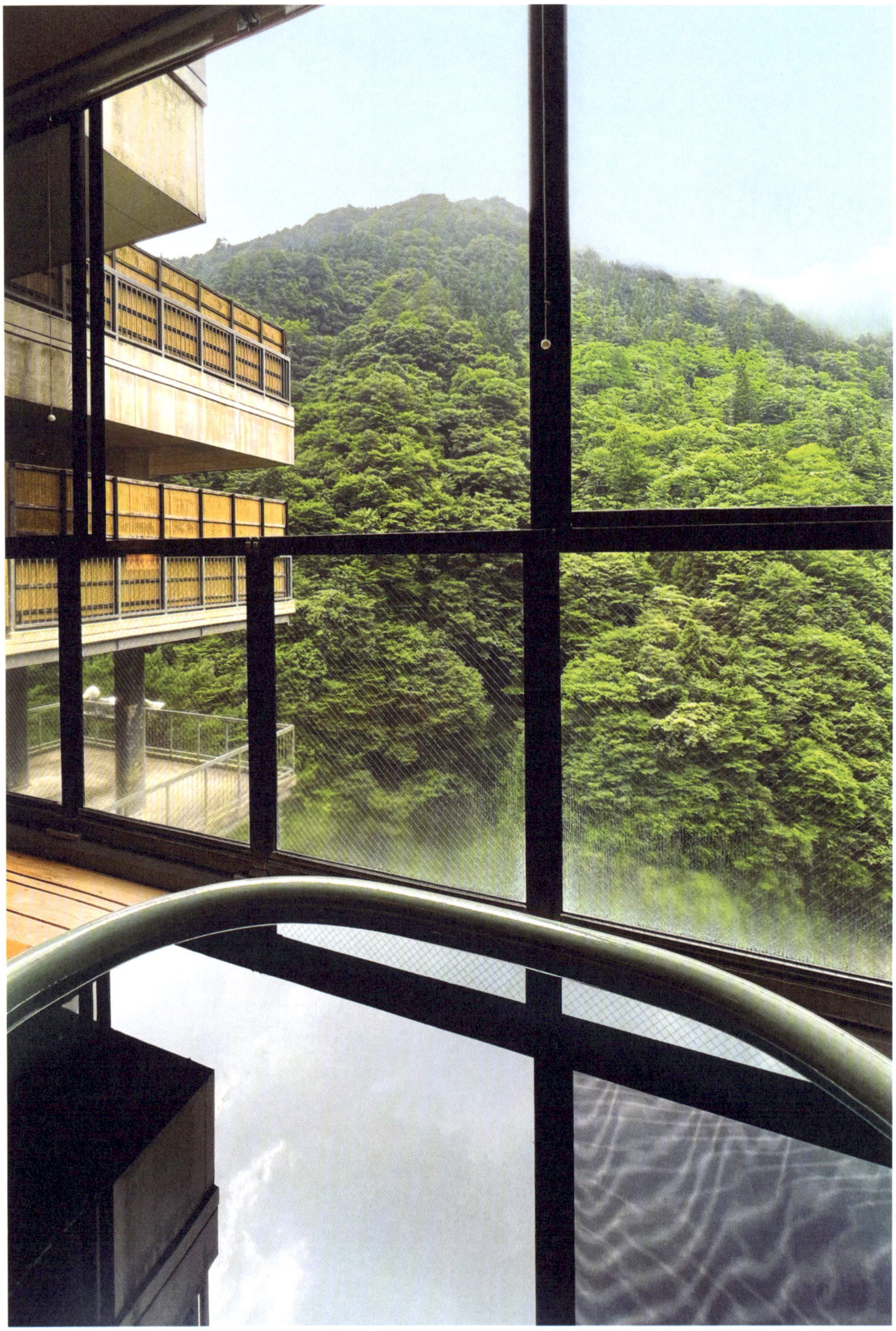

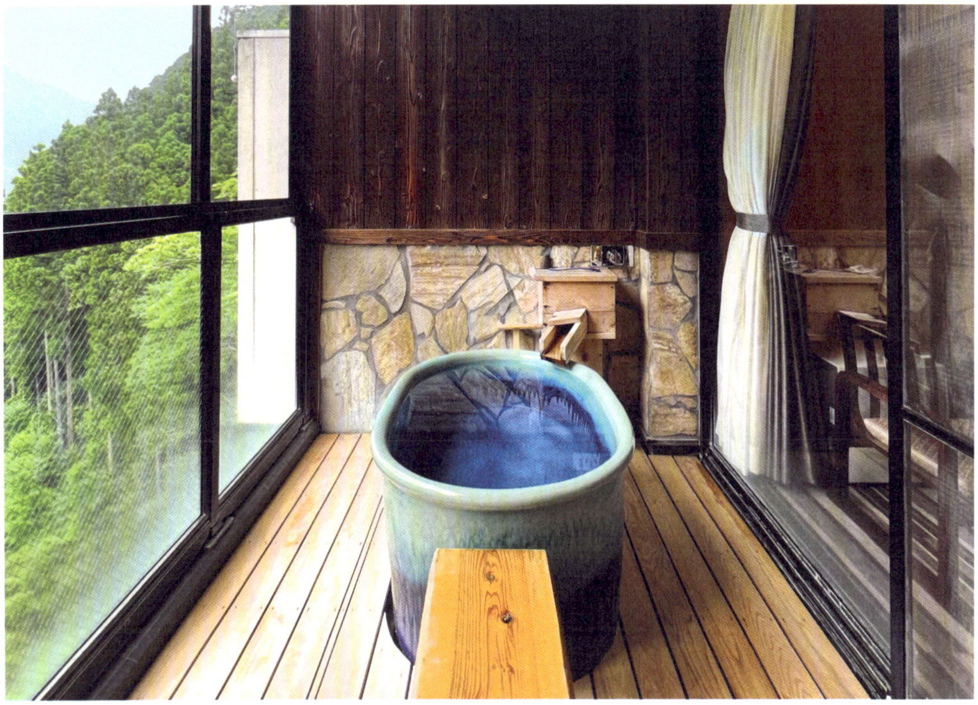

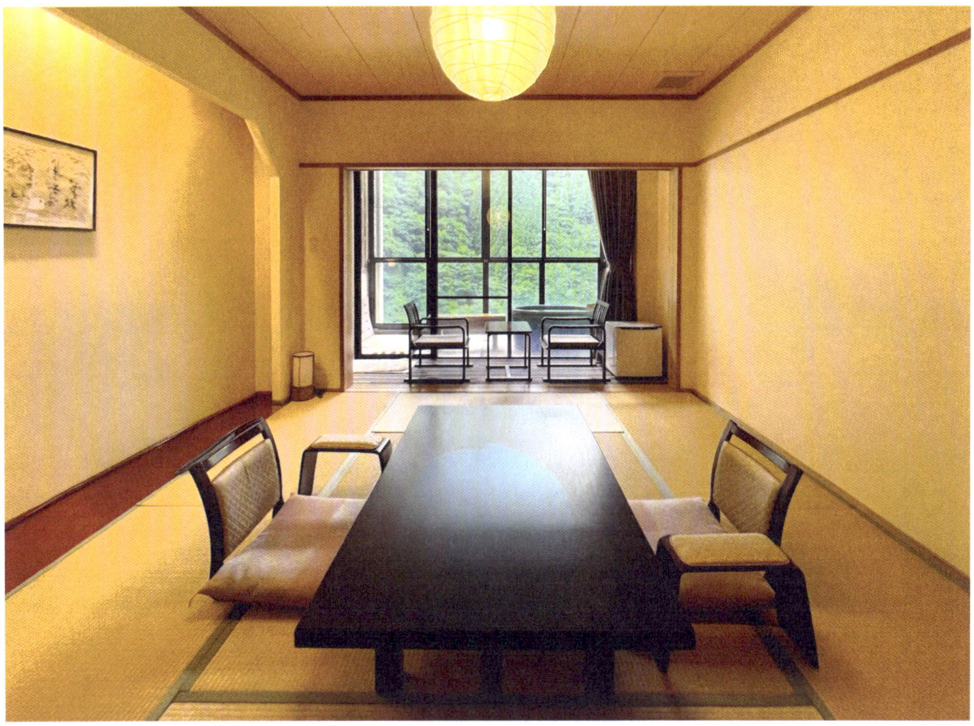

ABOVE AND LEFT One of Iya Bijin's nine rooms, each of which has a private, open-air onsen and wide views of the Iya Valley.

Unzen Onsen
Shimabara Peninsula • Nagasaki Prefecture

THE FIRST ONSEN TOWN TO ADMIT FOREIGN VISITORS

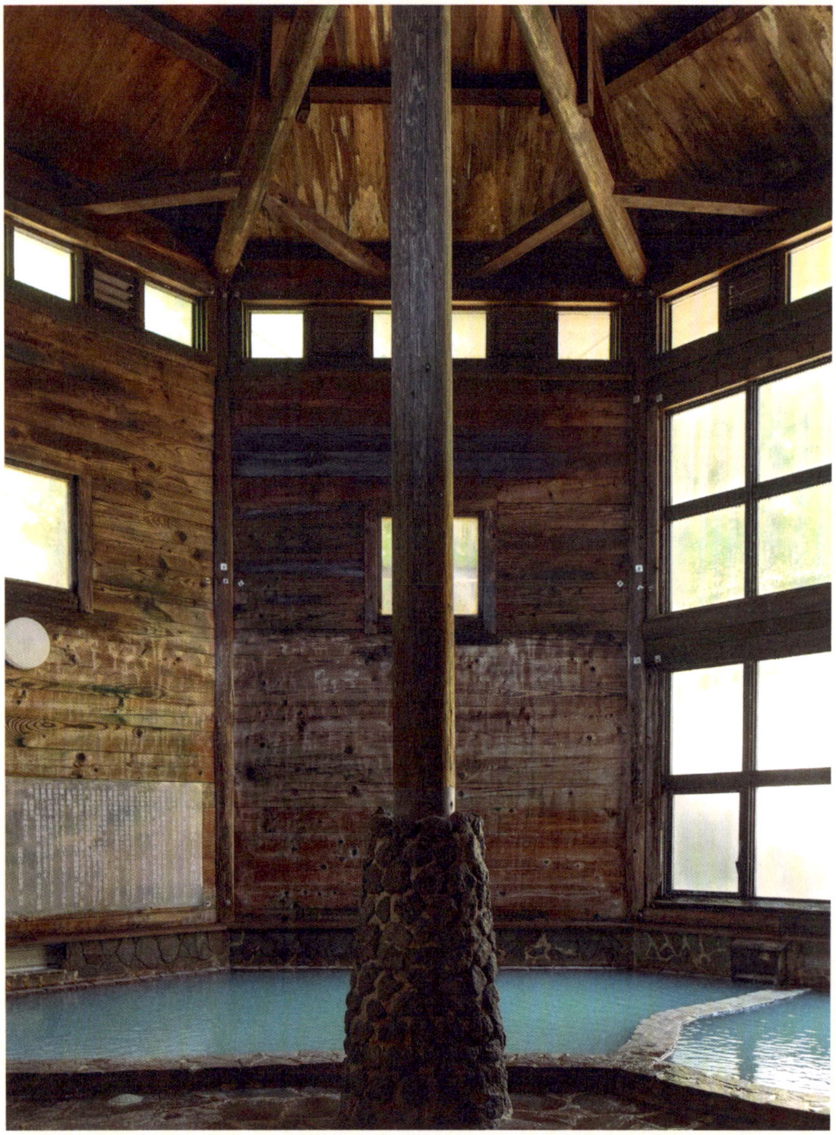

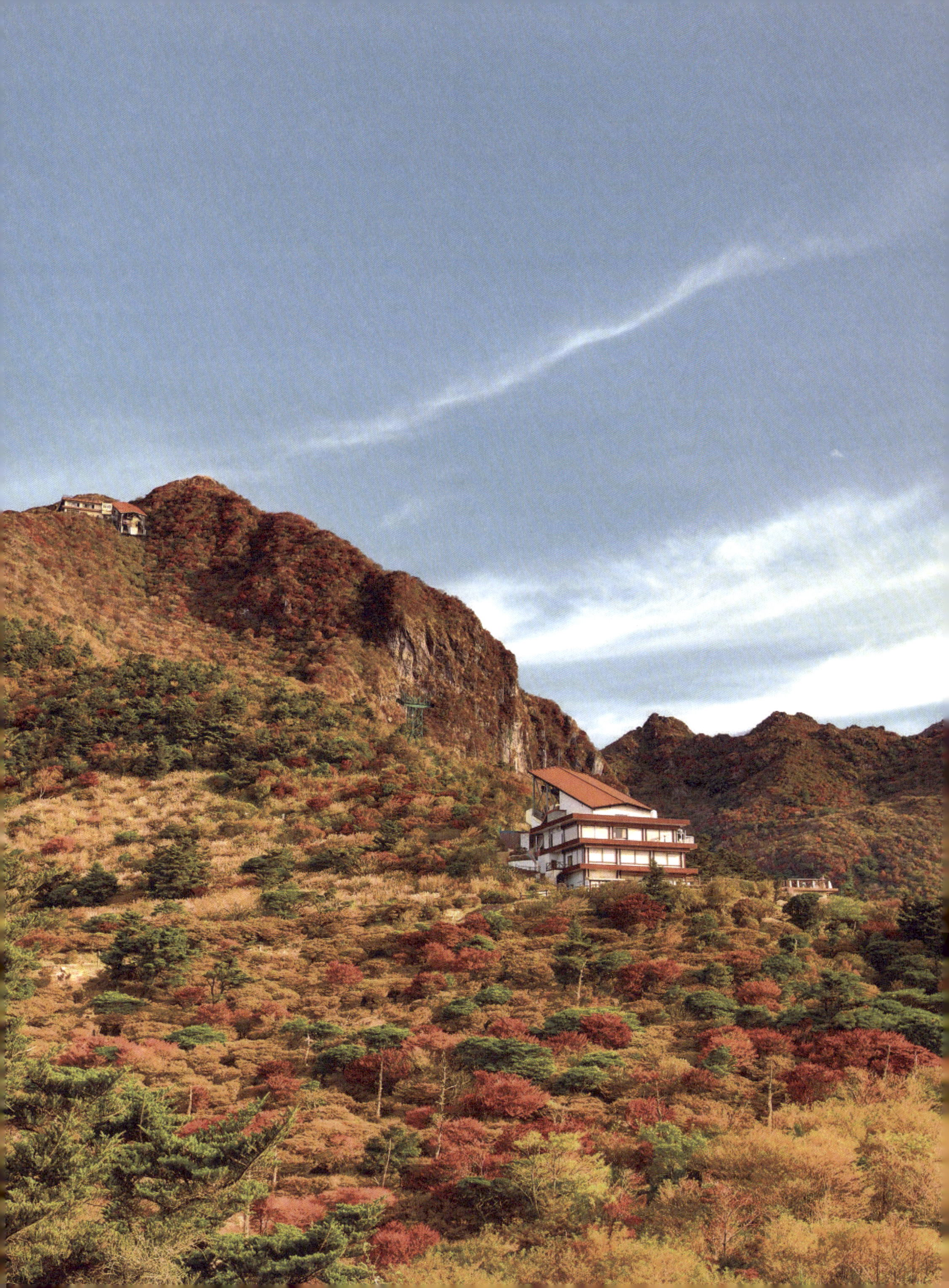

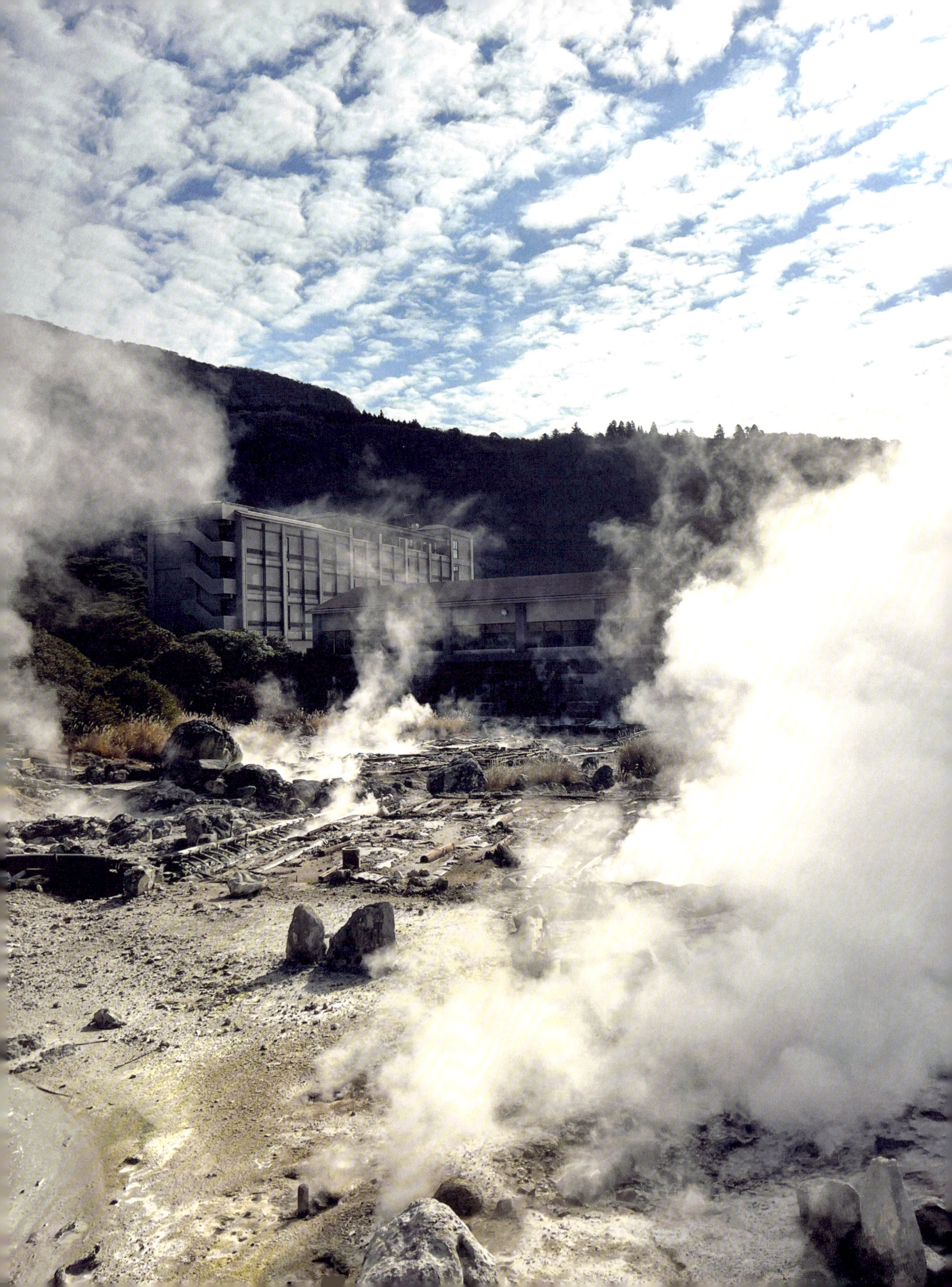

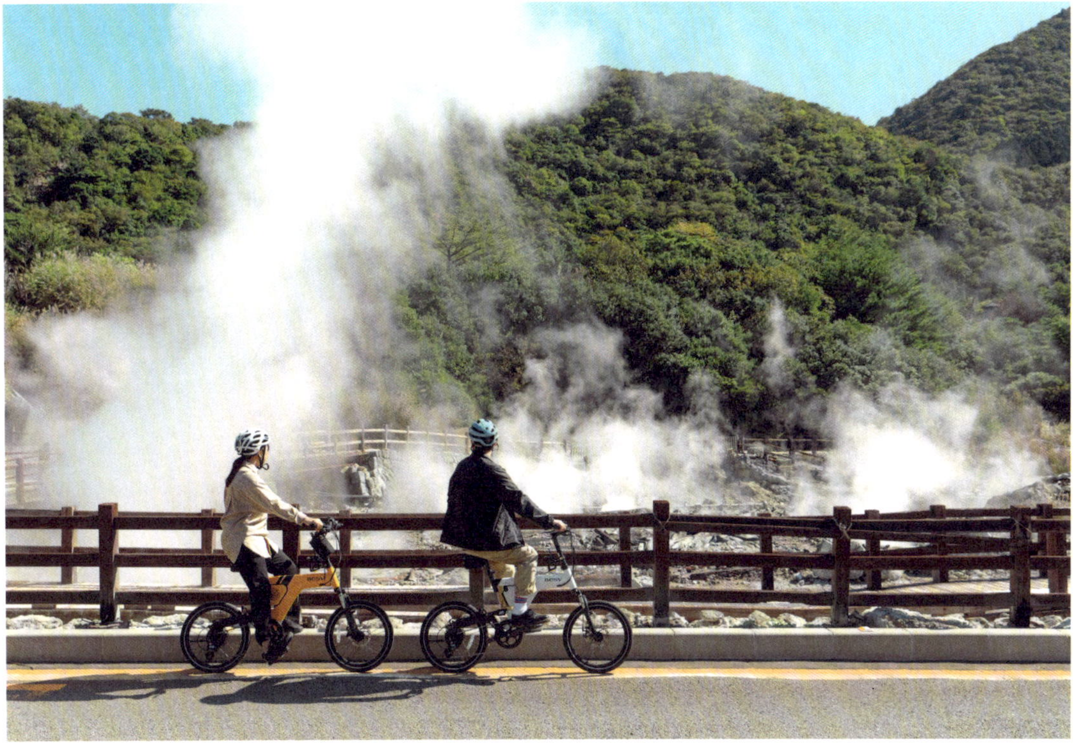

LEFT Onsen steam rising rapidly from Unzen Onsen's Jigoku Hell Valley.

This historic area lies in Japan's first-ever national park, where billows of onsen steam stream upward toward the sky.

Not far from Nagasaki is an onsen town affectionately known as the "cute cat kingdom." Situated near the peak of Mount Unzen, the aptly named Unzen Onsen was originally developed as a temple town and once rivaled Koyasan in size. During Japan's period of isolation (1639–1853), Nagasaki was the only Japanese port open to foreign trade, so when Japan reopened to the world it was Nagasaki that stood at the forefront of international relations. Through the last years of the Edo period and well into the Meiji period, Unzen Onsen became one of Japan's first tourist destinations, favored by visiting foreigners whose influence can be glimpsed in the town's architecture. This Western influence is especially evident in the iconic Unzen Kanko Hotel, one of nine "classic" hotels that first accommodated overseas dignitaries, celebrities, and regular guests when Japan opened its borders.

Unzen Onsen's Jigoku (onsen hell) lies in the heart of town; to one side of the main road one finds a tranquil atmosphere with walking trails leading to the beautiful Manmyoji Temple, while on the other, huge billowing steam clouds drift up from the eerie, rocky landscape. The land itself might be said to contain a few demons, as historically these grounds were the site of executions following the failed Shimabara Rebellion. Today, however, one finds only a walking area leading to the powerful onsen source, whose healing waters flow to the town's multiple ryokan and free onsen footbaths.

In contrast to Noboribetsu Onsen, where you can view the huge plumes of steam from afar on the wooden promenade, the duckboard paths of Unzen Onsen bring you right through the steam clouds as

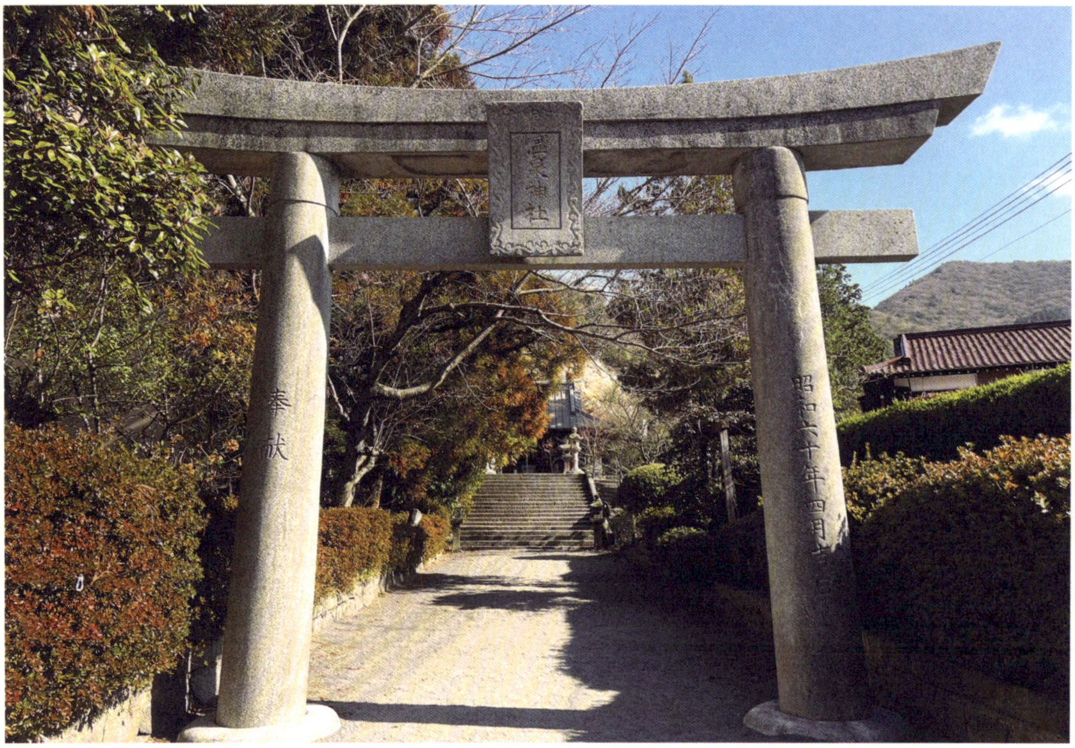

ABOVE A stone torii gate marks the entrance to Unzen Onsen's shrine.

you pass alongside the bubbling, milky, and sulfurous waters springing from the earth. Its snaking paths lead visitors around the grounds, offering several mountain viewpoints and rest areas so as to better take in the impressive sights.

In an unusual contrast, while strolling the paths, visitors will also encounter a variety of adorable local cats, either meandering around, having a snooze, or enjoying the warmth of the onsen-heated wooden boards. Inquisitive, yet happy to keep to themselves, the cats are a permanent fixture in the hell valley and are typically found in the central picnic area where, in addition to the mischievous cats, one can enjoy a snack of onsen *tamago*, or onsen-cooked eggs.

As in many other onsen towns, various small shrines are spread out across Unzen. Situated adjacent to the onsen hell valley, the main shrine, Shimengu—known simply as "Unzen Onsen Shrine" to the locals—is a pleasing, rustic wooden structure with two stone torii gates guarding its entrance. Unzen is an easily walkable town, and visitors can leisurely amble through the sights while stopping in its small cafes, restaurants, the onsen footbaths. Also popular is the traditional local handmade snack, *yusempei:* a thin, crispy wafer made from eggs, flour, and its most vital ingredient, the town's onsen water.

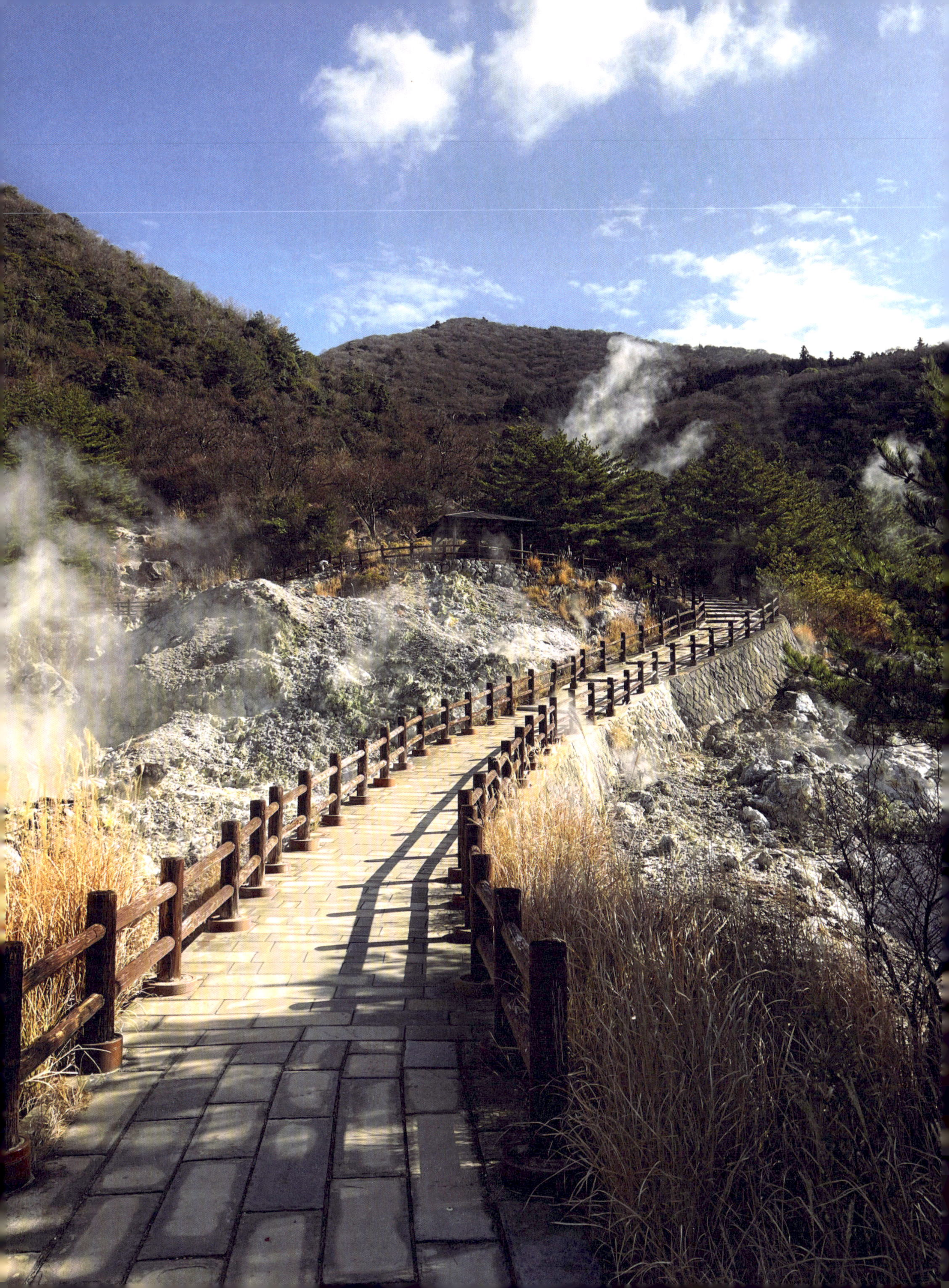

Sanso Yamanoiro
Kokonoe • Oita Prefecture

TRAVEL THE LESS-TROD PATH TO REACH THIS DREAM ONSEN REGION

The journey to this remote area—a haven for onsen lovers—takes time and patience, but visitors will be rewarded with a soothing stay.

"Good things take time" runs the old adage, and there's something extremely satisfying about the slow journey one takes to reach the onsen area known as Kokonoe "Yume Onsen" in Oita Prefecture. The area features 12 onsen, with three that are especially notable: Chojabaru, Ukenokuchi, and Sujiyu Onsen. Chojabaru feeds Sankei no Yu, an open-air bath within the Kokonoe Hosshou Hotel, and Ukenokuchi supplies water to the casual ryokan Shinseikan, whereas Sujiyu lies at the base of the Kuju foothills. Visitors to this area are rewarded with beautiful countryside vistas, friendly locals, and an atmosphere that inspires calm and thoughtful contemplation.

Sujiyu opened its first bath in 958, before growing into an onsen resort by 1658. Today, it's renowned for its strong water and four public onsen: Iwanyu, a stone *rotenburo;* Yakushi, an indoor hinoki onsen; Ikoi, an outdoor footbath; and the most famous, Utase-yu, where 18 onsen sources flow down into the bath from above to create a waterfall onsen. Sujiyu is considered Japan's best cascading onsen, offering relief to stiff shoulders, sore backs, and aching muscles onto which the cascading onsen pours down.

Among the town's ryokan, Sanso Yamanoiro stands out for offering a truly charming and intimate stay. The cozy, rustic inn has only eight rooms—essentially a row of private independent villas, connected by a covered outdoor corridor facing the garden. Five of these rooms have private, open-air onsen and two have semi-open-air onsen. Each of the rooms differ slightly not only in interior style but in its onsen design: elements of traditional Japanese aesthetics, antiques, tatami floors, and shoji doors typically feature, with only two rooms containing Western-style beds. The rooms' private onsen range from deeply embedded, cut-stone baths to curving rock *rotenburo* and aromatic hinoki wood baths, with many featuring gorgeous views of the mountain scenery.

There are three additional private, freely reservable onsen available to staying guests. Yamasowa no Yu is a large, open-air rock *rotenburo* with two pools and views of the Kuju Mountains. Saezuri no Yu is a semi-open-air hinoki bath, where sliding shoji doors reveal the nature outside. Both Yamasowa and Saezuri are private until 7:00 am, whereupon they become *konyoku* (mixed bathing onsen) until 10:00 am. Hogure no Yu is a smaller, indoor stone onsen that remains private all the time.

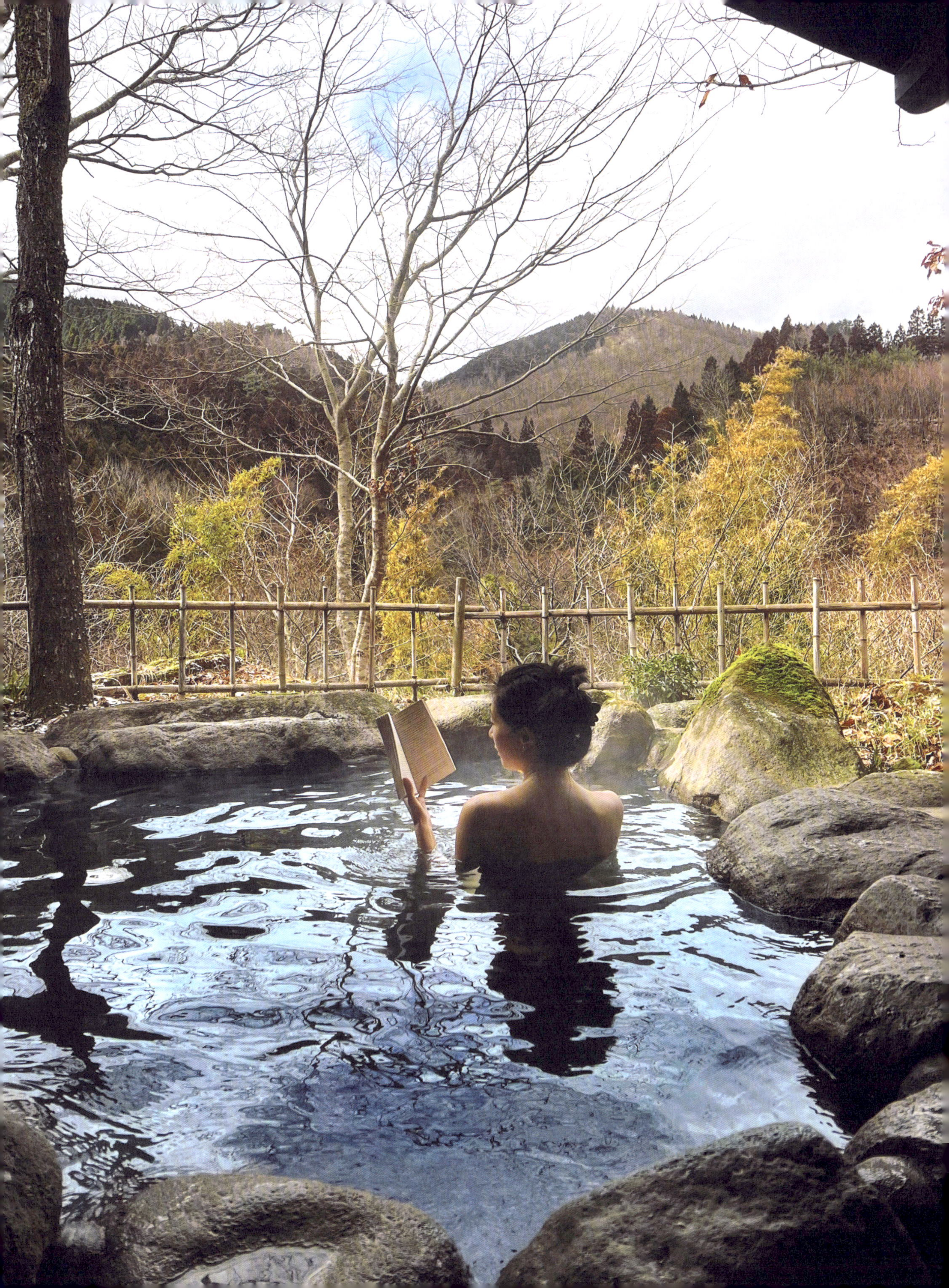

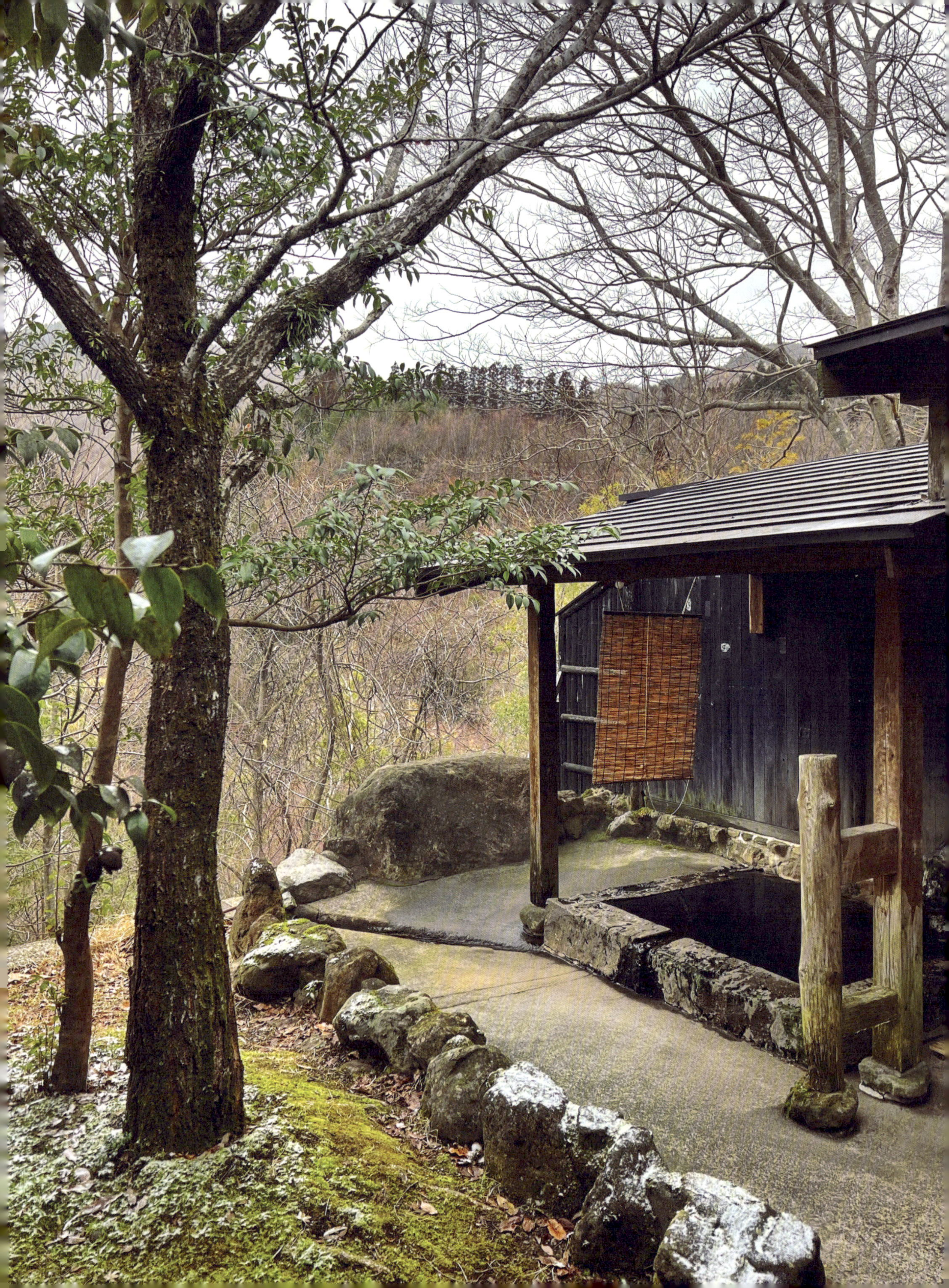

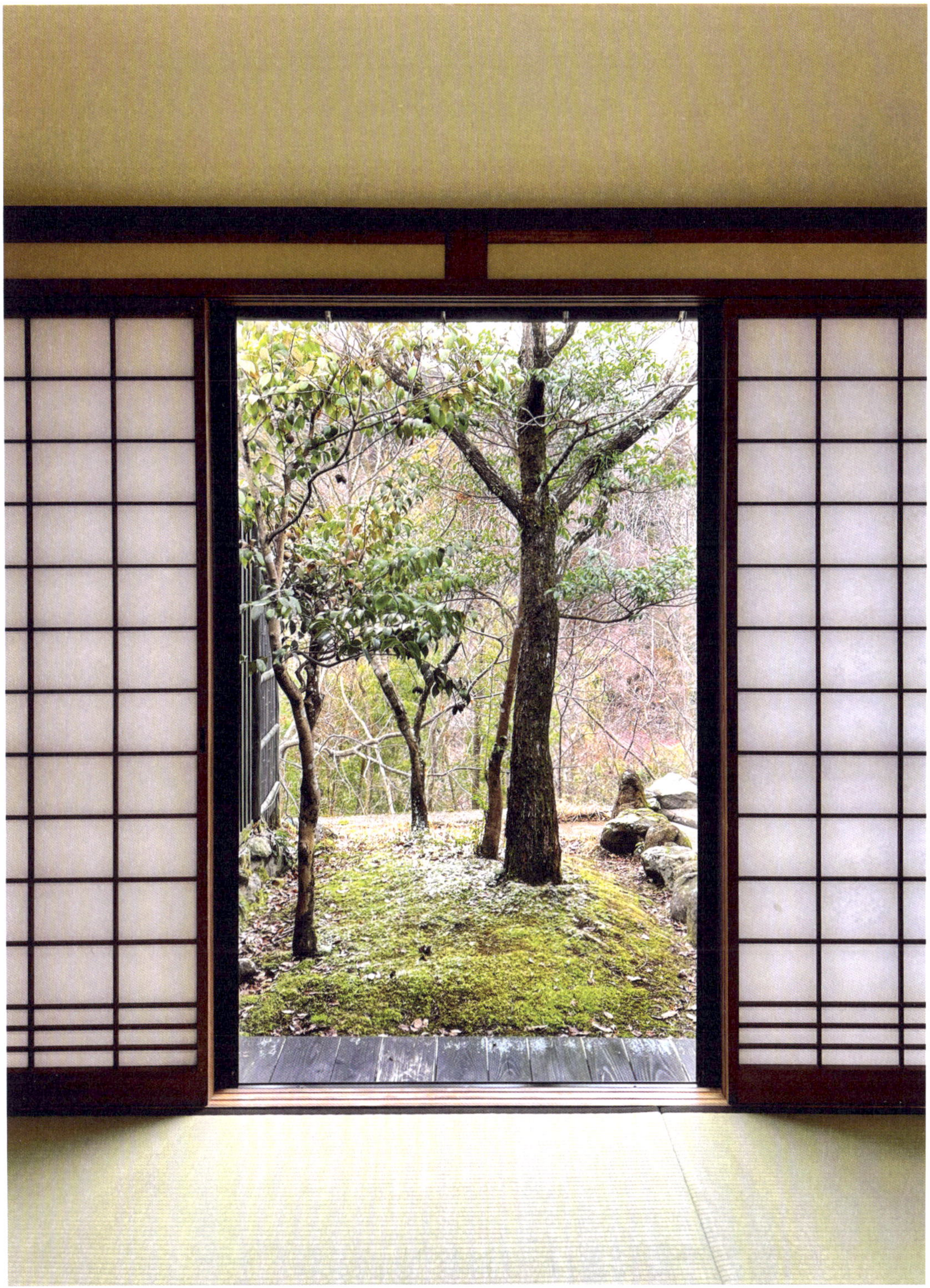

ABOVE Sliding shoji doors offer garden views in many of the private villas of Sanso Yamanoiro.

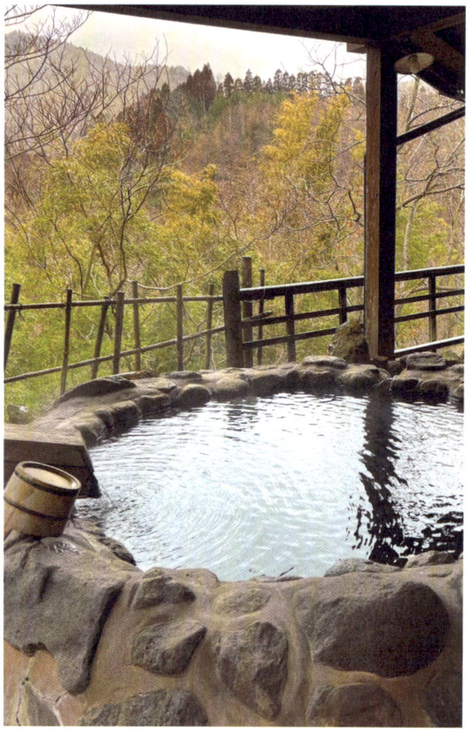

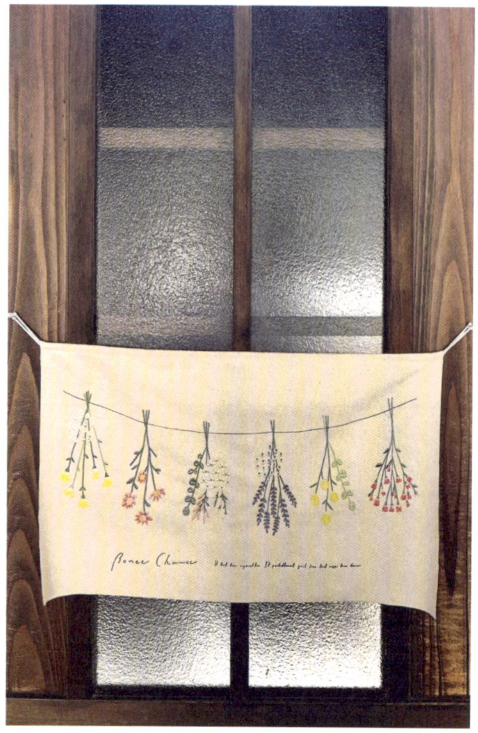

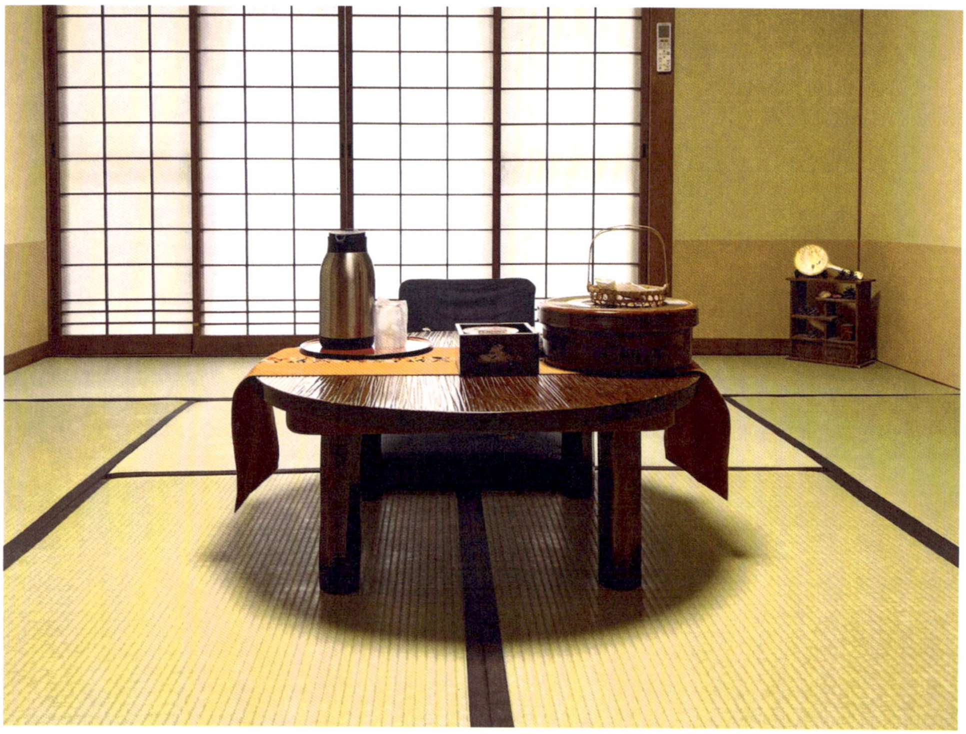

RIGHT One of Sanso Yamanoiro's three freely reservable private onsen baths for staying guests.

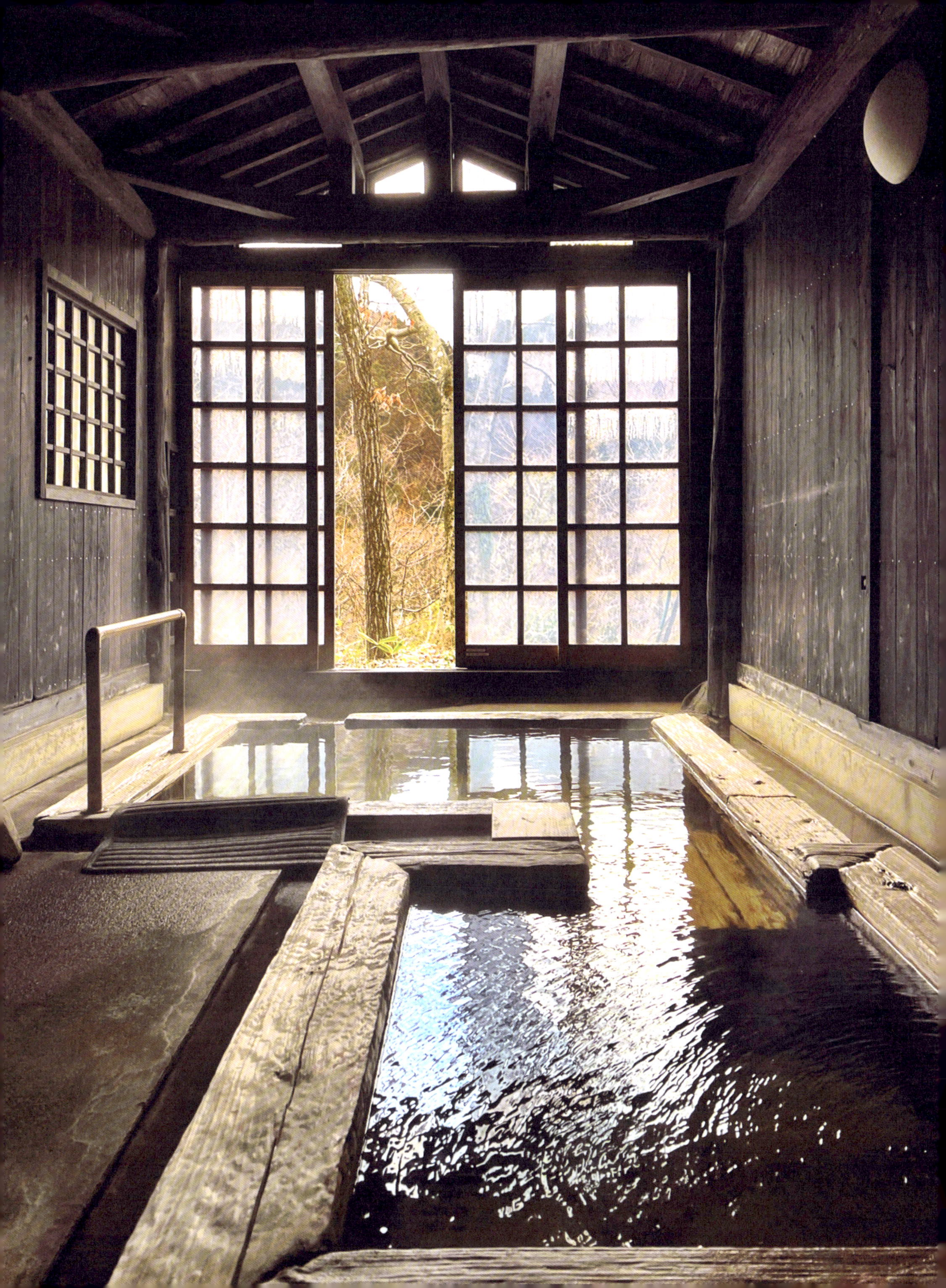

Haiya Ryokan
Awara • Fukui Prefecture

LEISURELY ENJOY THE SLOW PASSING OF TIME

Within the elegant, beautiful rooms of the Shofuan Annex, one can experience the breathtaking skills of Japan's *shokunin*.

Along the Sea of Japan lies Fukui Prefecture, home to the charming onsen town of Awara. In 1883, a farmer discovered the first onsen source while digging an irrigation well, and by the following year numerous onsen ryokan and inns, including Haiya Ryokan, began establishing themselves in town.

The inn's name (Haiya means "house of ash") honors the owners' ancestors, who produced the fine, artisanal ash once used in the dyeing of Kabuki and Noh theater costumes. Haiya is currently helmed by Okami Makita-san, the matriarch and *yondaime*, or fourth-generation family head.

The onsen ryokan's 50 beautifully appointed rooms are distributed across three main buildings, each offering its own distinct charm and ambiance, and all overlooking a quintessential Japanese garden. The main building, Jyurakutou, holds 17 traditional, simply-styled rooms, whereas the newest annex, Kangetsutei, possesses eight spacious, light-filled suites of differing design and layout, each incorporating both Japanese and Western elements.

Shofuan, the original 1884 annex, features 15 distinct rooms, each with its own traditional garden. Several rooms in this annex also have private, open-air onsen baths to enjoy, while the largest room even holds a gorgeous koi pond. A stay in Shofuan evokes an atmosphere of the bygone feudal era, with low ceilings, earthen walls, and subdued lighting, and gives the feeling of having entered the secret world of Miyazaki Hayao's *Spirited Away*. Detailed Sukiya architecture, beautiful shoji doors, high ceilings, and tasteful antiques fill these original rooms, while the ryokan's mossy gardens encourage the practice of *shinrin-yoku*.

Haiya boasts its own private onsen source right on the property, allowing guests to relax in the gender-separated public baths—Hidamari no Yu and Komorebi—each offering both indoor and open-air bathing experiences. Hidamari no Yu is the larger of the two public onsen and features a delightful reclining bath, while its outdoor *rotenburo* has a tiny stone bridge connecting the two pools. Komorebi's indoor onsen is crafted with hinoki cypress, and its outdoor *rotenburo* has a cascading waterfall feature. There is also an onsen bath perfect for families, which is free to use on a first come, first serve basis.

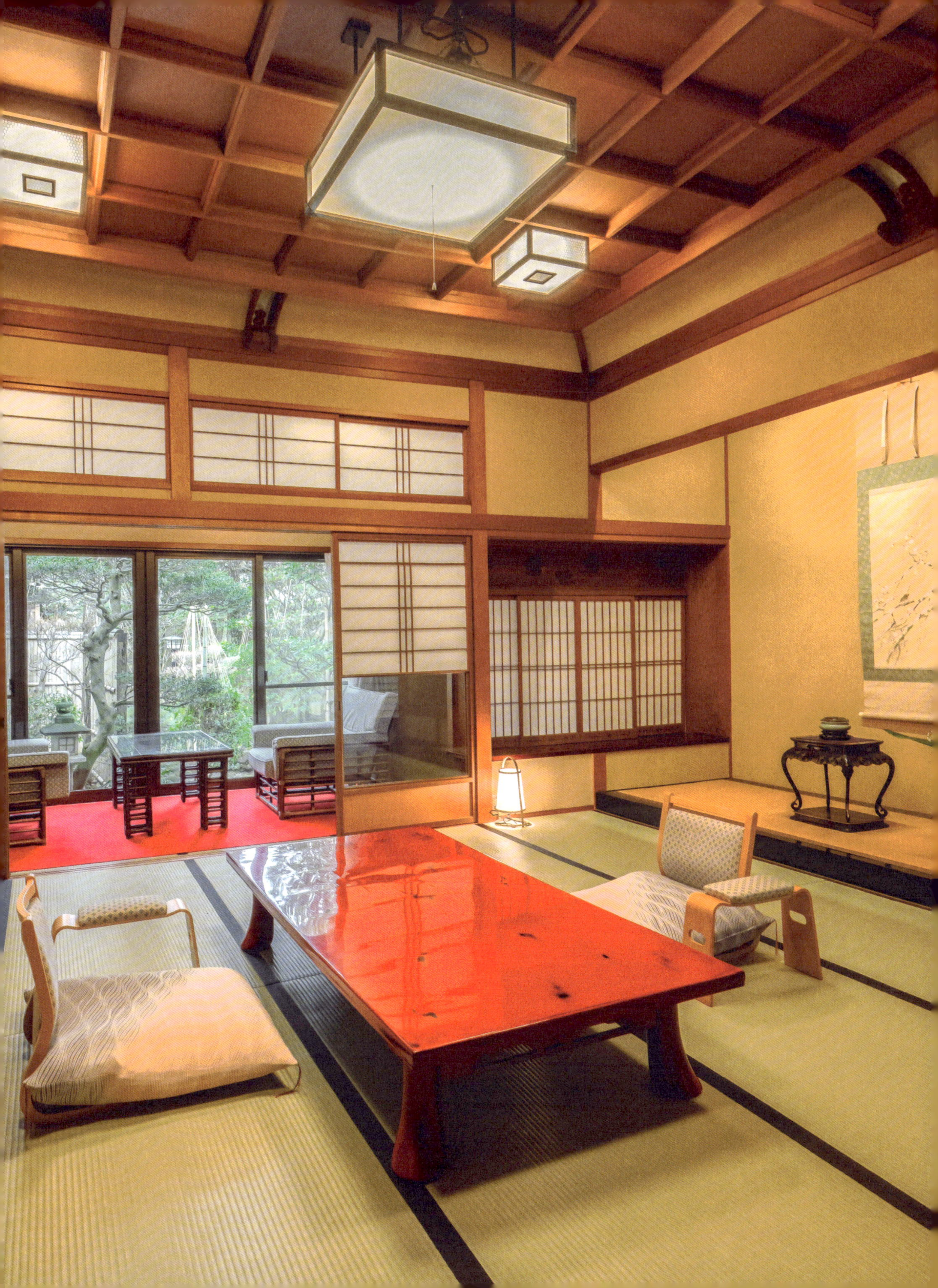

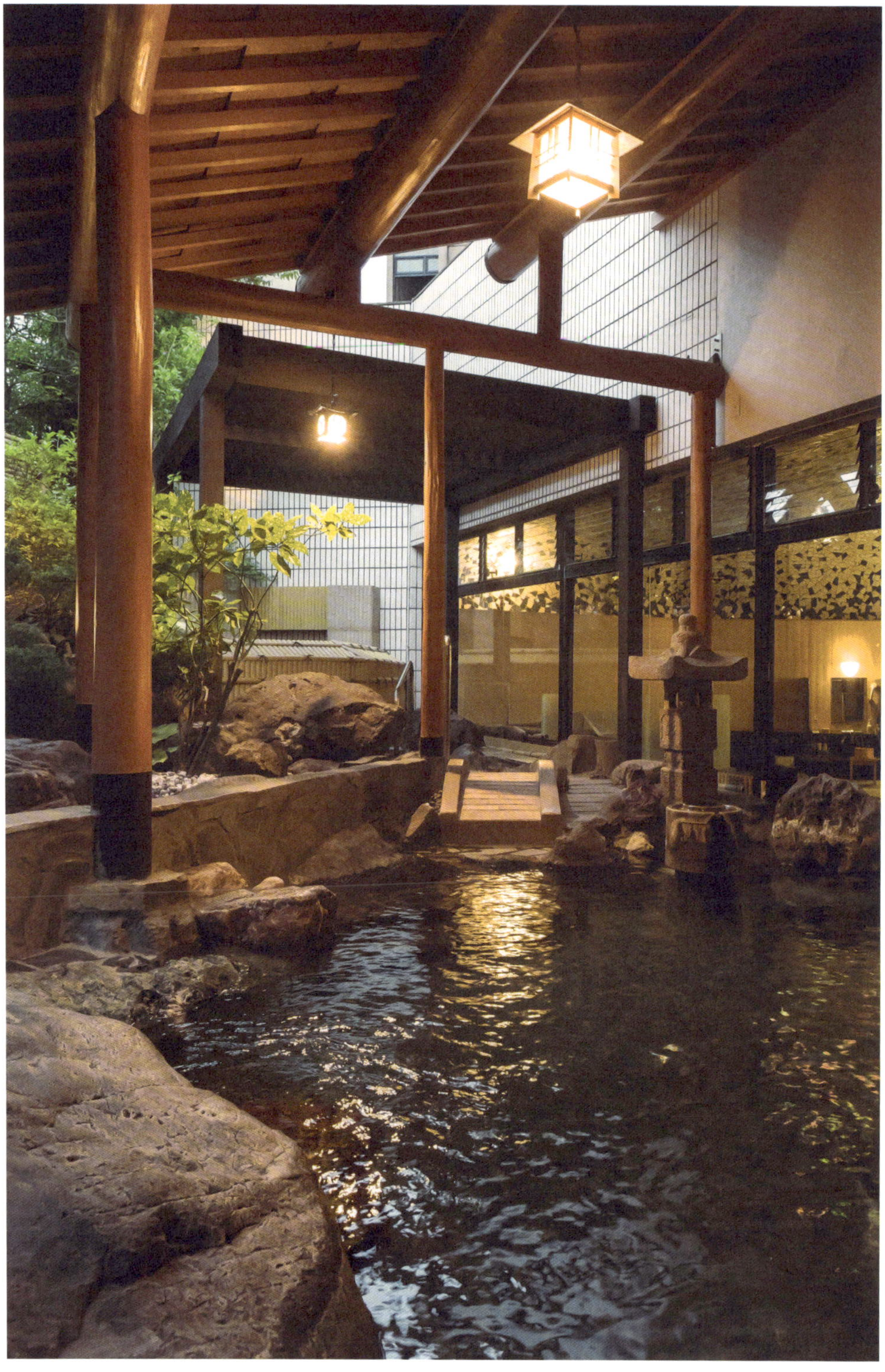

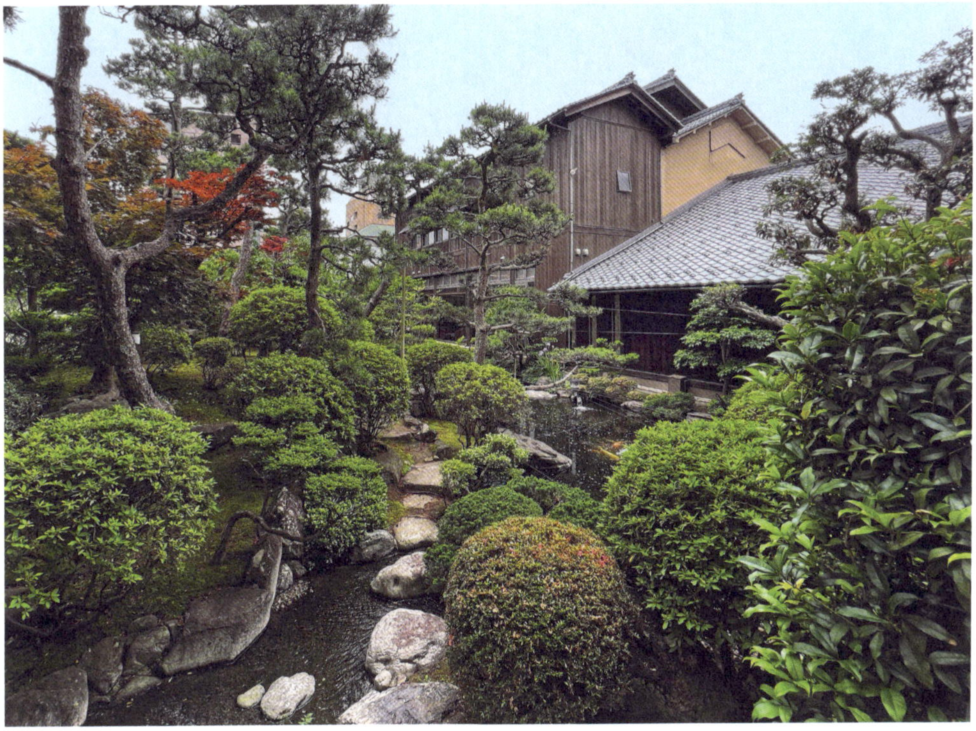

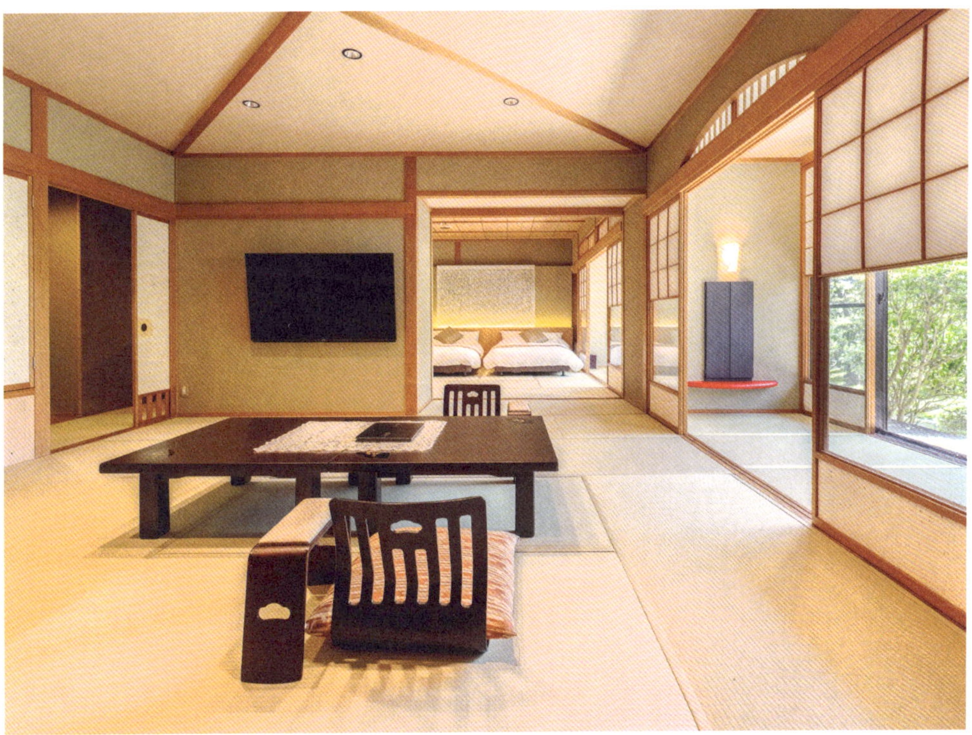

LEFT One of Haiya's public onsen baths, where guests can experience the benefits of its silky, *bijin-no-yu* waters.

Taigakukan
Hakuba • Nagano Prefecture

STAY IN ONE OF THE COUNTRY'S FIRST *MINSHUKU*

Cozy, wooden lodgings sit at the foot of a mountainous region beloved for its snowy white winters and summer hiking trails.

The village of Hakuba, in the Nagano mountains, is the birthplace of the *minshuku:* affordable "private residence" lodgings that feature a small Japanese guesthouse with communal bathhouses, often run by a local family. These *minshuku* provide intimate, traditional hospitality in a more relaxed atmosphere than one finds in an onsen ryokan. Generally found in rural villages and mountain areas, *minshuku* are a wonderful way to experience authentic local culture.

The concept of *minshuku* began in the village of Hosono (now Hakuba Happo-one), and is deeply intertwined with the practice of mountain climbing. Historically, Happo-one's Mt. Shirouma (part of the Hida range) was considered sacred, and climbing was forbidden until the end of the Edo period. Restrictions were loosened after the Meiji Restoration, and the mountains were opened up to explorers, geologists, botanists, and famous mountaineers. As there were few affordable accommodations for the new travelers, local guides offered them the opportunity to spend the night at their own houses instead of staying at a ryokan. In 1937, 16 of these houses were given formal permission to provide private travel lodging, signaling the beginning of *minshuku* accommodation. Out of these 16 houses, Hotel Taigakukan still exists today.

Steeped in the nostalgic charm of the Showa era, Taigakukan is a family-run chalet *minshuku* located in the heart of Happo Village. Welcoming wooden interiors, with soft lighting and an open brick fireplace, create a warm, soothing ambiance for guests to relax in after a day on the mountain. Upstairs, one finds a spacious tatami rest area, as well as a small private museum depicting the history of Hakuba and its mountain adventurers.

Rooms are cozy and inviting, with sliding shoji-covered windows and seating areas with traditional *zabuton* cushions. Guests can select either simple tatami rooms with futons—a throwback to the past—or rooms with Western-style twin beds and floral-covered duvets that were popular during the Showa era.

Among the *minshuku,* Taigakukan is also a rarity, as it has its own natural onsen on-site, where guests can soak their aching, tired bodies in either the indoor or outdoor hinoki bath. Hakuba's onsen water is also unique: holding an extraordinarily high pH value of 11.2, the water has a silky, smooth, luxurious, almost lotion-like quality that promotes beautiful skin.

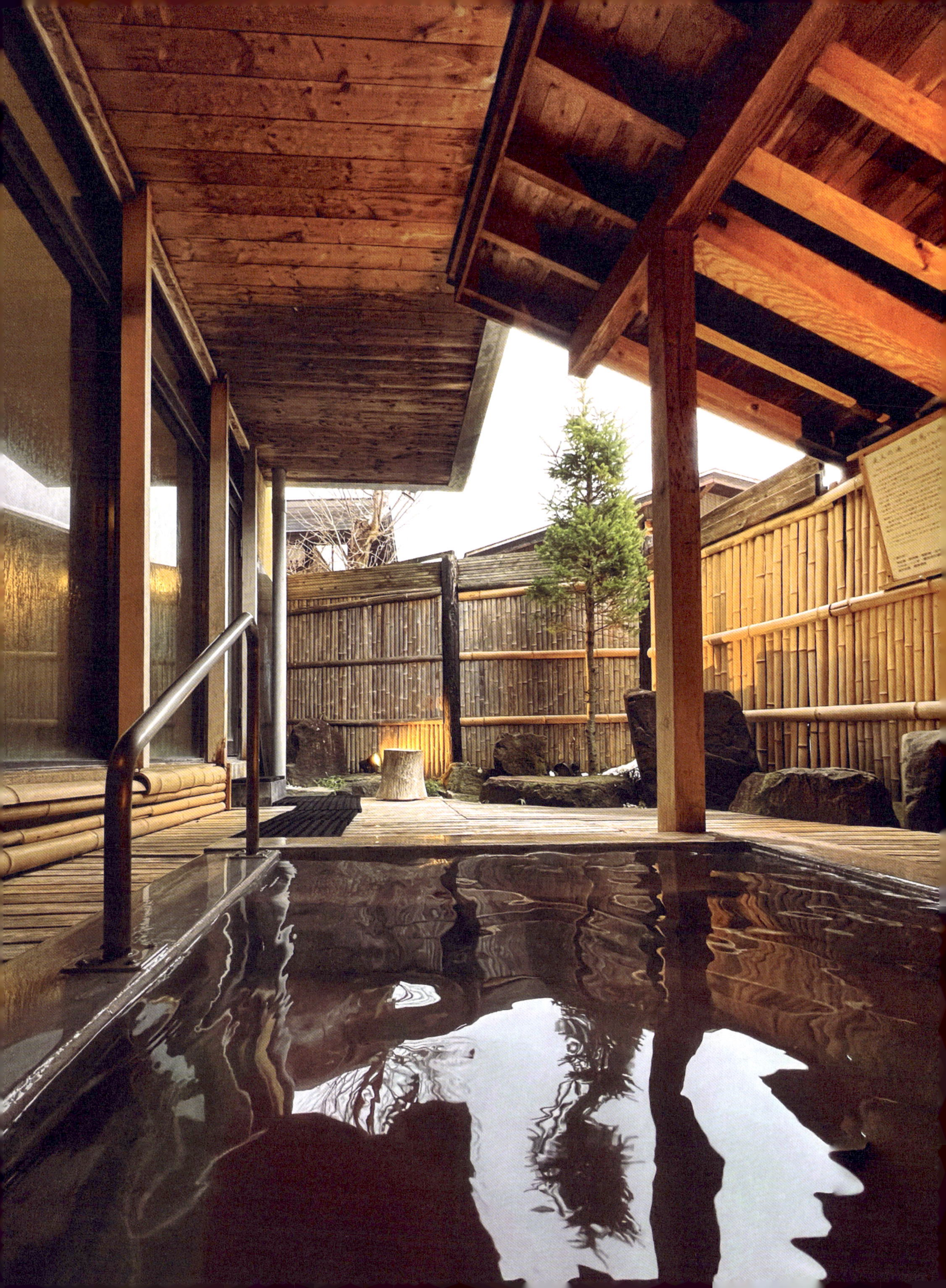

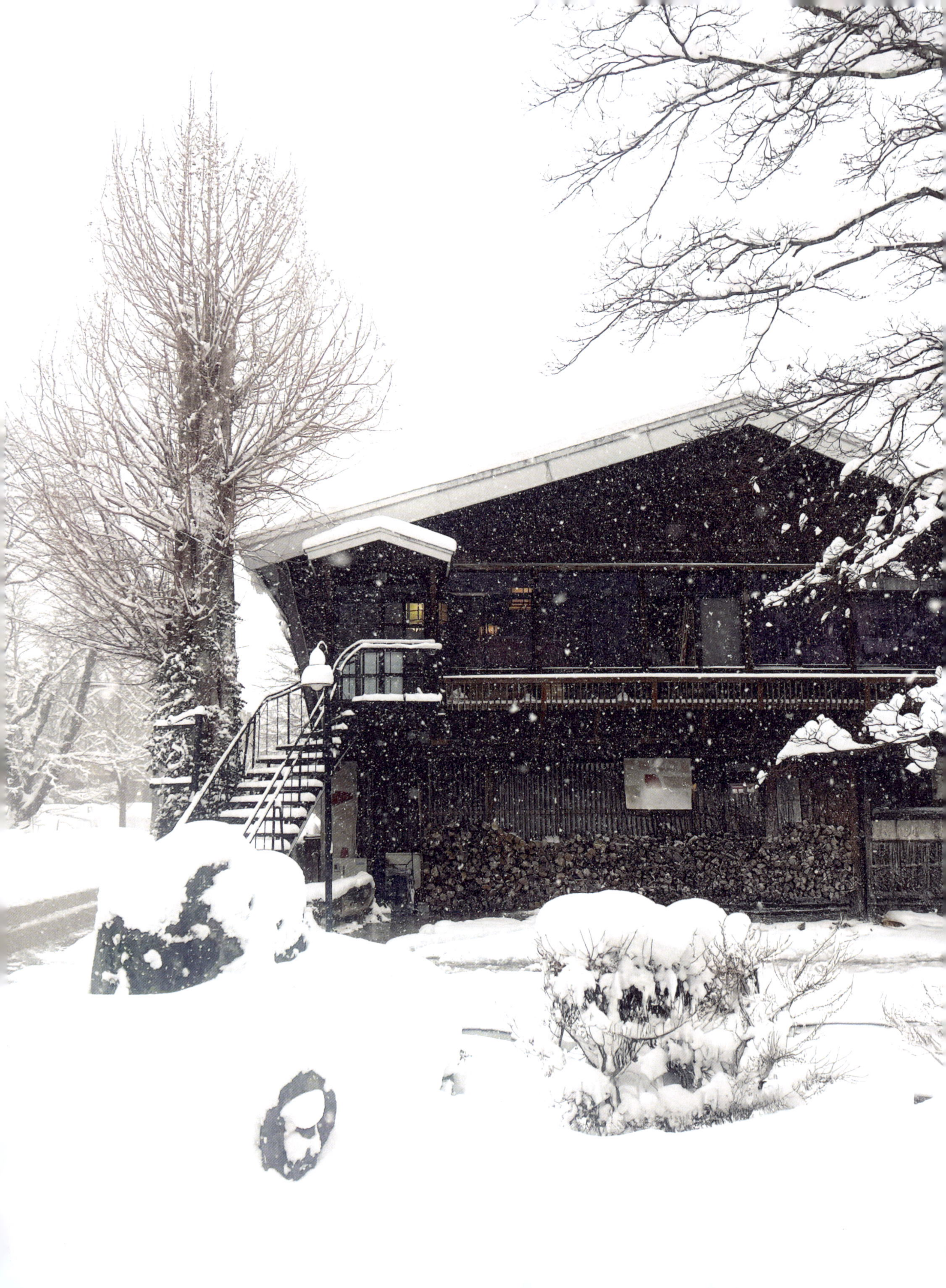

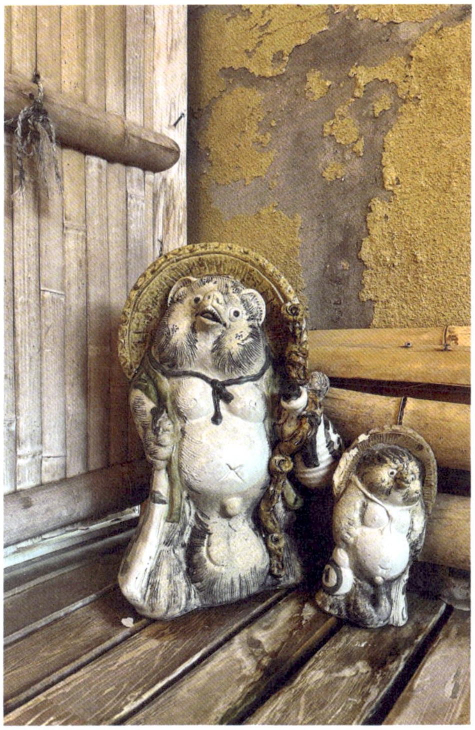

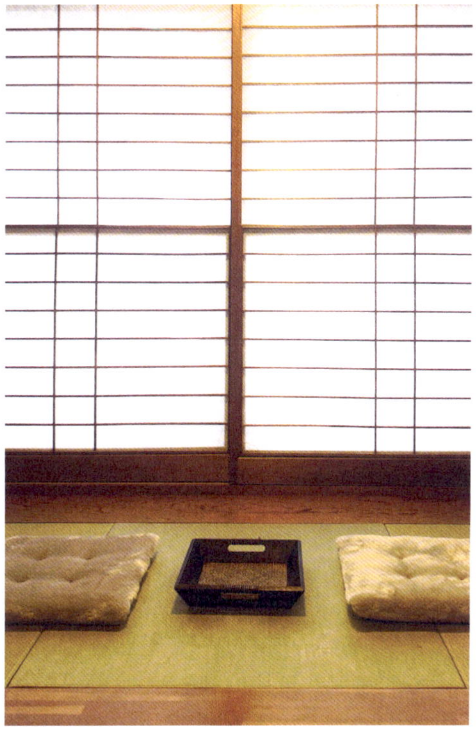

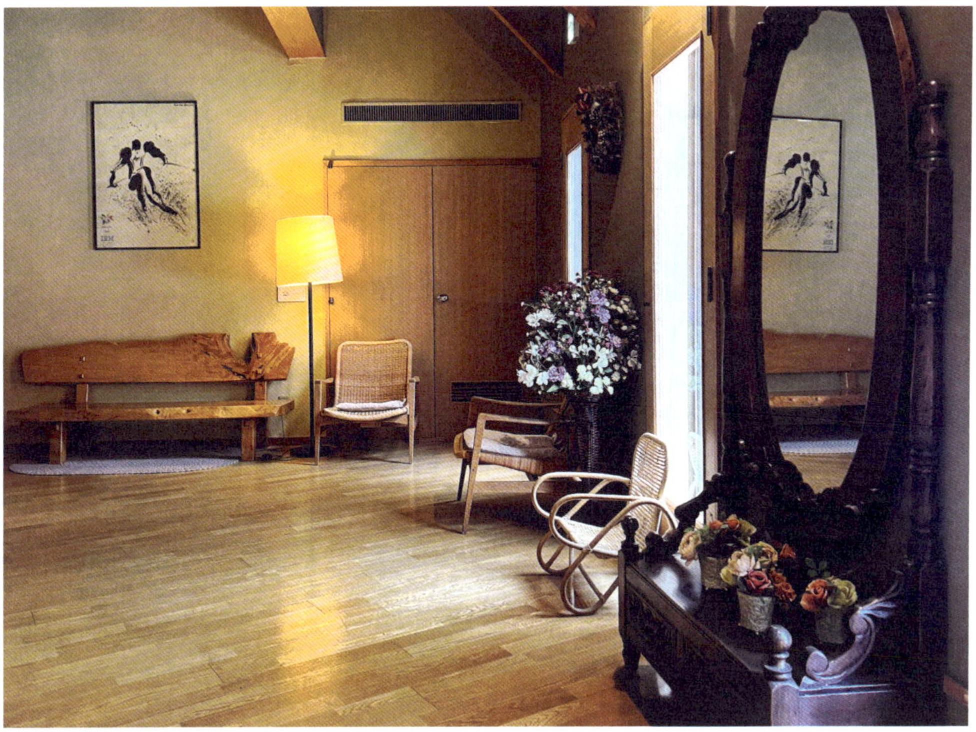

ABOVE An elegantly rustic aesthetic makes this historic Showa-era *minshuku* a cozy lodge experience.

KAI Sengokuhara
Hakone ● Kanagawa Prefecture

A SERENE WEEKEND RETREAT IN THE HEART OF THE HAKONE REGION

Embrace your inner creativity at this luxury onsen ryokan, where one is surrounded by the works of Japanese and international artists.

For a stunning getaway a short distance from Tokyo, no place is more beloved than the mountain-surrounded onsen region of Hakone, where visitors can glimpse the majestic Mt. Fuji across Lake Ashi and the famed red torii gate of Hakone Shrine. Many first-time visitors will base themselves around the main Hakone-Yumoto Station or Gora area, where the Hakone Open Air Museum and the Owakudani Valley (another onsen hell) are located. However, for those who prefer a quieter, more tranquil site, one need only travel a little further to Sengokuhara in the Hakone highlands.

These highlands are renowned for their walking paths through the vast, tall pampas grass (*suzuki*) field, with views of Mt. Kintoki and the wetlands further down. The best time to see the pampas field is during the fall season, but no matter when one visits, the scenery of Sengokuhara is always magnificent—visitors can spend time meandering through the many small museums and art galleries in the area, including the Hakone Venetian Glass Museum (Glass Forest) and the Pola Museum of Art. If the highlands happen to beckon you for a bit longer, spending a night or two at KAI Sengokuhara provides an ideal and rejuvenating retreat after one's inspiring outdoor adventures.

An advocate for Sengokuhara's rich artistic history, this KAI property was designed around the concept of an atelier, where guests are invited to surround themselves with nature and celebrate art. A select 12 artists, hailing both from within Japan and overseas, were invited to stay at KAI Sengokuhara before it officially opened and, while there, they were commissioned to create artworks inspired by Hakone—these are now showcased not only throughout the guest rooms, but the entire onsen ryokan.

Guests can also nurture their own budding creative talents by participating in KAI's *tenugui* workshop, decorating a traditional Japanese towel while taking inspiration from the local scenery.

Following a day of creative exploration, KAI Sengokuhara's 16 rooms offer a truly relaxing atmosphere—each features its own private outdoor onsen with exceptional views of the Hakone landscapes. The ryokan's slightly cloudy, acidic onsen water (pH 2.0) is drawn from Owakudani Onsen and filled with copious mineral deposits known as yu-no-hana (onsen flowers). One can also enjoy soaking in the public onsen, where the outdoor *rotenburo*'s scenery changes dramatically with each season.

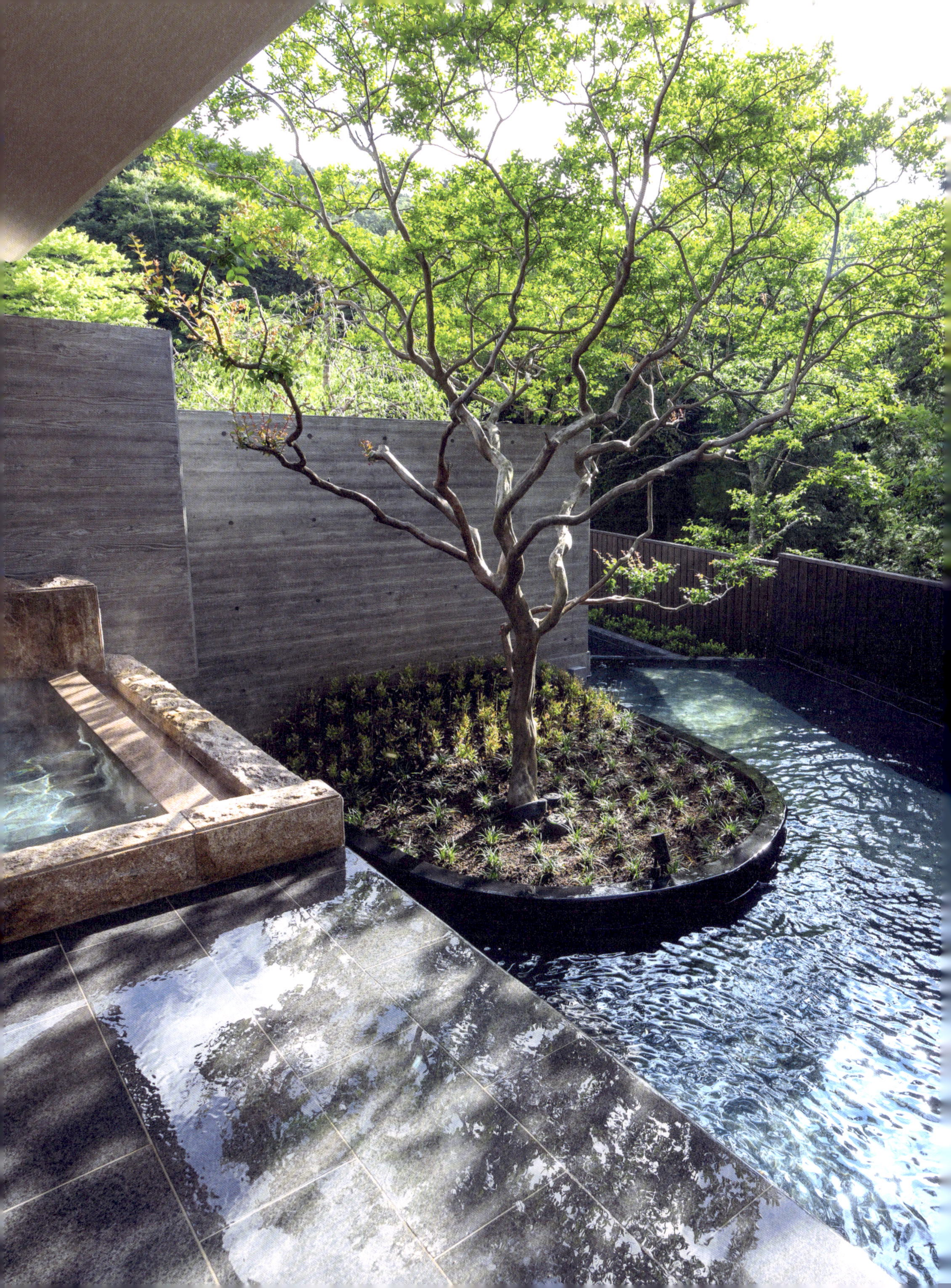

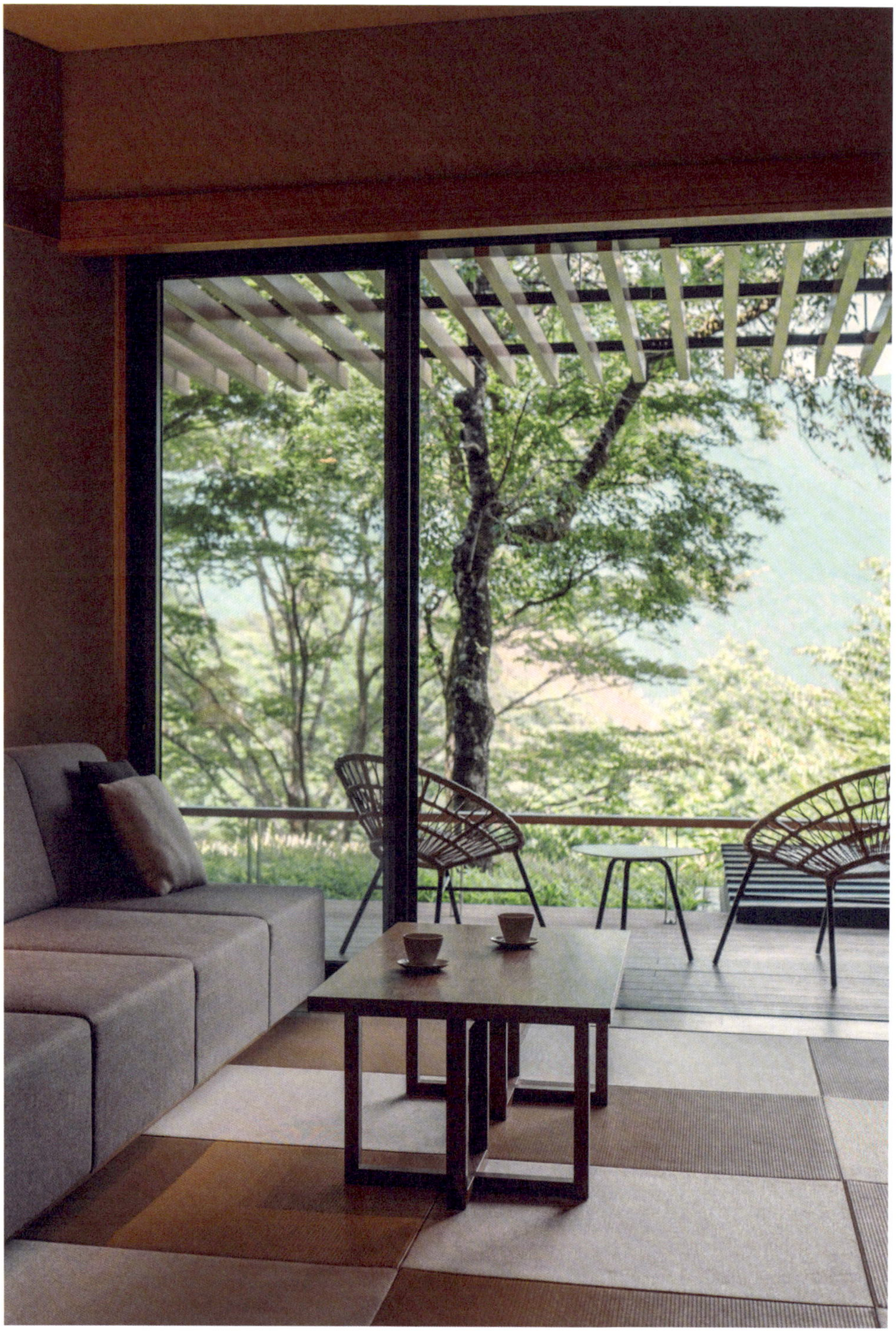

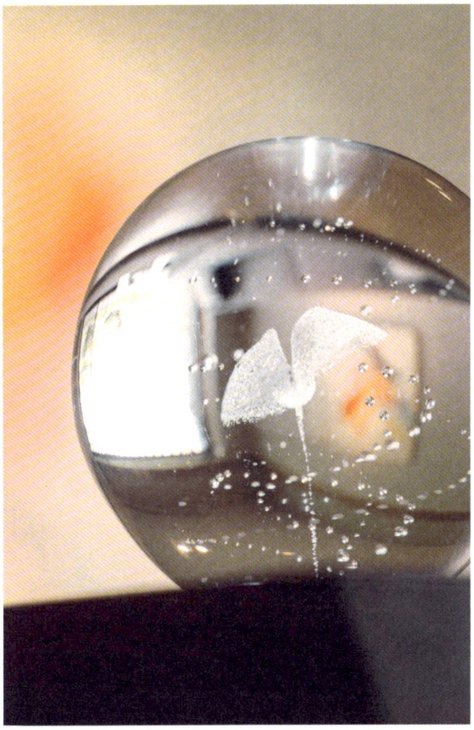

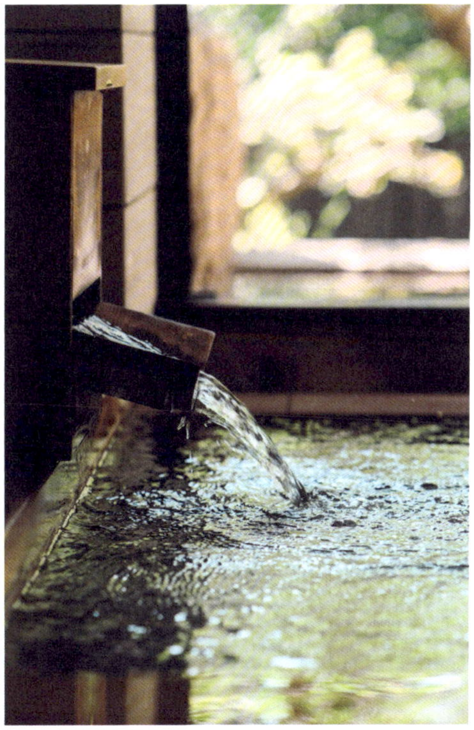

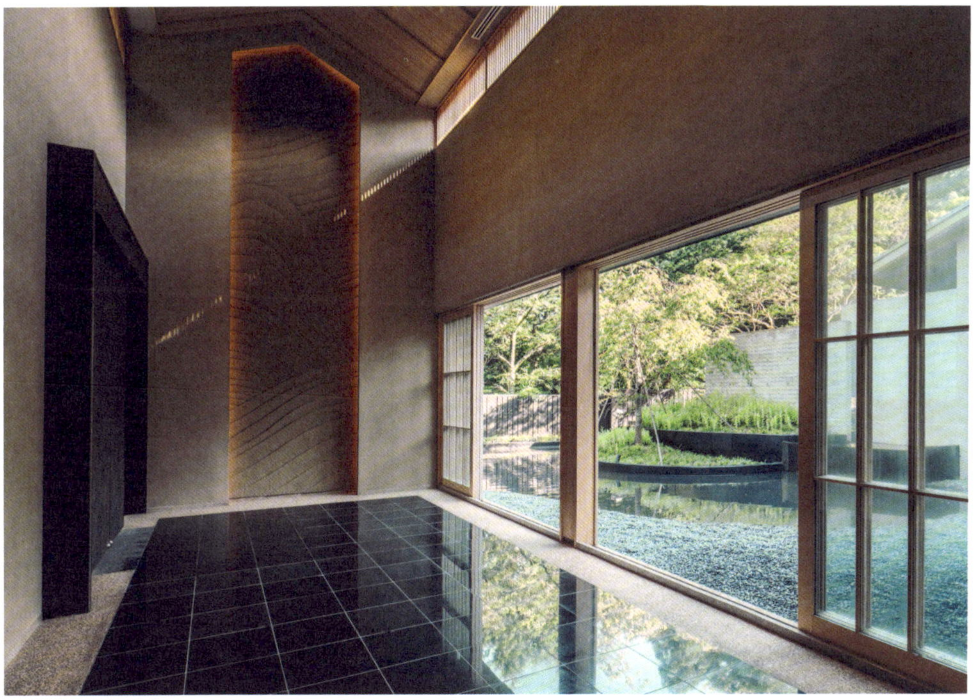

LEFT Modern minimalism and traditional Japanese design sensibilities make for a luxurious stay at KAI Sengokuhara.

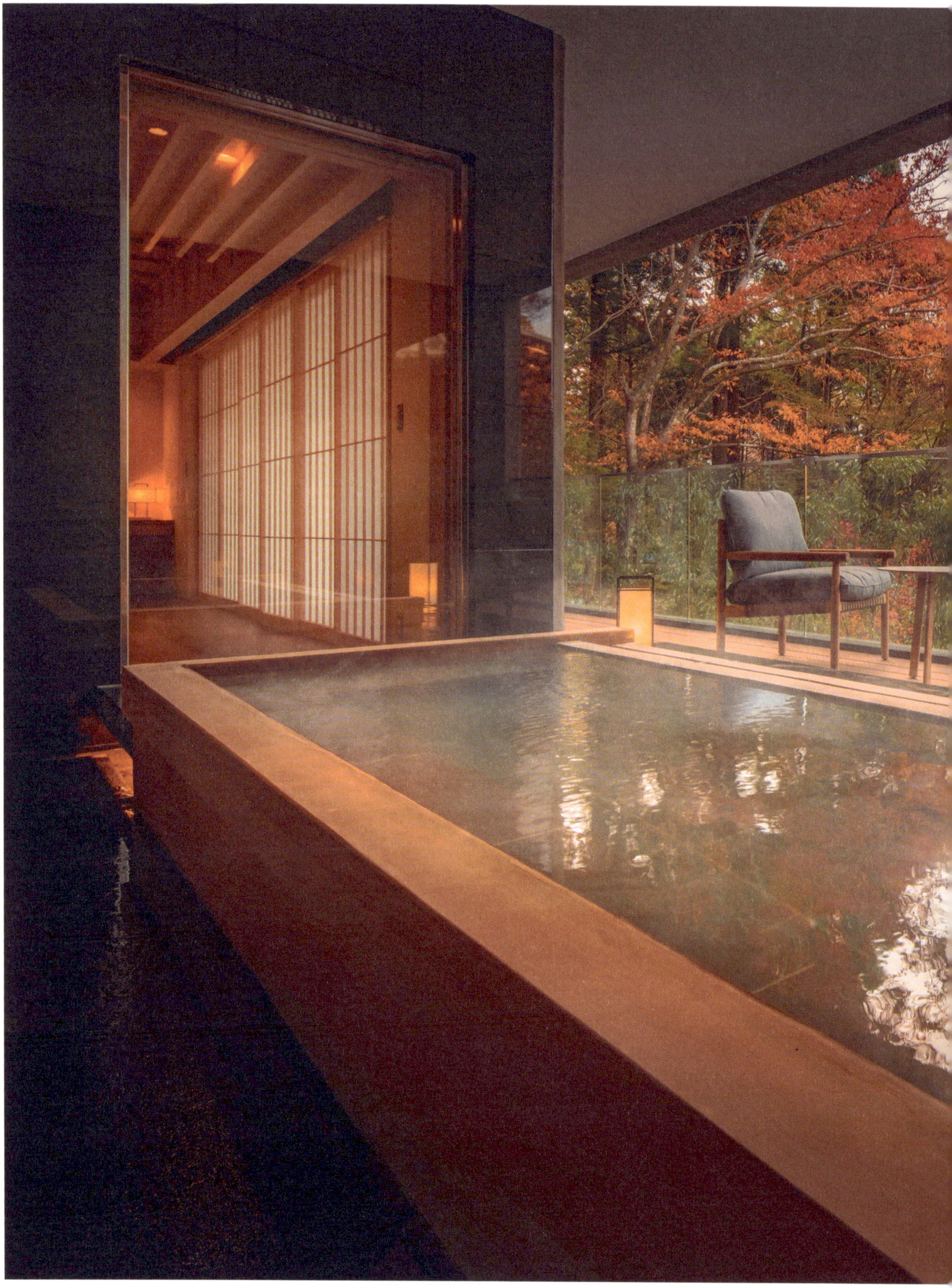

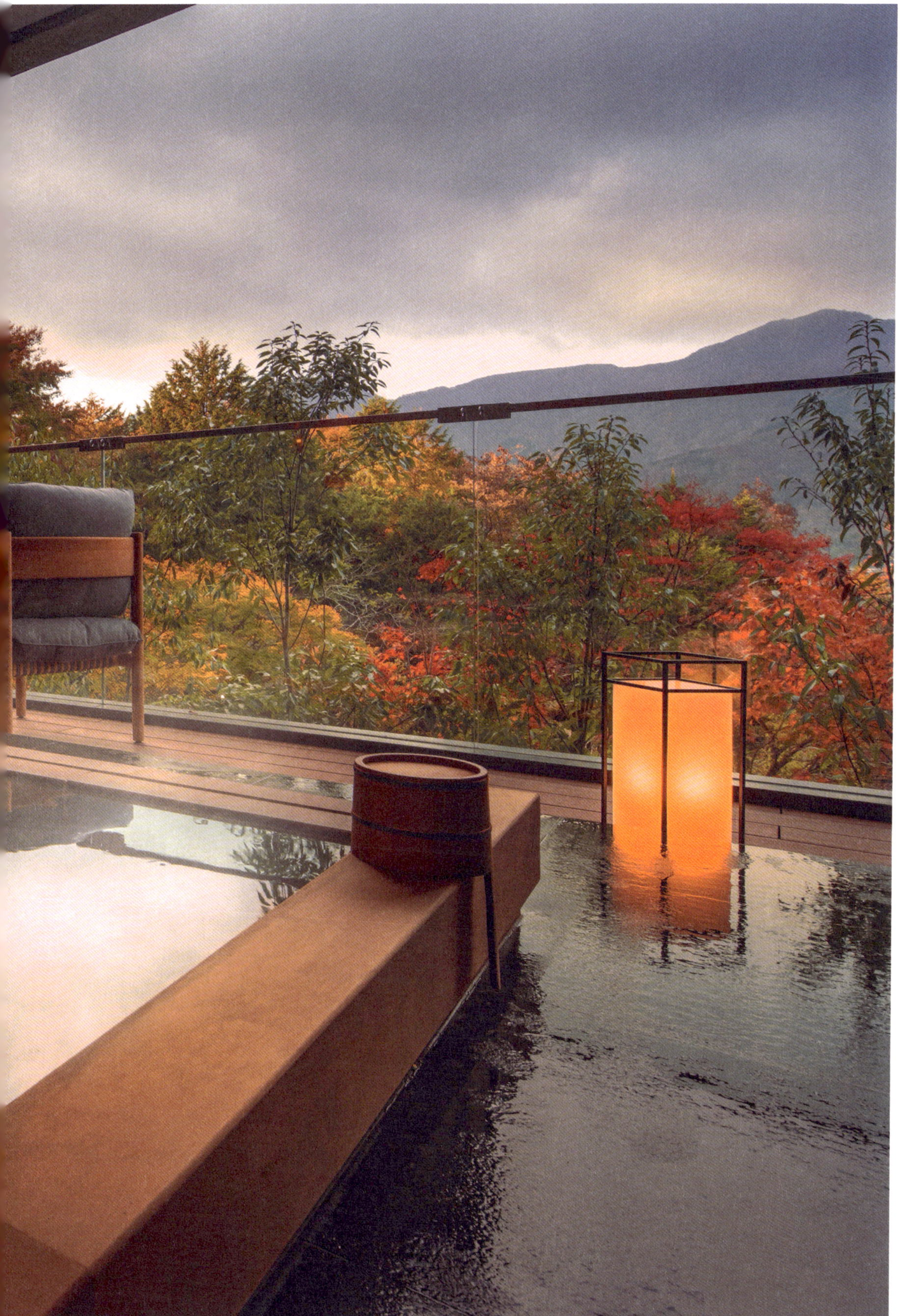

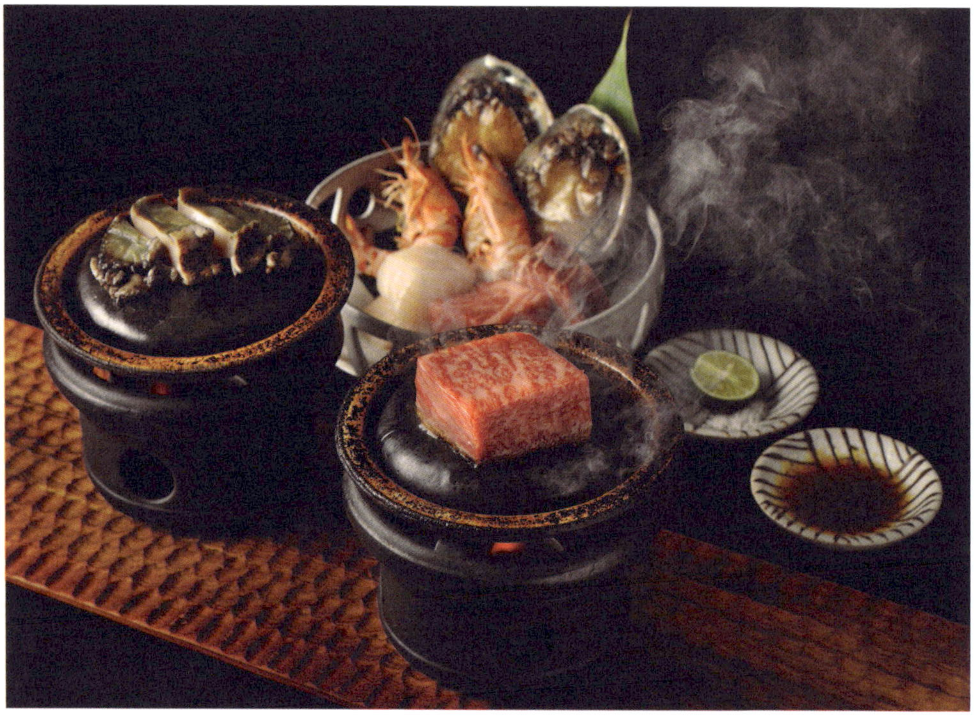

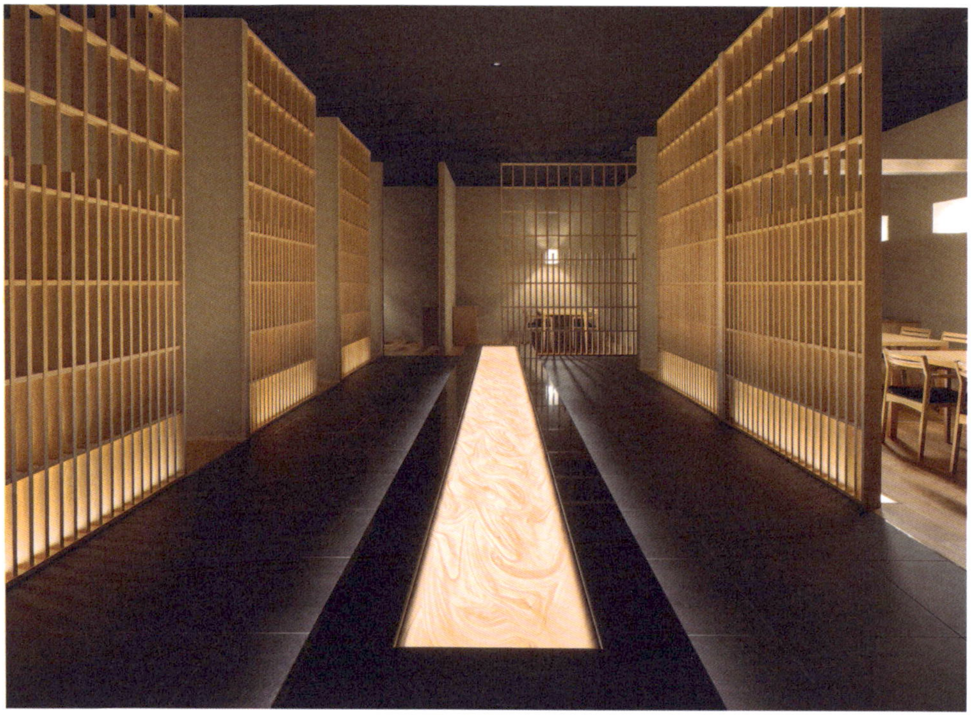

ABOVE AND TOP Indulge the senses with seasonal *kaiseki* meals in your own semi-private dining room within the restaurant.

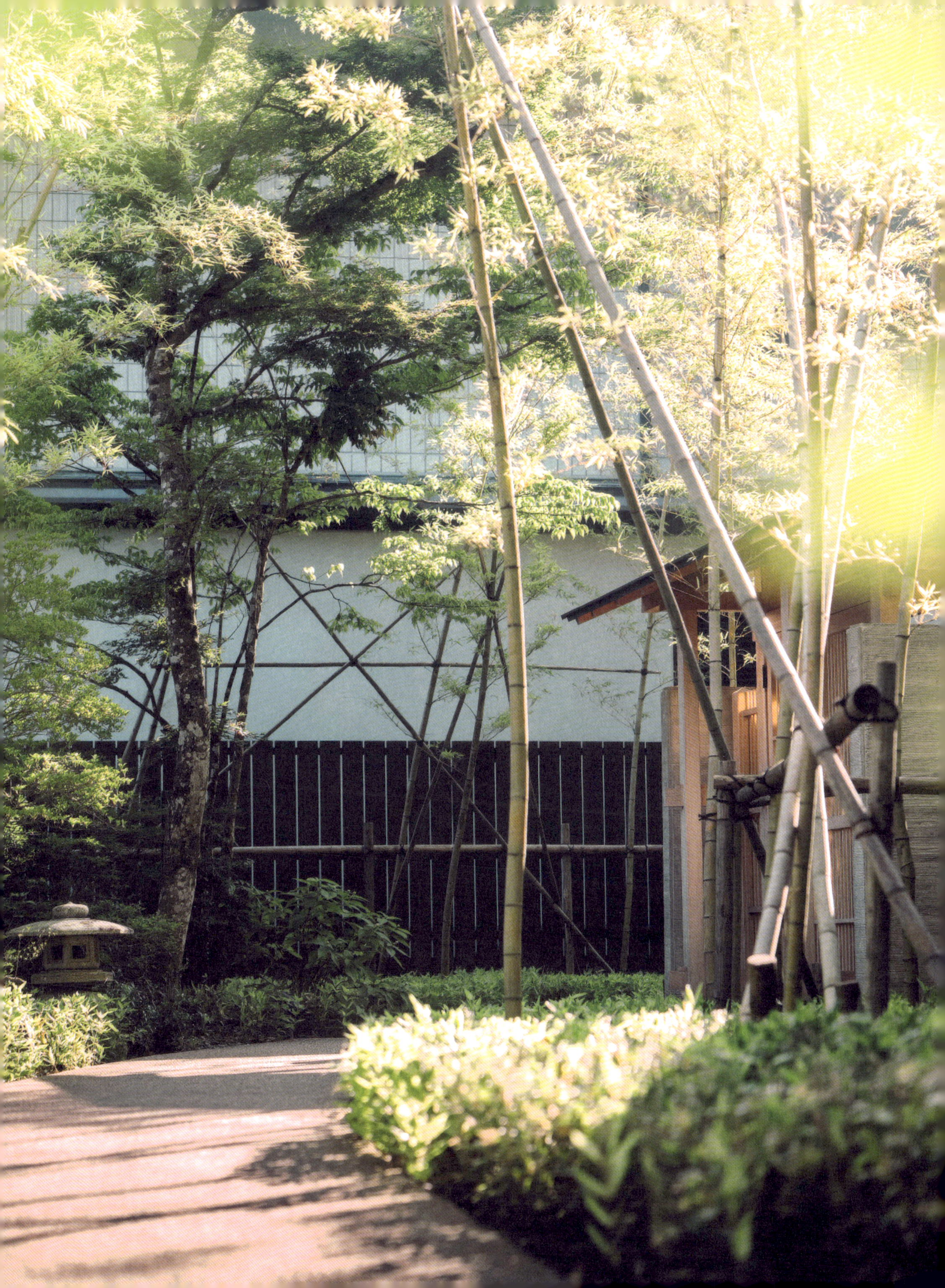

Tsubame Onsen
Sekiyama • Niigata Prefecture

A BELOVED, COST-FREE *HITOU* IN THE MOUNTAINS

The vivid turquoise of the onsen waters provides a striking contrast to the forest's seasonal backdrop.

Along the scenic winding roads to Mt. Myoko in southern Niigata one finds Tsubame Onsen, a local secret beloved by hikers and mountaineers—and those seeking out remote onsen. The journey to Tsubame is startlingly picturesque, the scenery resplendent with the changing seasons. The onsen can be somewhat difficult to reach at times, as roads may be blocked with fallen trees, or tunnels closed due to heavy snowfall, so an alternate route can come in handy.

Upon arrival, one's gaze will be immediately drawn upward toward the towering mountains, lush with vivid foliage. Against such a backdrop, one can't help but feel that an extraordinary discovery is imminent and that time in the traditional sense no longer applies. Walking up the relatively steep road into town lets one acclimate to the stunning location, as the scenery deepens and mist rises from the nearby waterfall.

Passing through the small town, with its few onsen lodgings and local shops, one continues to the trailhead of Mt. Myoko—the highest mountain in the Hokushin area and part of the Myoko Togakushi Renzan National Park, encompasses both Nagano and Niigata prefectures.

Travelers will next encounter Ougon no Yu, an outdoor *rotenburo* with milky, almost pale-blue onsen water protected by a wall of trees. Ougon no Yu has baths for men and women, separated only by a large boulder and thin bamboo mats. Kawahara no Yu is a free, mixed-gender *rotenburo* reached by another short hike from Ougon no Yu. One must cross a small suspension bridge in order to arrive at this scenic onsen with views of the waterfall.

Authentic and traditional, these baths are for those who truly wish to experience the way of onsen in all its pureness. No showers or washing area can be found at either public onsen, only a simple changing hut to provide privacy when disrobing. To cleanse one's body before entering the baths, take the *yu-oke* (the small wooden or plastic bucket), scoop the onsen water, and pour it over the body three times before entering. Both *rotenburo* at Tsubame can be enjoyed until early November. A donation box accepts contributions for continued upkeep and maintenance, but the baths are free to enter.

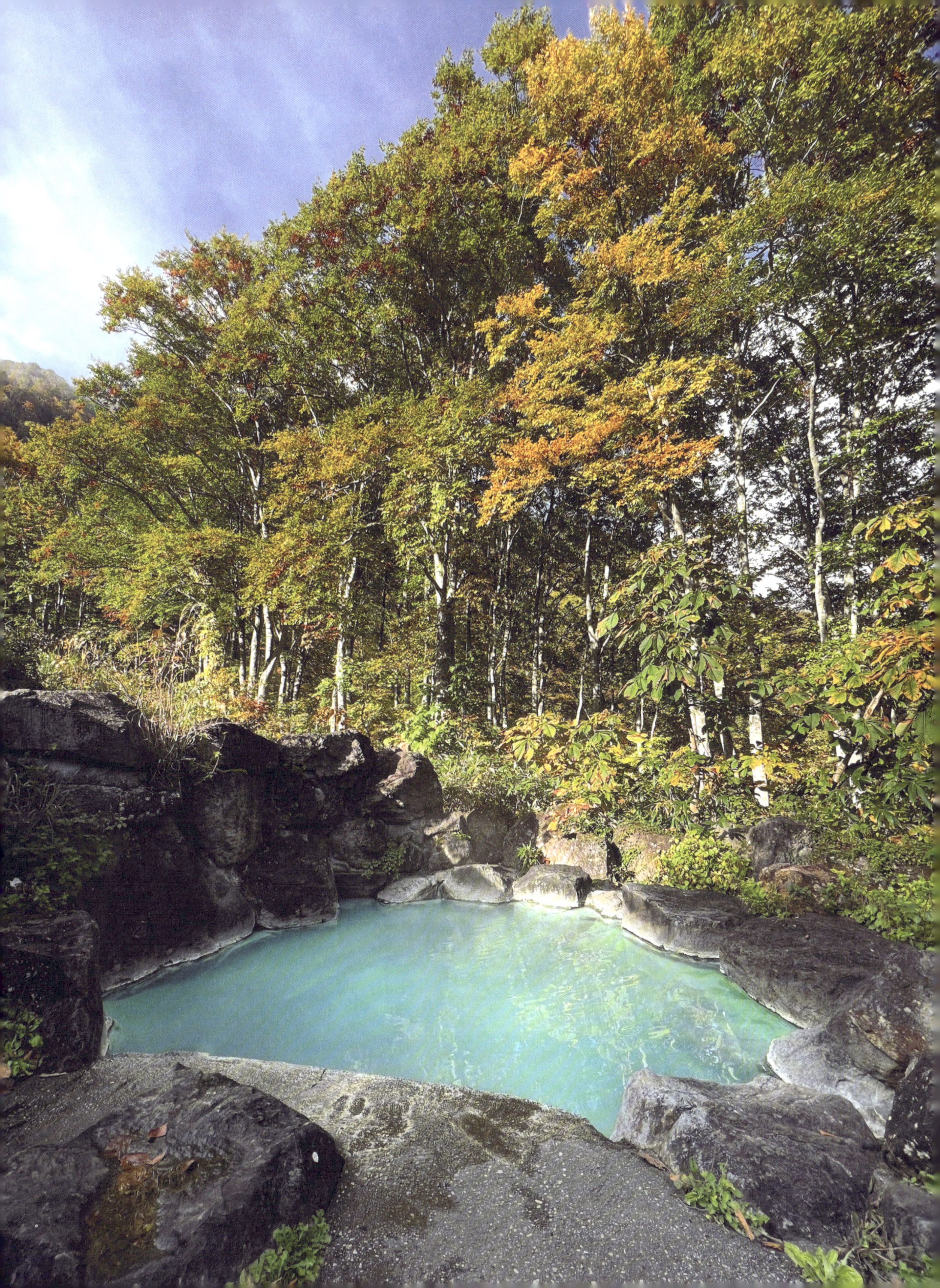

Shuzenji Onsen
Tagata District • Shizuoka Prefecture

A DELIGHTFUL ONSEN TOWN EASILY ACCESSIBLE FROM TOKYO

Take a leisurely stroll around this quaint, pleasing onsen town, filled with history, charm, and lovely natural scenery.

Surrounded by the volcanic Amagi Mountain Range, the quaint onsen temple town of Shuzenji beckons. With a history that can be traced back to the 800s, it is one of the oldest and most famous onsen havens on the Izu Peninsula. Local folklore tells of the legendary monk Kukai (later known as Kobo Daishi) who, while taking one of his many treks across the country, stumbled on a boy bathing his sick father in a cold river. Using one of his ritualistic instruments, the compassionate monk struck a river rock, out of which flowed streaming onsen water. To honor this gift from the gods, Kukai founded a temple nearby, marking the humble beginnings of Shuzenji town.

The onsen that Kukai discovered became famously known as Tokko no Yu, which is located in the riverbed running through the center of town. Once an actual bathing area, it is now used exclusively as an onsen footbath.

Though one can see all the sights of Shuzenji and indulge in an onsen on a day trip, to fully appreciate its numerous charms, many visitors will stay a night or two in one of several onsen ryokan encircling the town. Days can be spent strolling through the town's promenade, which runs alongside the river and Tokko no Yu. Many will also pay a visit to Hie Shrine, which looks especially sweet when the late-blooming *yaezakura* are in bloom, then climb the steps to the historic Shuzenji Temple, around which the town was built.

Further past Tokko no Yu on the other side of the river, one finds an unexpected sanctuary in peaceful, picturesque Shuzenji's small bamboo forest, where a stone path and circular rest area give visitors space to quietly unwind. One of the town's five wooden bridges can be found at one end of the bamboo forest; the beautiful red bridge offers scenic views of the foliage shadowing the Katsura River. The backstreets of the town have a retro, Showa ambiance, where cute boutiques, *kissaten,* and restaurants mingle in between old soba shacks, antique and secondhand shops, and charming snack bars. After exploring, take a moment to soak your feet in the onsen footbaths or head back to your ryokan to immerse yourself in Shuzenji's nourishing waters.

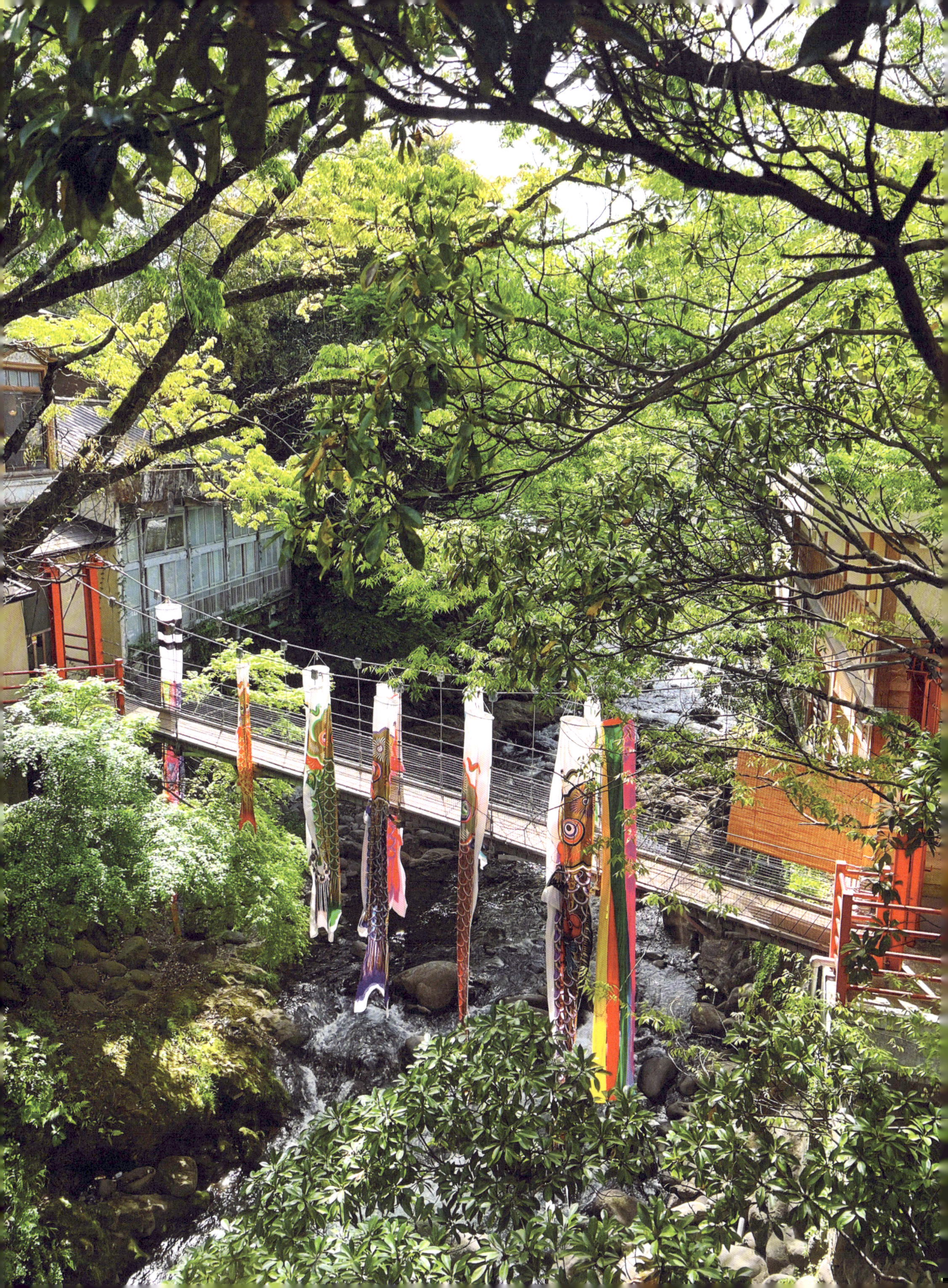

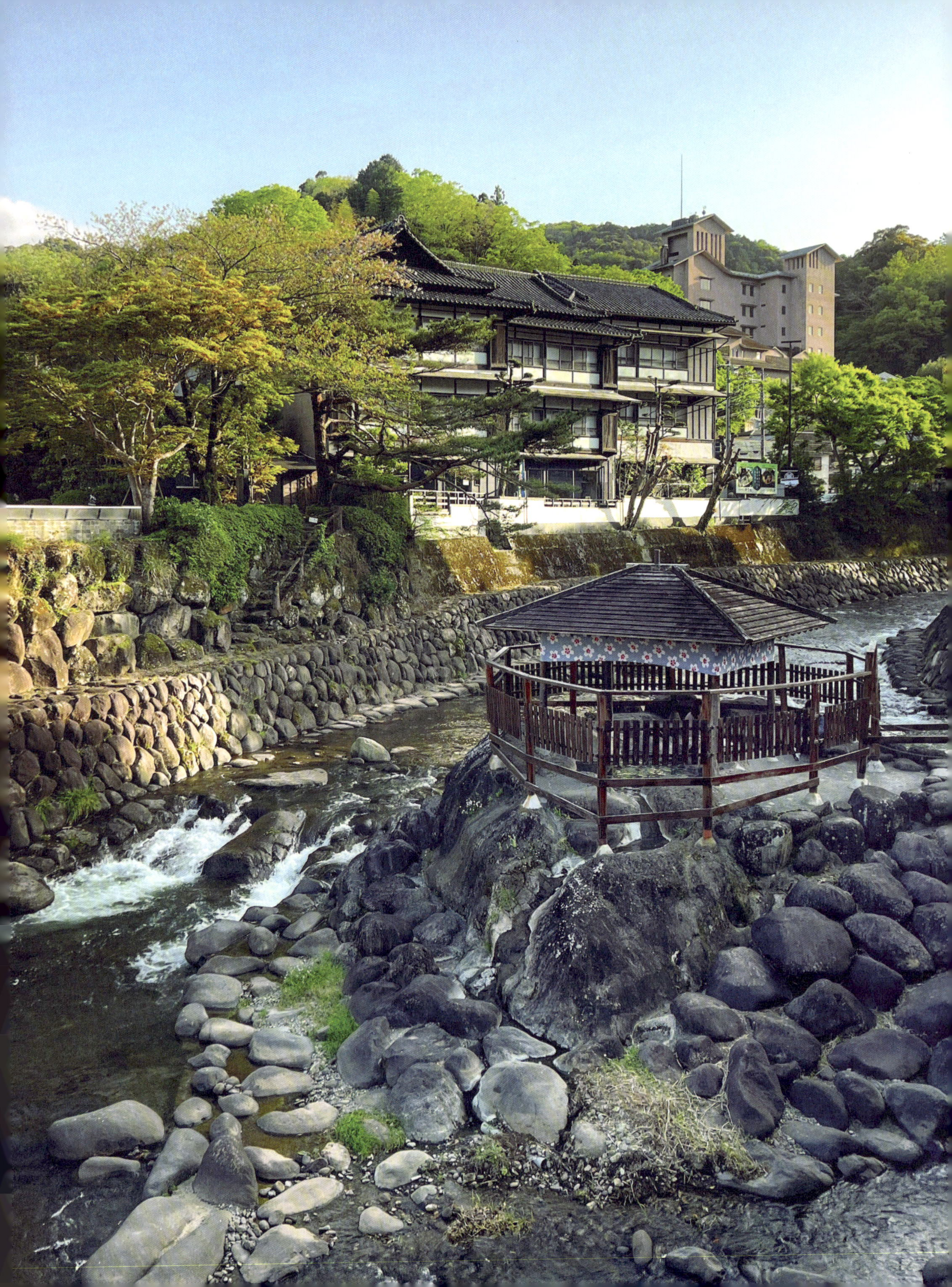

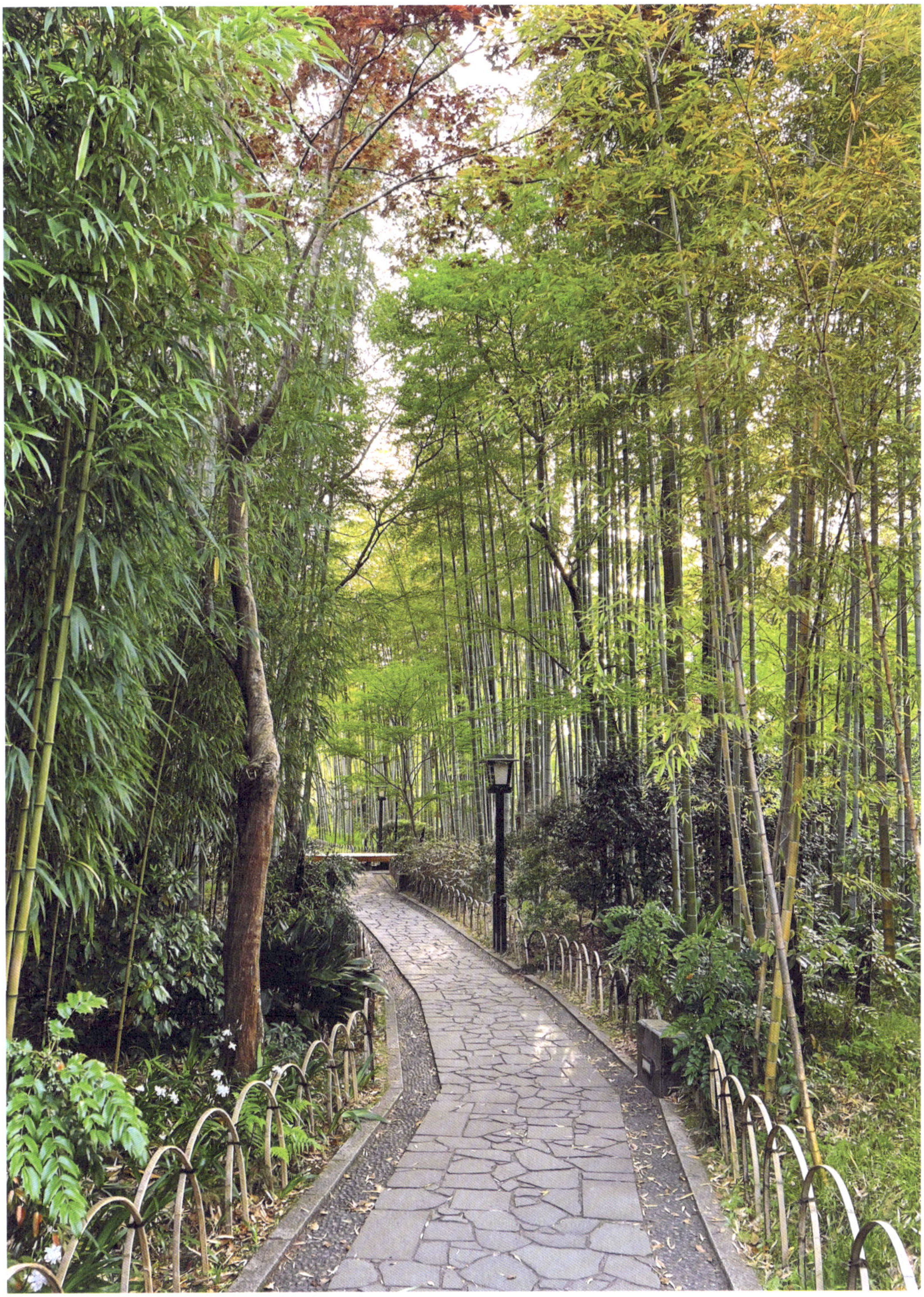

ABOVE Wander through the peaceful grove of bamboo trees in Shuzenji Onsen town.

Yamashiro Onsen
Kaga • Ishikawa Prefecture

THE BIRTHPLACE OF JAPAN'S MODERN ALPHABET

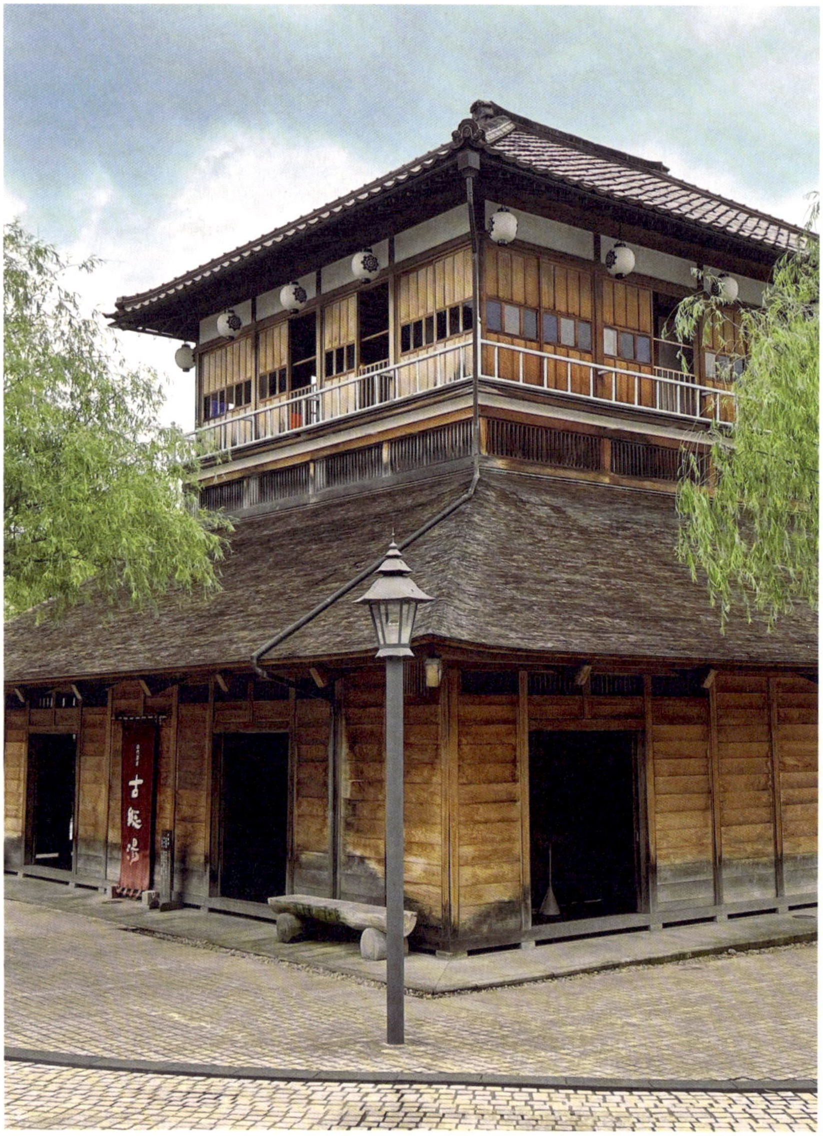

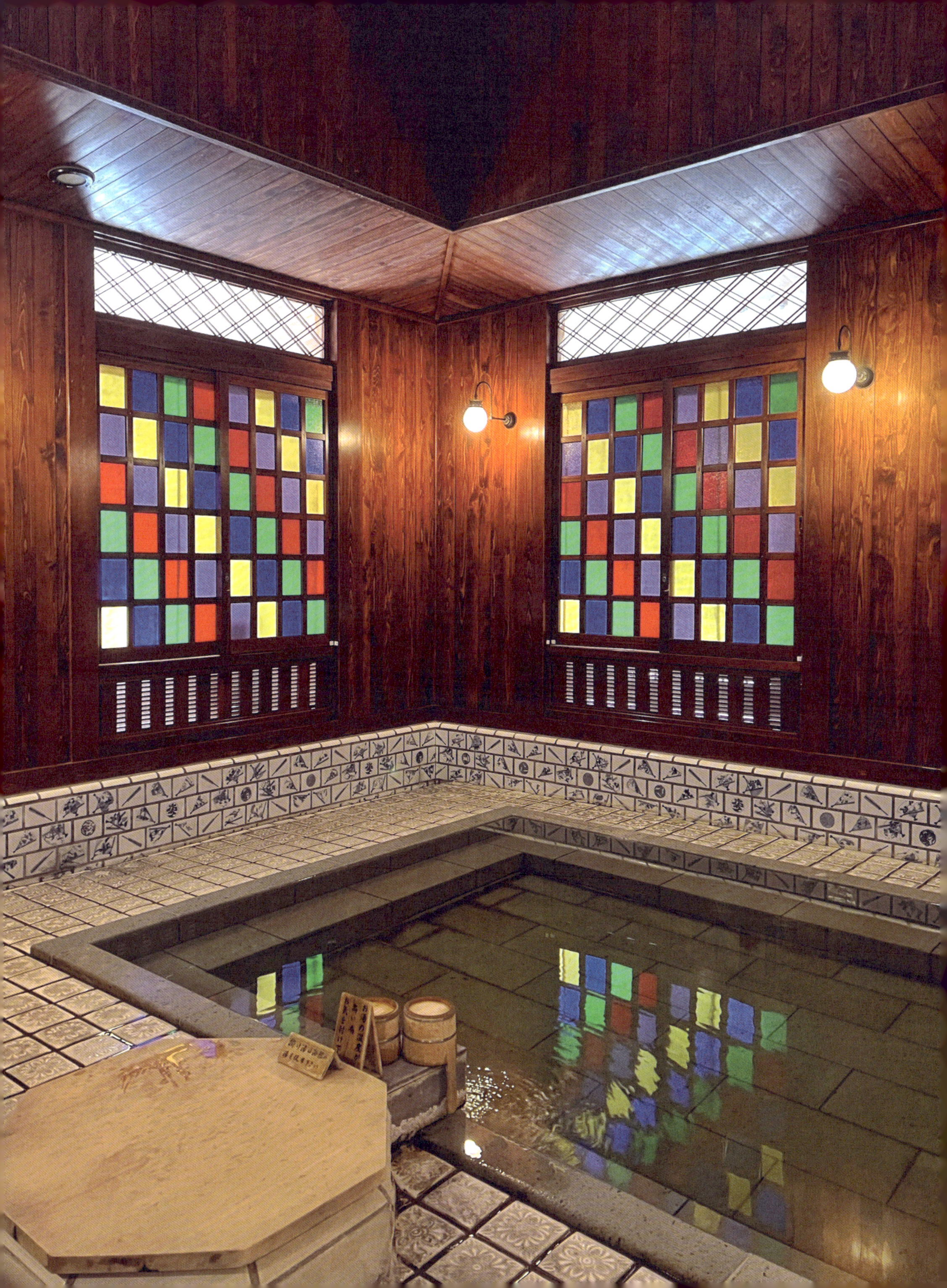

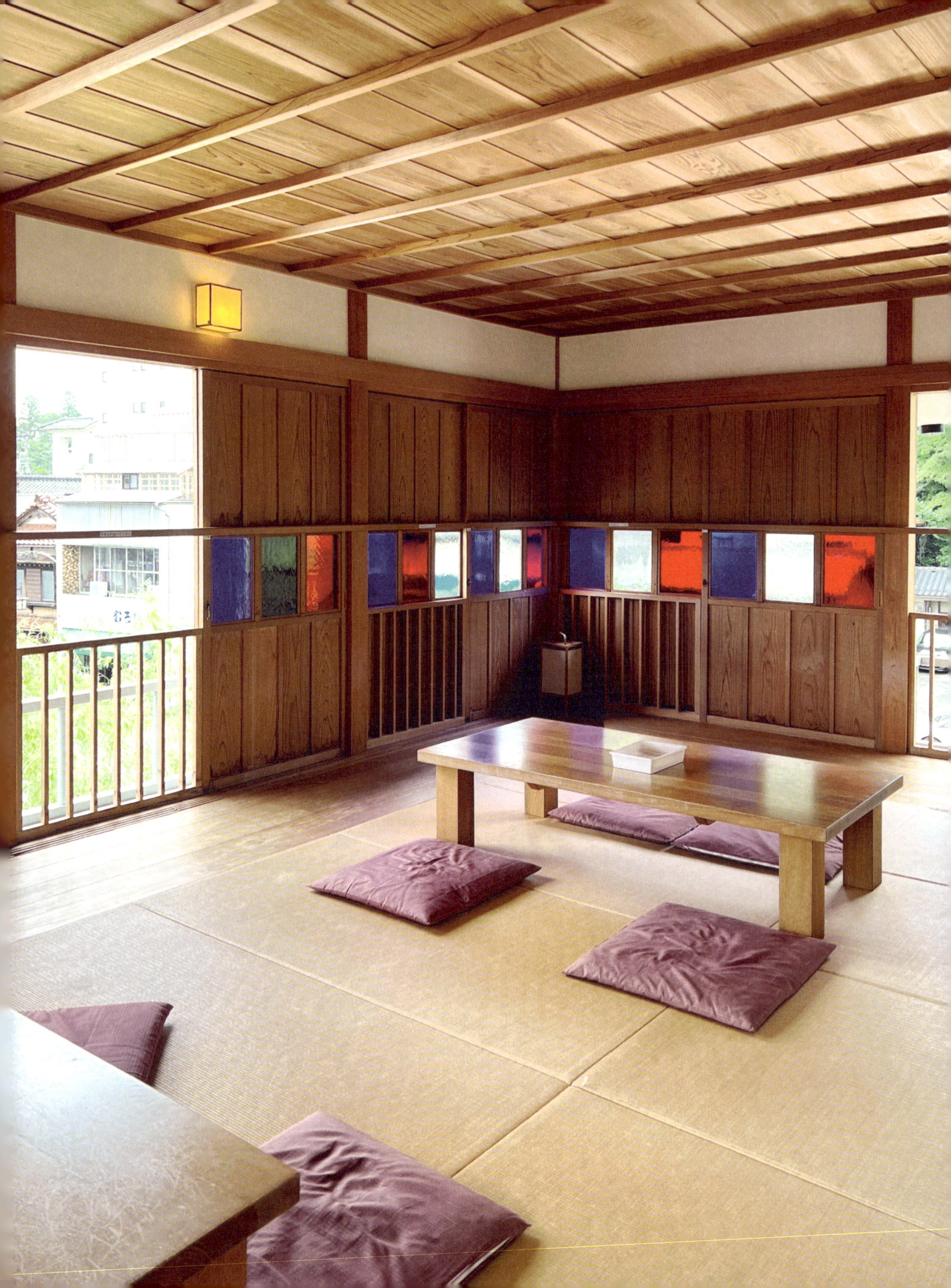

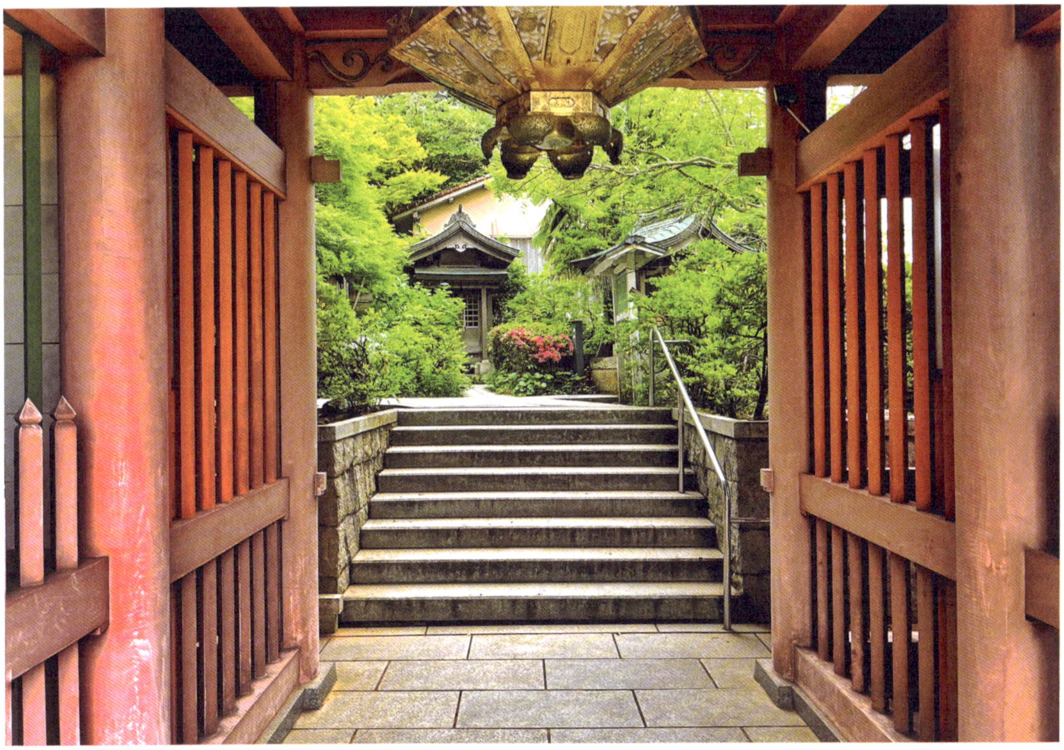

ABOVE The faded red entrance gate leads the way to Yakuoin Onsenji Temple, birthplace of Japan's modern alphabet.

Flourishing around its central iconic bathhouse Kosoyu, where both locals and travelers intermingle, this onsen town offers a relaxing weekend escape.

This onsen, located on Japan's main island of Honshu, is thought to have been founded around the year 725. Legend tells of the wandering high priest Gyoki, who was making a pilgrimage to the sacred Mt. Haku-san when he stumbled upon the giant three-legged crow Yatagarasu. The crow was bathing its injured wing in a pool of onsen water, and Gyoki observed how Yatagarasu's wing miraculously healed.

The site of Gyoki's discovery would eventually become Yamashiro Onsen, and the hot spring pool is affectionately known among locals as Karasu no Yu (crow's bath). Over time—particularly during the Edo period—the town of Yamashiro grew, as it was common for places to develop around castles, shrines, and onsen bathhouses.

In the Hokuriku region where Yamashiro is located, a public onsen bathhouse was more commonly known as a *soyu,* whereas the surrounding town was known as *yunogawa.* Yamashiro Onsen's original public bathhouse was an elegant, Meiji era construction that acted as the town's main landmark and social hub—the community gathered at Kosoyu to bathe, socialize, and relax together.

Rebuilt in 2010, Kosoyu (old bathhouse) is an exact restoration of the original. Framed by weeping willow trees, this delightful wooden structure is decorated with colorful stained-glass windows in the famed Kaga-gosai colors that are also integral to the Kaga-yuzen kimono dyeing method and Kutani pottery: indigo, crimson, ochre, dark green, and royal purple.

Crossing the threshold of the swaying *noren* curtains, the visitor is greeted by warm wooden interiors, whose rich, fragrant hinoki walls intermingle

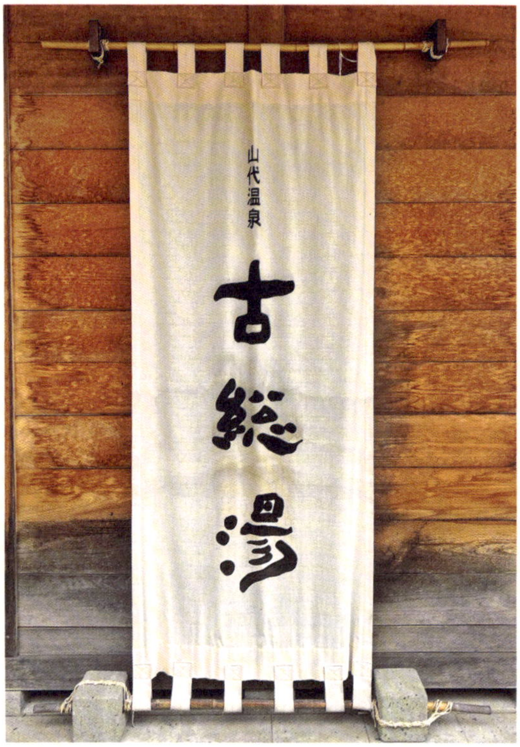

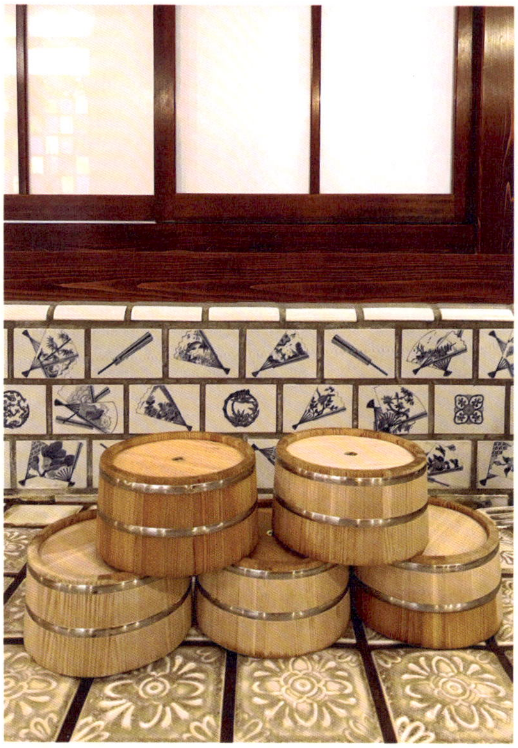

RIGHT Duckboard paths make for a pleasant walk through Yamashiro Onsen to Kosoyu, the beating heart of the town.

with stained-glass windows in the Kaga-gosai hues. Kutani porcelain tiles in indigo shades adorn the floor and lower walls with local motifs.

Opposite Kosoyu is the newer Soyu public bathhouse, which sits just beyond the entrance gate of the former Yoshinoya Ryokan. Soyu offers a larger, more spacious indoor onsen for locals and visitors to take pleasure in the healing waters. The nearby cobblestone path is lined with giant stone lanterns, each featuring a decorative piece of Kutani porcelain in varying designs. Both the lanterns and Kosoyu are aglow at night, exuding a colorful, comforting warmth.

The stone lanterns lead to the steps of Yakuoin Onsenji Temple, one of the Hakusan Five Temples that play a central role in the local people's reverence of Mt. Haku-san. Completed in the Heian period, they are strategically placed at equal distances from Gozenga-mine, the highest peak of Haku-san.

Yakuoin Onsenji Temple is also revered as the place where the modern Japanese language was born, as both the hiragana and katakana phonetic alphabets were created by the temple's chief priest, Myokaku Shonin. The peaceful grounds of the temple are a tranquil sanctuary, where every step on the moss-covered path has been embellished with a Kutani pottery tile, each featuring a colorful letter from the hiragana alphabet in the vibrant colors of the Kaga-gosai.

Adjacent to the temple is Hatori Shrine, another serene retreat where a large stone torii gate at the foot of the stairs leads up to the main structure. Dedicated to the god of traditional weaving, today's modern interpretation focuses on the interconnectedness of individuals woven together through our increasingly complex social worlds.

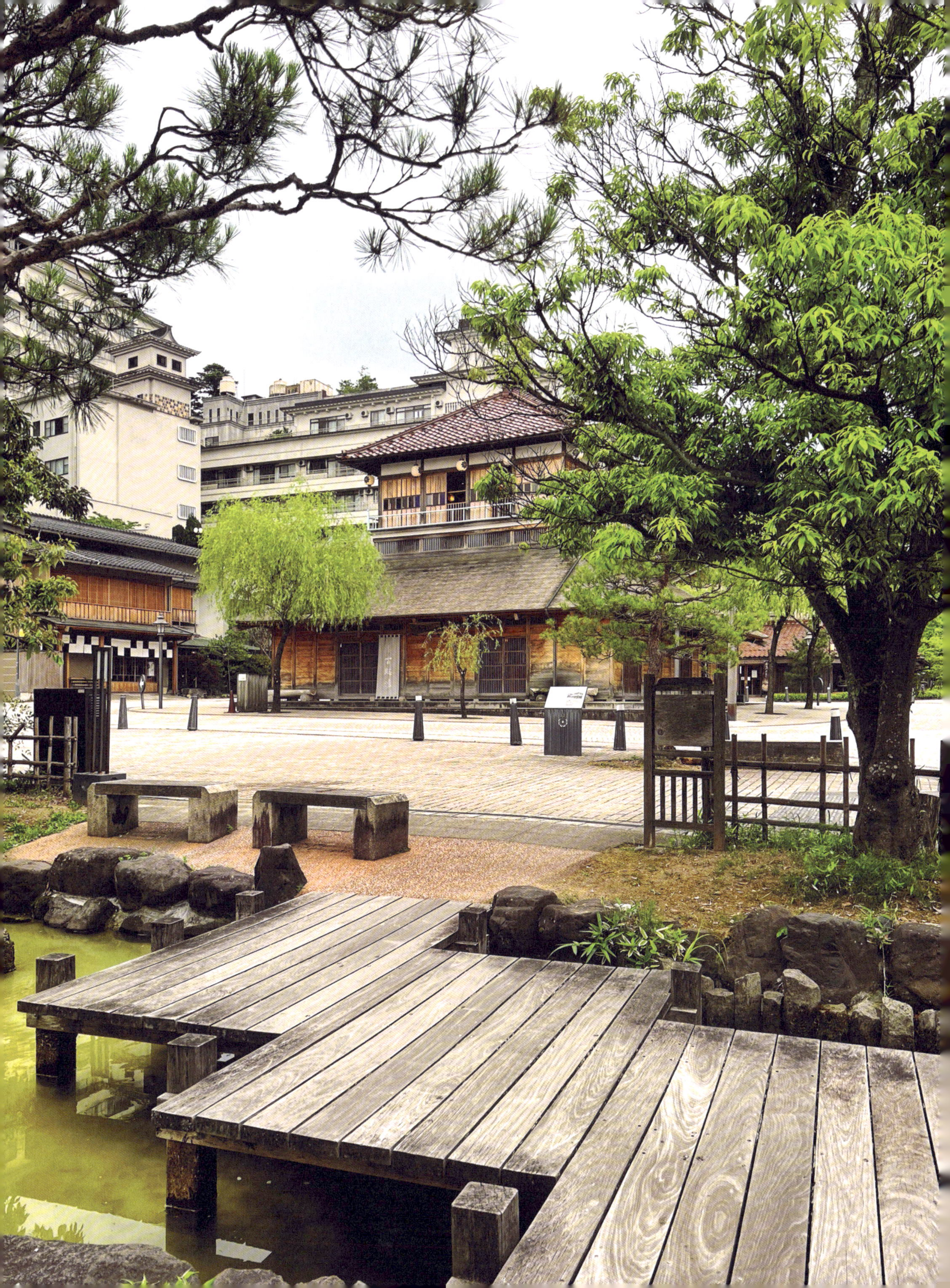

Nanadaru Onsen
Kawazu • Shizuoka Prefecture

IMMERSE THE BODY AND SOOTHE THE SOUL IN THIS STUNNING OPEN-AIR RIVER ONSEN

One of the country's most impressive public onsen features a crashing waterfall, superb baths, and a gorgeous riverside setting.

Nature lovers truly have their pick in Shizuoka Prefecture, where one's options include the rugged Jogasaki coastline, the cinder cone volcano Mt. Omuro, rows of early blooming *sakura*, and hikes through mountains to magnificent waterfalls.

Several well-known onsen are scattered around Shizuoka's Kawazu region, a place also famous for providing the setting for Kawabata Yasunari's short novel *The Izu Dancer* (*Izu no odoriko*); a bronze statue inspired by the novel can be found at Shokeidaru Falls. In another fitting homage, the express train that arrives at Kawazu station from Shinjuku or Tokyo is called Odoriko after the novella's Japanese title.

Shokeidaru is one of the seven stunning waterfalls that make up Kawazu's Nanadaru Falls, whose waters flow down the Kawazu River from the Amagi Mountain Range. Beloved by hikers and nature aficionados, the trail leading to all seven waterfalls is spectacular. The waterfalls themselves—known as Kamadaru, Ebidaru, Hebidaru, Shokeidaru, Kanidaru, Deaidaru, and Odaru—vary in size and height, with Kanidaru being the smallest at 6.5 feet (2 meters) and Odaru the tallest at 98 feet (30 meters).

Travelers aim to finish their hike at Odaru, where the powerful deluge pools magnificently into a turquoise basin before flowing into the river. Summer sees people swimming in the crisp, fresh waters; however, just as powerful a draw is the stunning rock *rotenburo* along the riverbank, where many hikers soak their sore limbs after their mountain trek. Though the onsen is located at the Odaru waterfall, the baths themselves are collectively known as Nanadaru Onsen.

Visitors enjoy moving from onsen to onsen, with one located to the side of the waterfall, offering majestic views, while others are found further along the bank, offering different yet equally stunning sights. The baths vary in size, some shallow and some deeper, some hotter and some colder, while several are set in the mountain's rock face where there is also a dimly lit cave onsen to explore. Rustic changing areas are available for both men and women, but as there is no shower, make sure to rinse by pouring onsen water over your body before entering. Note also that Nanadaru Onsen is a mixed onsen that allows guests to wear swimsuits, so be sure to have one packed.

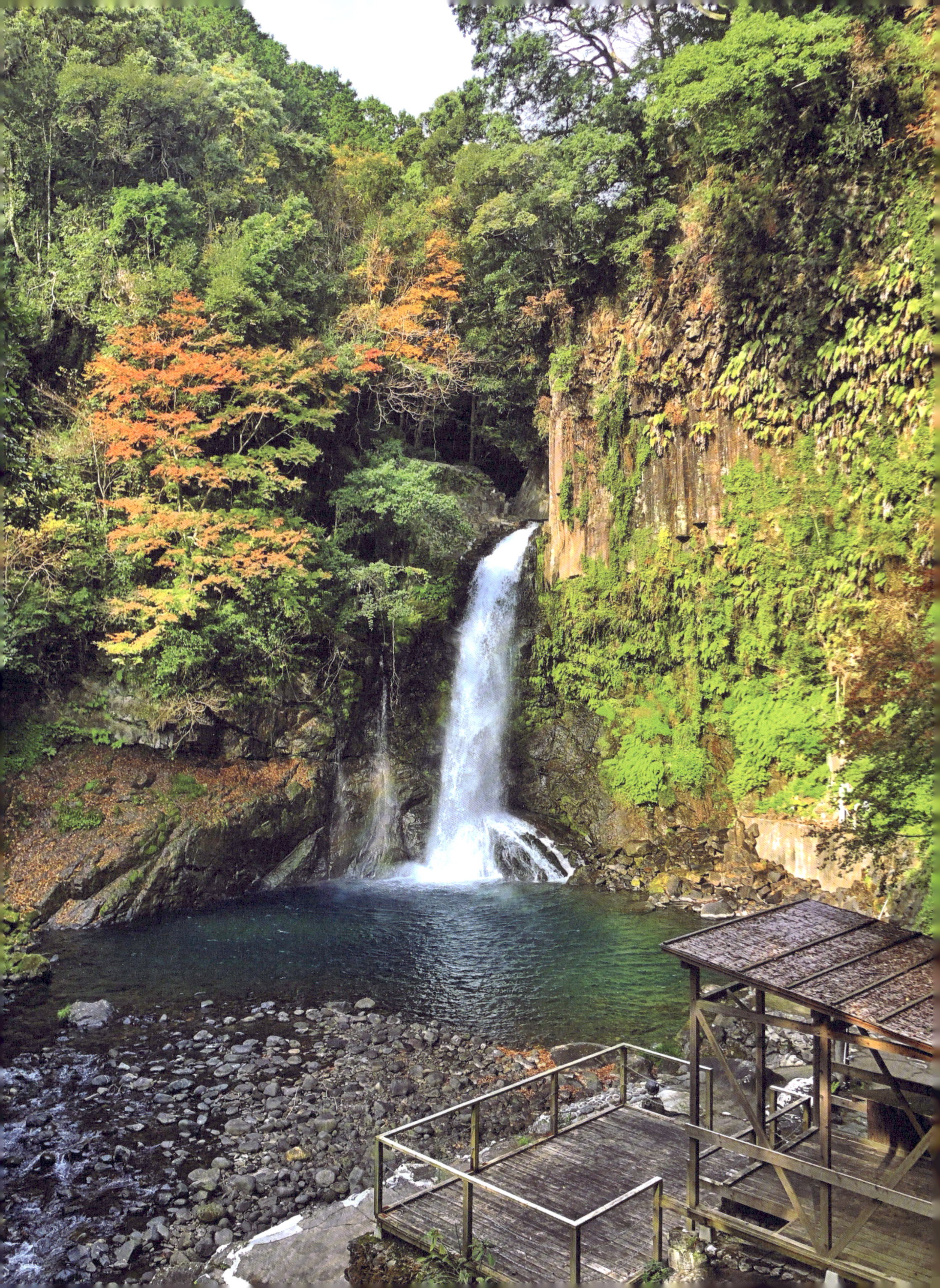

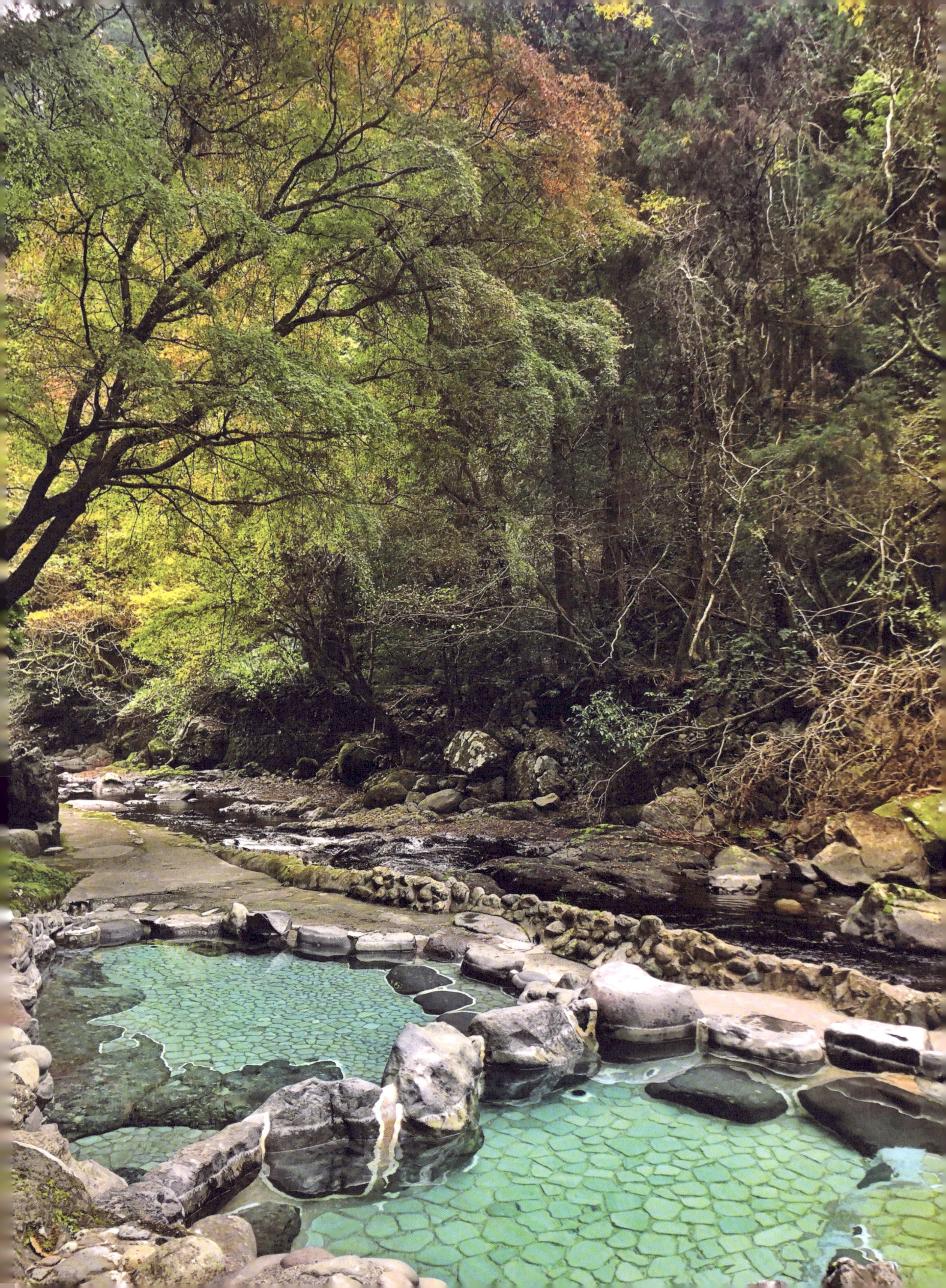

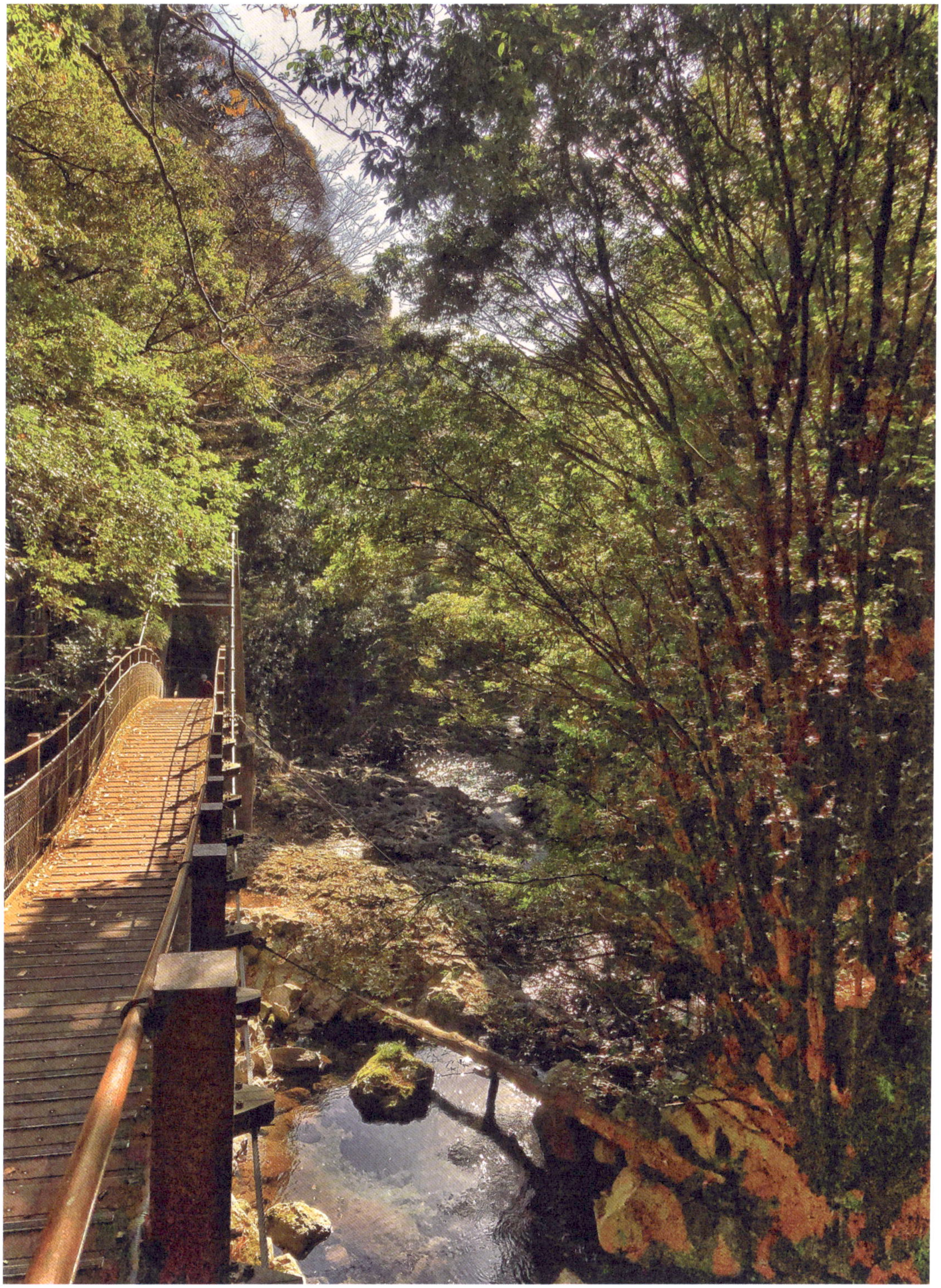

ABOVE Lovely in any season, the hike along Kawazu's seven waterfalls is especially breathtaking in autumn.

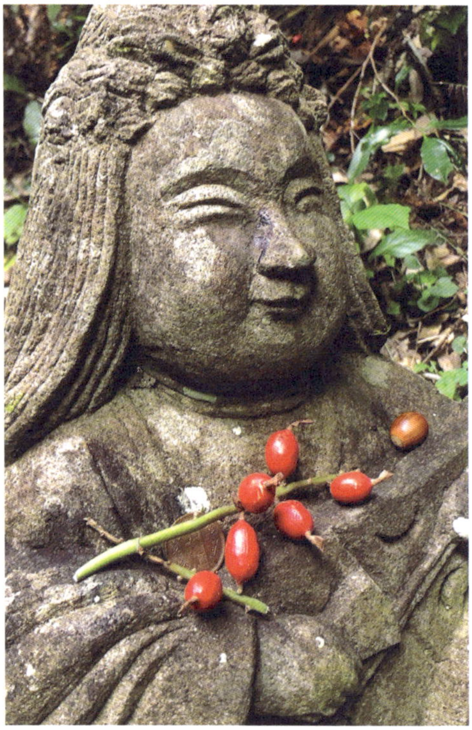

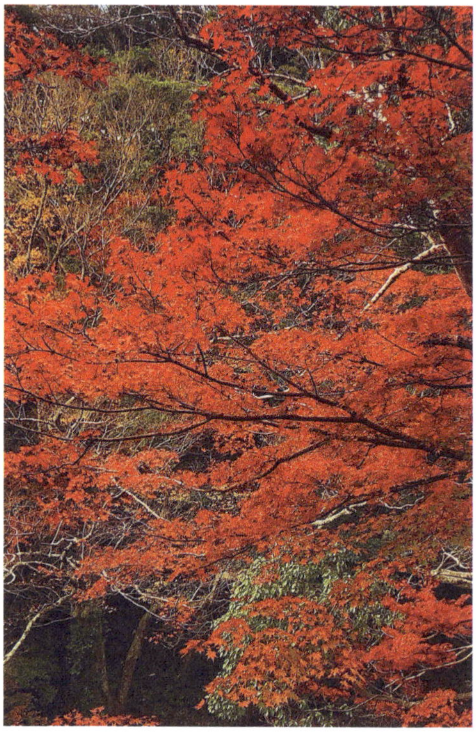

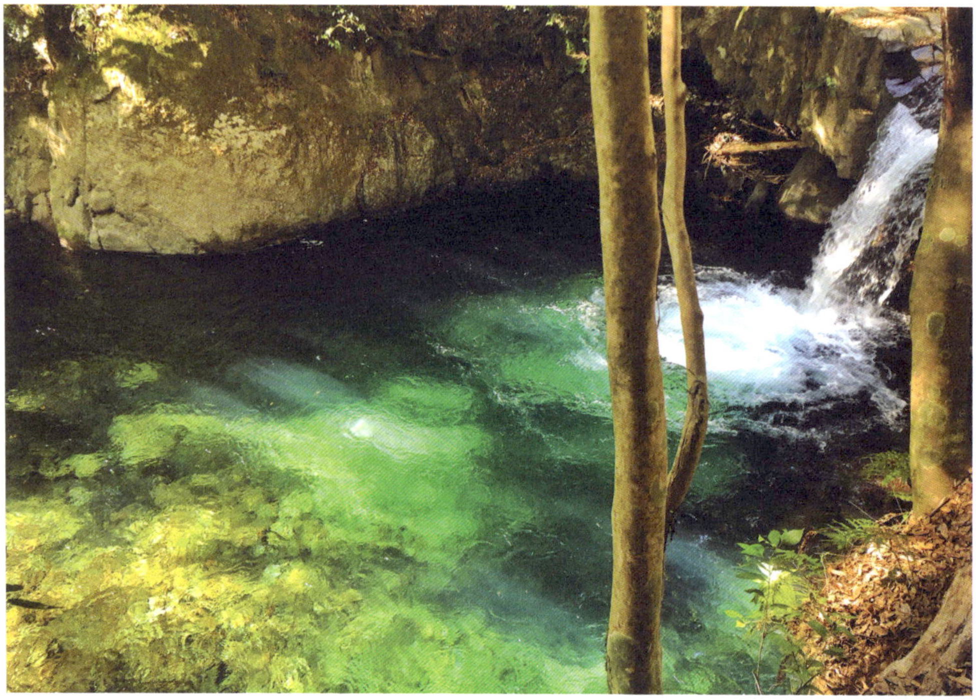

RIGHT Odaru, the final and largest waterfall of the Nanadaru Taki (Seven Waterfalls), where several *rotenburo* onsen await.

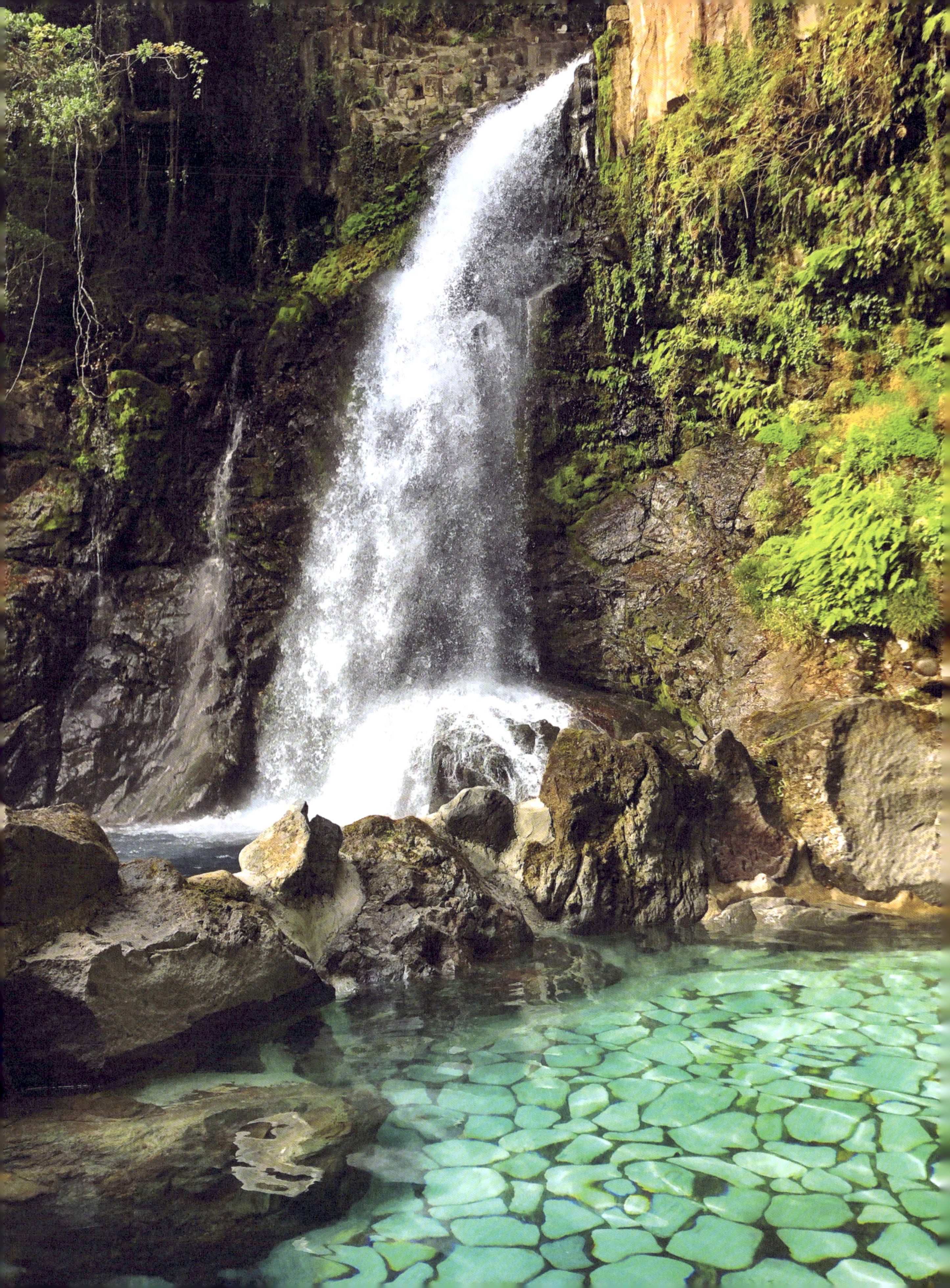

Takamiya Ryokan Miyamaso
Zao Onsen • Yamagata Prefecture

THE MOST HISTORIC ONSEN RYOKAN IN ZAO ONSEN

Stay in a place of living history: a traditional onsen inn that has watched over Zao for centuries.

Zao Onsen's history dates back 1,900 years to when Kibi no Tagayu, a retainer of Prince Yamato Takeru, was injured by an enemy's arrow. Fleeing to the top of Mt. Ryuzan, his gaze fell upon a surging flow of onsen water streaming from the rocks. Quickly descending the mountain, the vassal healed himself in the warm, medicinal waters, whose curative powers are still revered today.

The town is renowned for its imposing juhyo (snow monsters), snow-encased trees created by the region's unique geological conditions and specific type of fir. Unsurprisingly, these strange and gorgeous "monsters" make winter one of the most popular times to visit, when travelers glide down the powder-soft slopes surrounded by the impressive phenomenon. Yet regardless of when one visits, Zao Onsen is beautiful throughout the year and there is no better place to stay than the historic Takamiya Ryokan Miyamaso.

Spanning nearly 17 generations, the Okazaki family has been deeply intertwined with Zao Onsen. Takamiya Ryokan Miyamaso was established in 1717 by Okazaki Yaheiji, making it the oldest onsen ryokan in town. It is currently helmed by the 16th-generation family head (*jurokudaime*) who is also named Okazaki Yaheiji and whose son will one day take the name Yaheiji to signify his role as head of the family.

Stone steps lead the way to a fluttering *noren* curtain and hanging lanterns that beckon toward the historic buildings. Inside, the traditional wooden architecture, reflective of a bygone era, is accented by cozy *tokonoma* alcoves, sliding shoji doors, and comfortable tatami floors. The soft rustle of cotton *yukata* accompanies visitors as they move between the rooms and baths, the sound evoking a sense of refuge and healing. The ryokan's three private onsen sources can be experienced in the semi-open-air "longevity tub" onsen, the Zao stone onsen, and the Seseragi no Yu hinoki onsen.

For travelers in search of complete privacy and tranquility, Miyamaso's detached villa Hinakura offers its own private, open-air onsen. Once a traditional storehouse, Hinakura has been lovingly renovated and restored, making for a luxurious stay that maintains the beauty of traditional Japancse design.

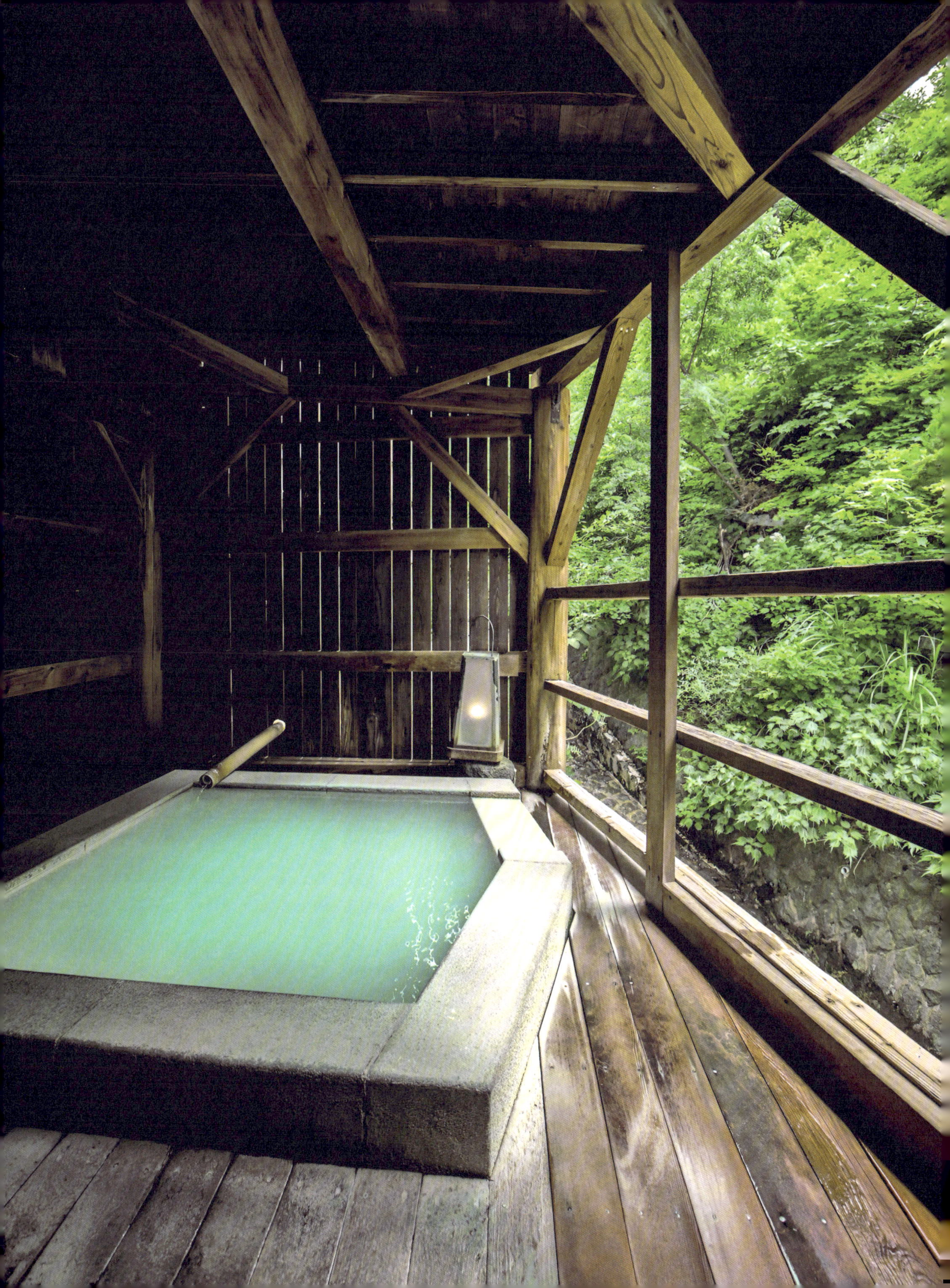

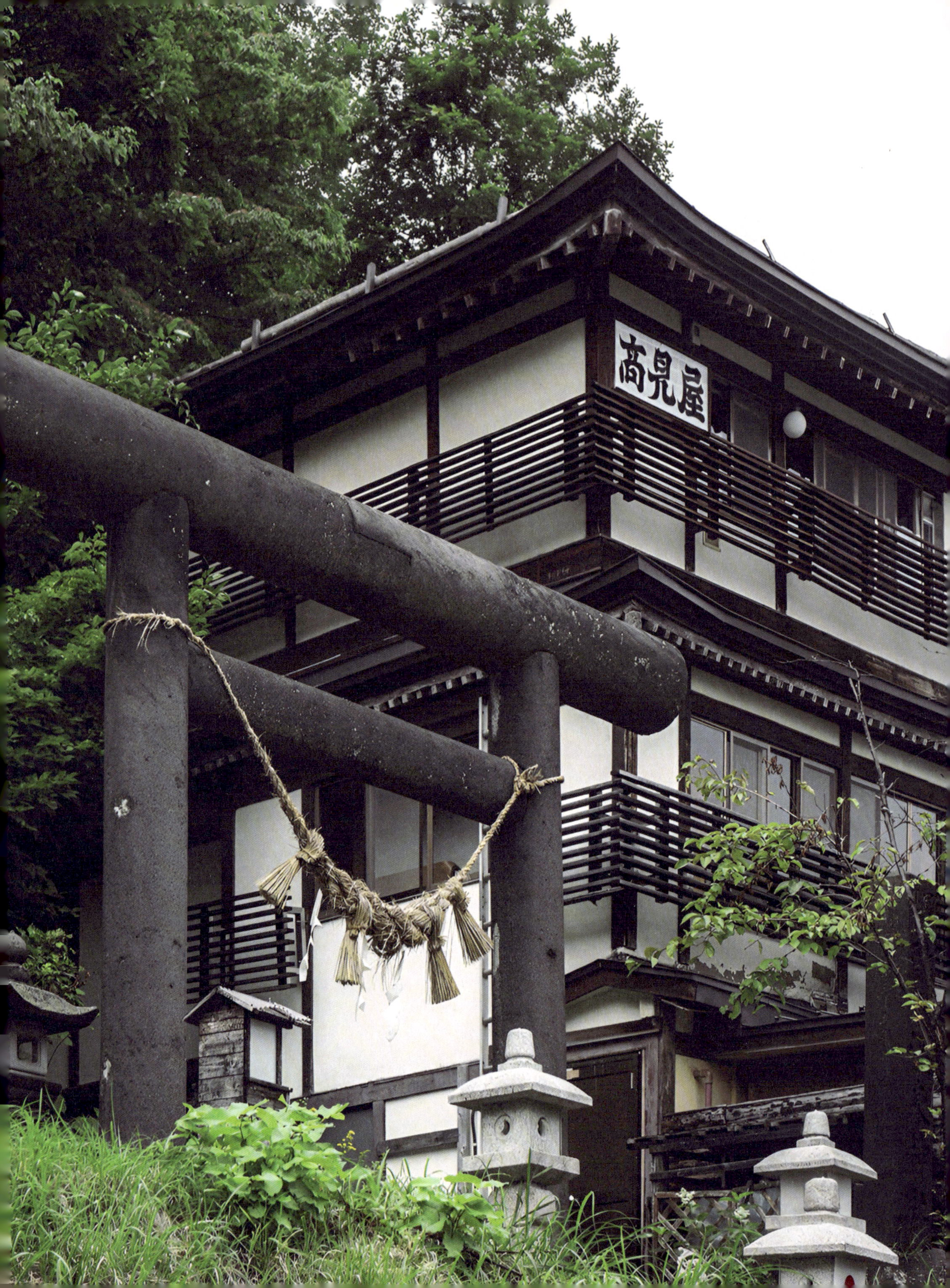
高見屋

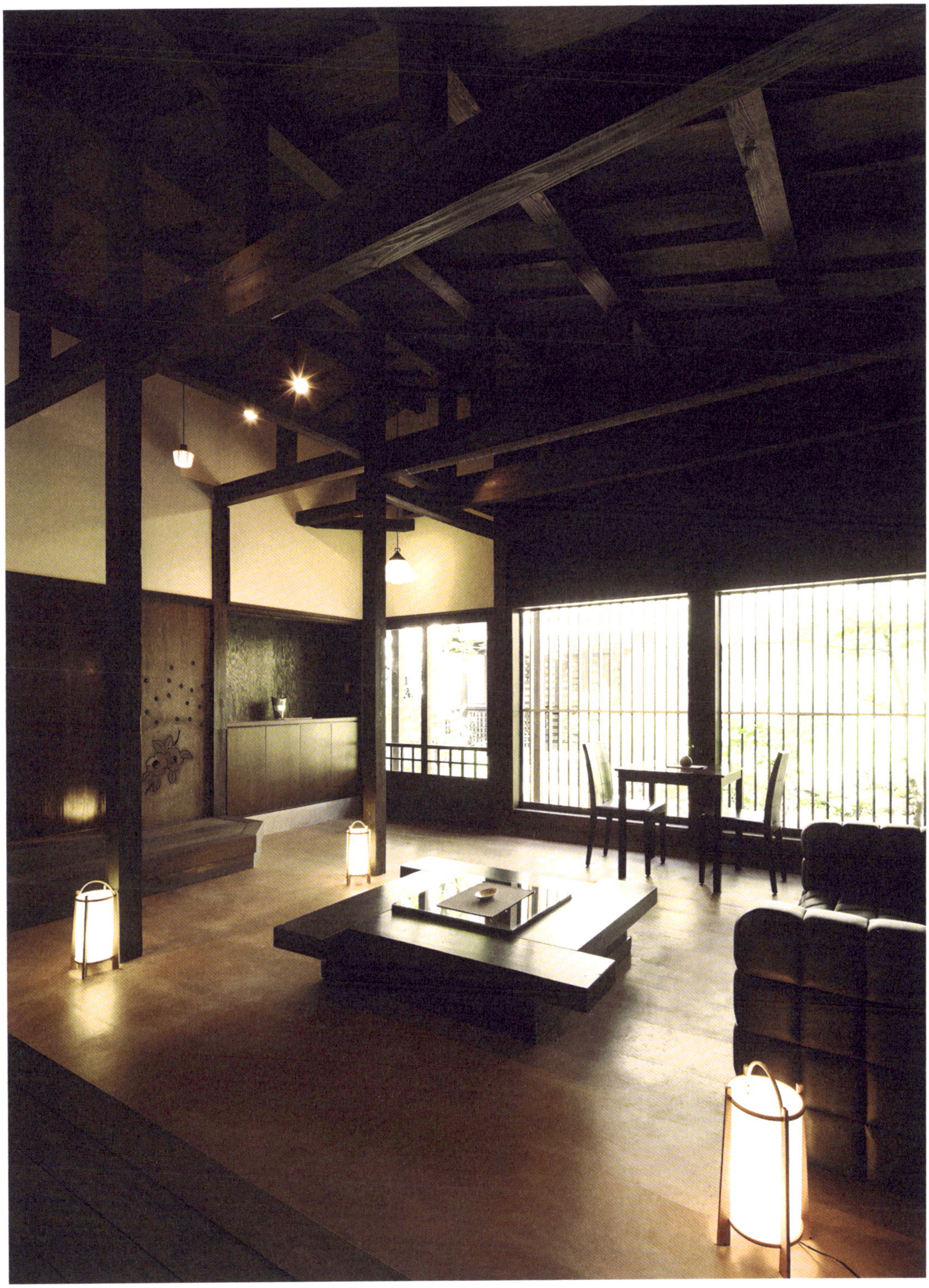

ABOVE Dark wooden beams and pillars highlight the traditional architecture of Takamiya Ryokan Miyamaso.

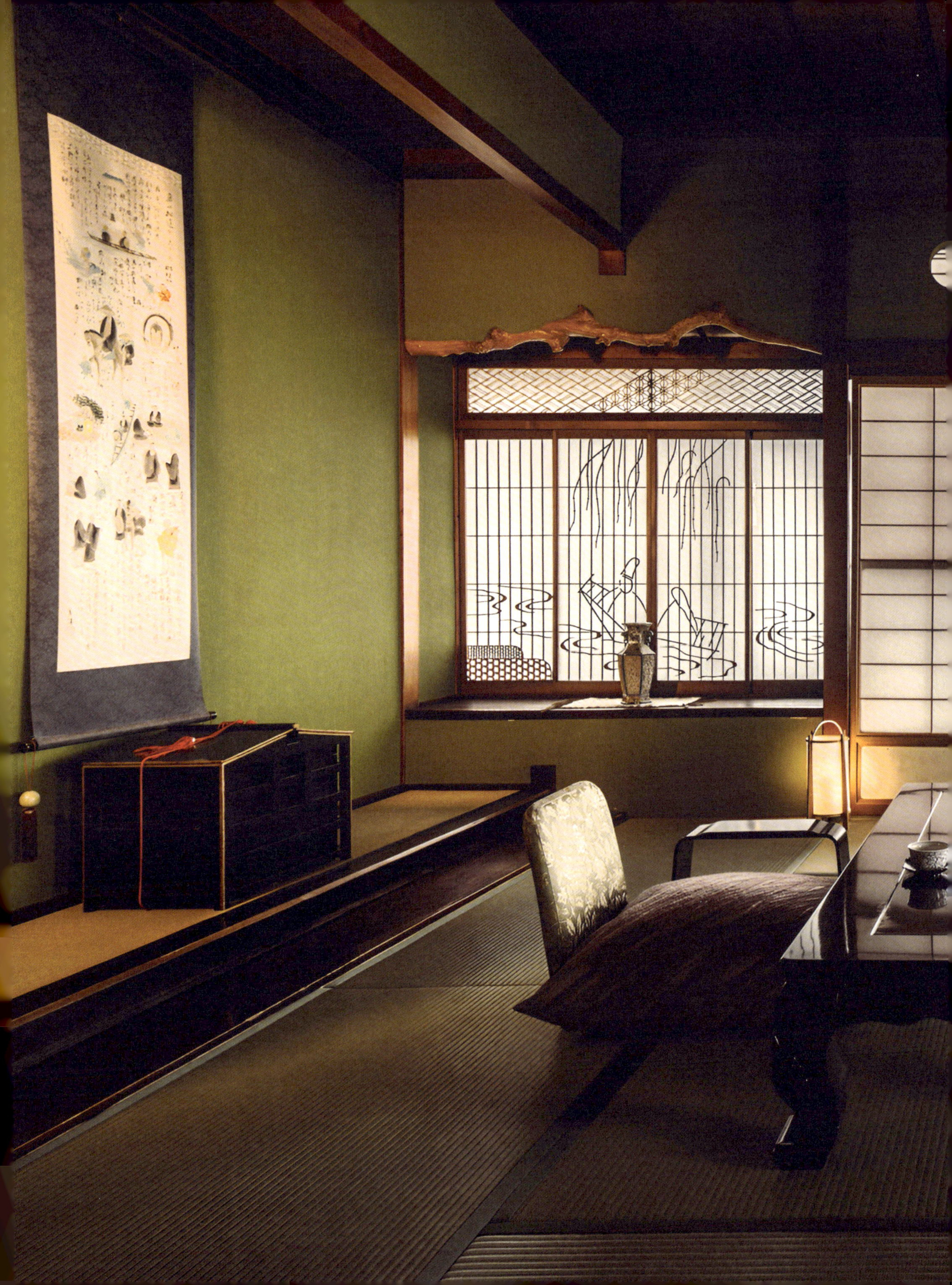

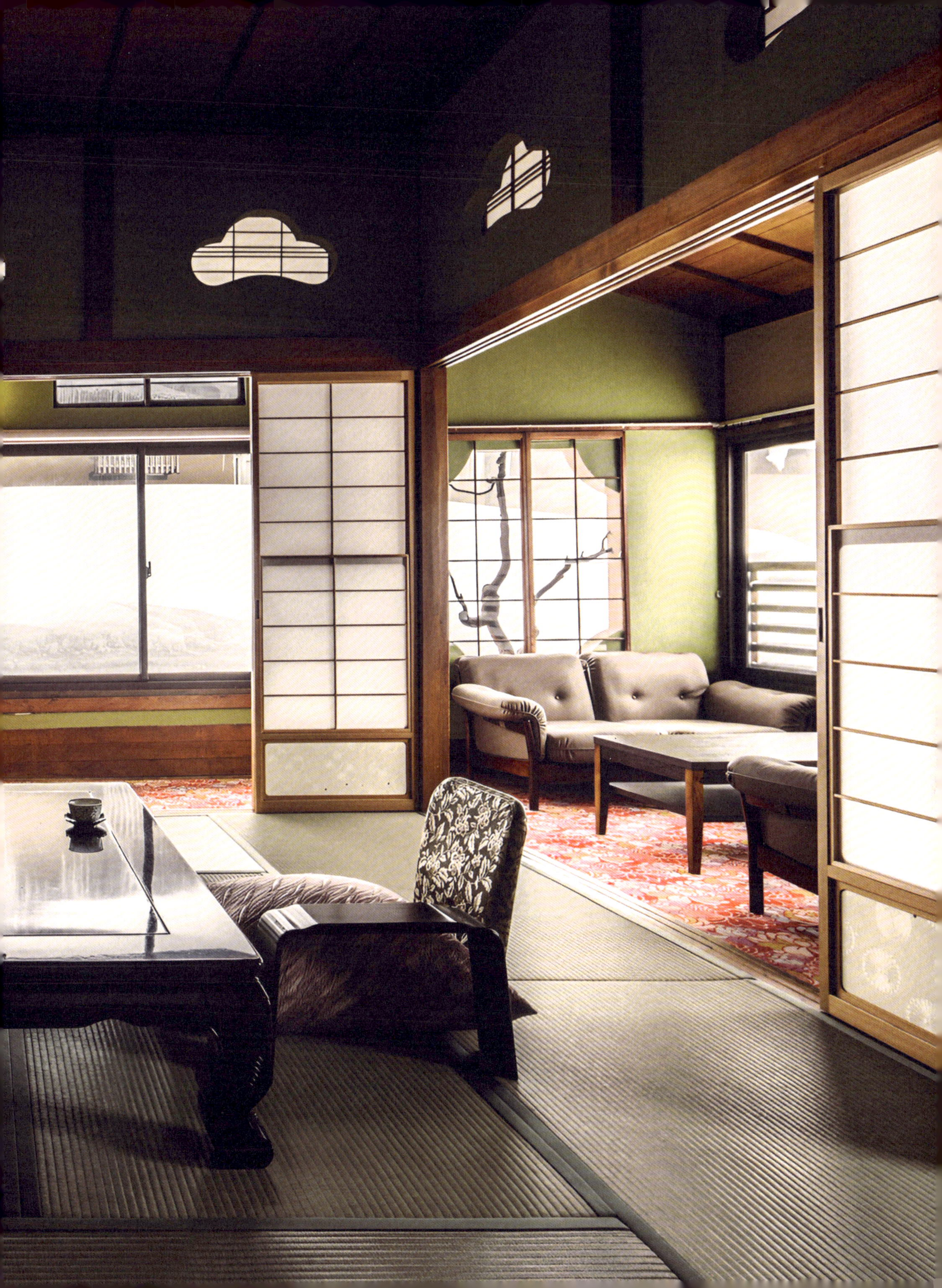

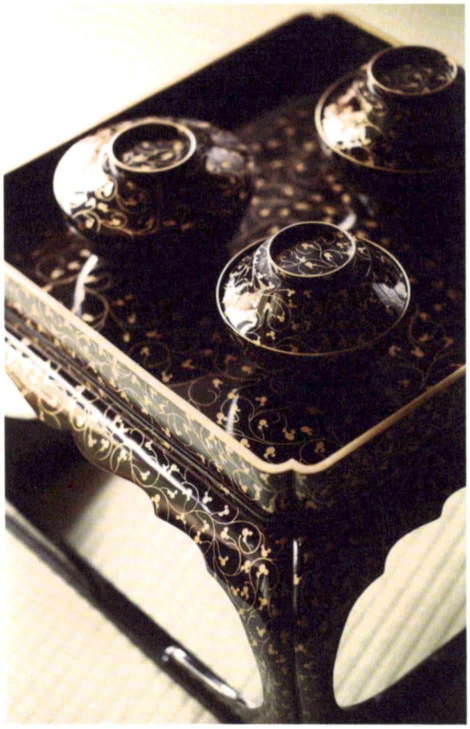

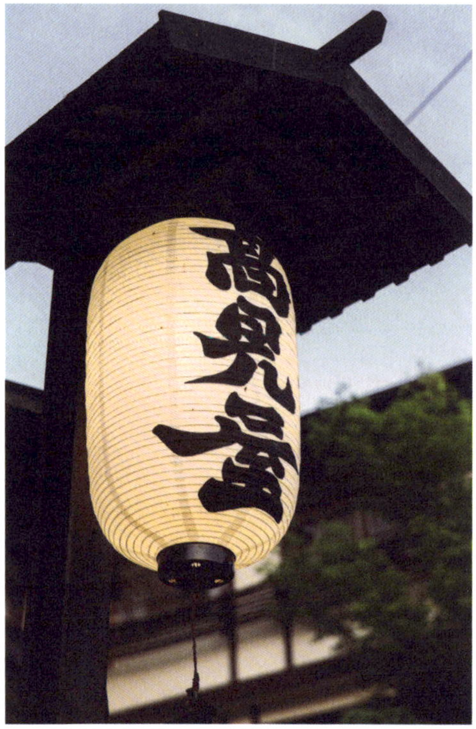

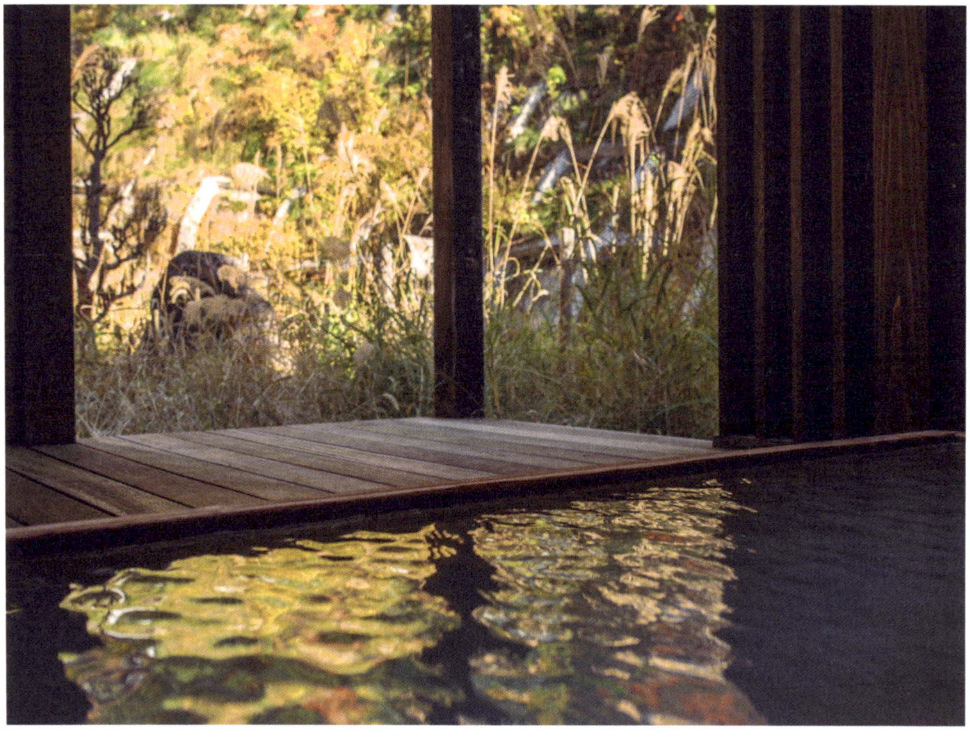

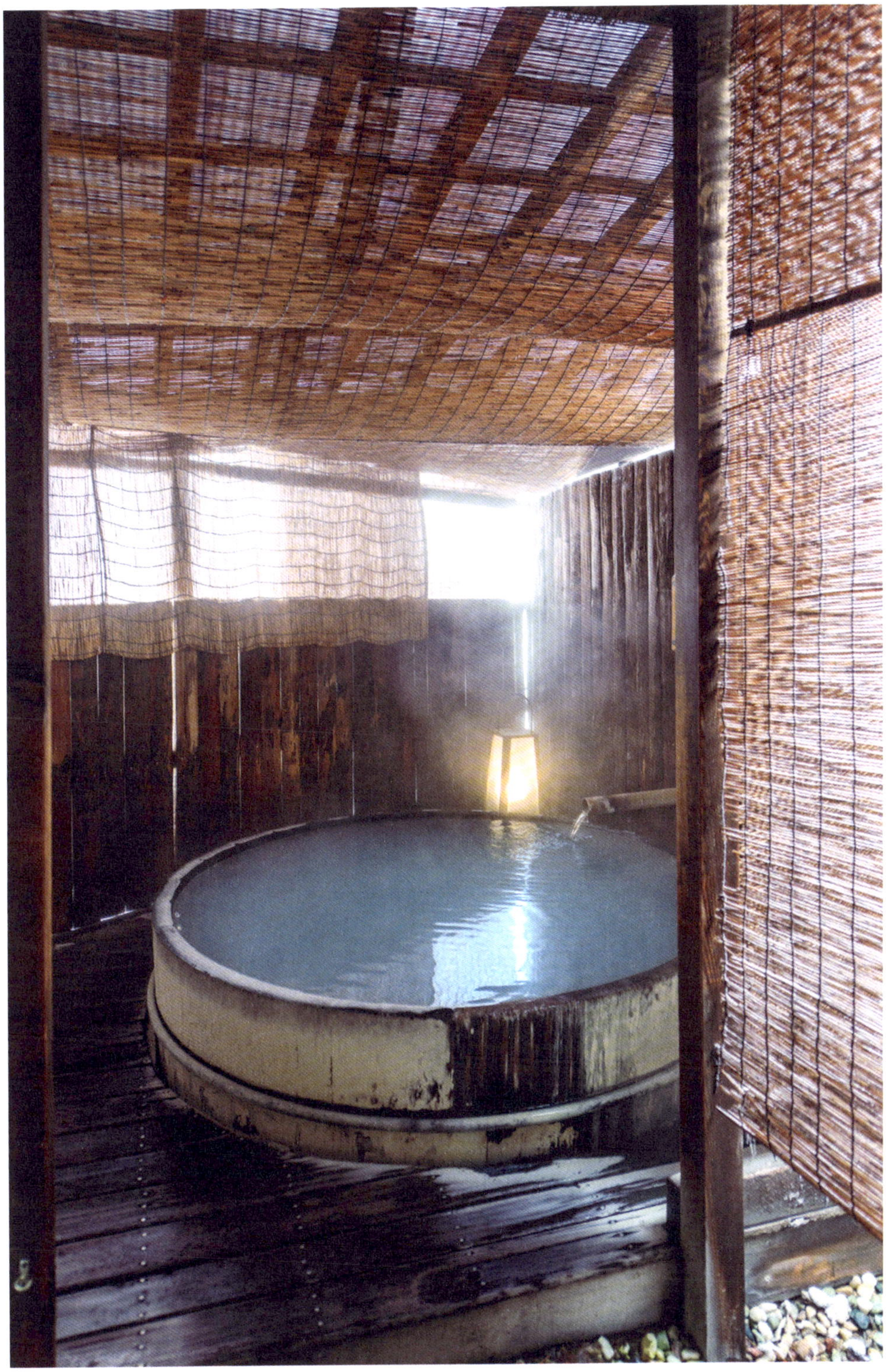

ABOVE Experience the pure *gensen-kakenagashi* waters of Takamiya Ryokan Miyamaso in one of their many baths.

Ginkonyu
Yakumo ● Hokkaido Prefecture

A SECLUDED, TRANQUIL, TRADITIONAL ONSEN RETREAT

In rural, forested Hokkaido, explore this unique mini *meguri* of several secluded onsen baths found in the forest and by the riverside.

Enveloped by mountains in a secluded valley, the remote Ginkonyu Ryokan is found in the pristine natural surroundings of Kamino-yu Onsen, a famous hot spring flowing from an island in the middle reaches of the Otoshibe River which, for hundreds of years, served as a hunting and healing retreat for the Indigenous Ainu people.

One of the few traditional onsen ryokan in Hokkaido, Ginkonyu's wooden interiors—in daytime lit by gorgeous, dappled sunlight—and sliding shoji doors create a peaceful respite away from the distractions of the modern world. Set in a lush natural environment, the inn is a serene escape, featuring vivid greenery in spring and summer, vibrant foliage in fall, and snowy landscapes in winter. At Ginkonyu, one is invited to embrace the Japanese way of *shinrin-yoku* (forest bathing) as much as the way of *toji*.

Ginkonyu, which translates to "Silver Wedding Bath," was named in honor of its auspicious beginnings. In 1925, a man named Kawaguchi Fukutaro began digging in search of the Otoshibe River's onsen source, as he had always dreamt of building an onsen getaway. He struck the spring's source on May 10th of that same year, a date coinciding with the "silver," or 25th, wedding anniversary of the Emperor Taisho. At his wife Tono's thoughtful suggestion, they named the bathhouse Ginkonyu, which officially opened in 1927. Today, Ginkonyu is celebrated as a "Bath of Marital Harmony," attracting many couples who visit to mark their own anniversaries, especially the silver year.

Kawaguchi Yohei, the fourth-generation owner, proudly manages Ginkonyu with his family, paying homage to its past while growing the legacy left by his ancestors. Just as the *katsura* seeds planted by his ancestors have now stretched to full-grown trees, Ginkonyu too has evolved.

The family now own five onsen sources, which provide the pure *gensen kakenagashi* water (continuously flowing onsen water) throughout their 11 baths. Communal public onsen are available for both men and women, and feature indoor and outdoor baths, as well as a reservable indoor family onsen and outdoor footbath. The highlight, however, is the onsen *meguri* experience the Kawaguchi family has built. Five hidden, private onsen are spread out across the vast forest grounds, with three of them remaining open even during the winter months.

At Ginkonyu, visitors are offered a mini pilgrimage through the forest or across the swaying suspension bridge over the Otoshibe. One can soak in the onsen treehouse Katsura no Yu, meander across the bridge to relax in the stunning rock *rotenburo* of Donguri no Yu, or head in the other direction to Tochi no Yu, where one finds both a giant, hollowed-out tree trunk onsen bath, and a square, wooden bath built into the rockface, both with different river views.

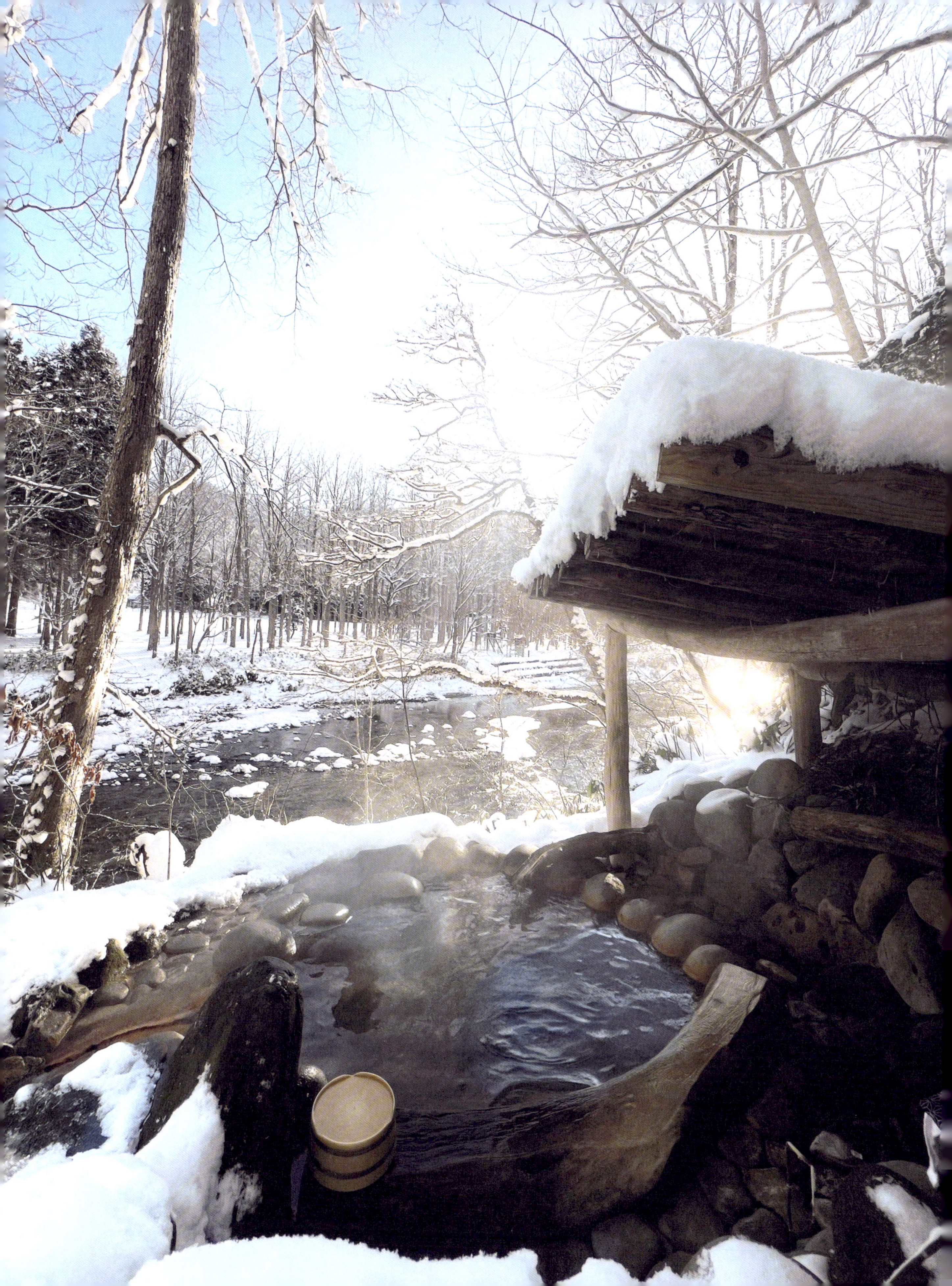

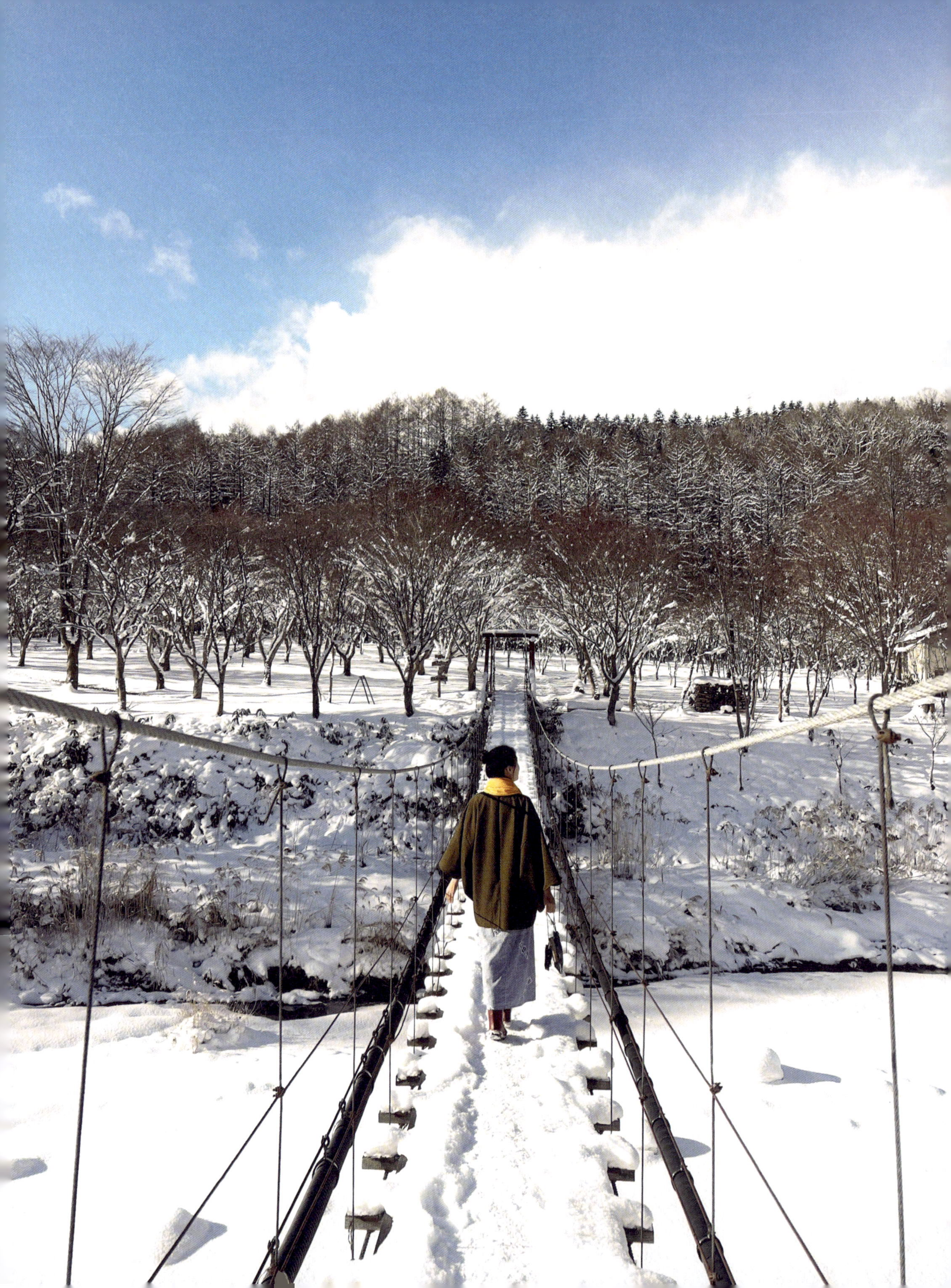

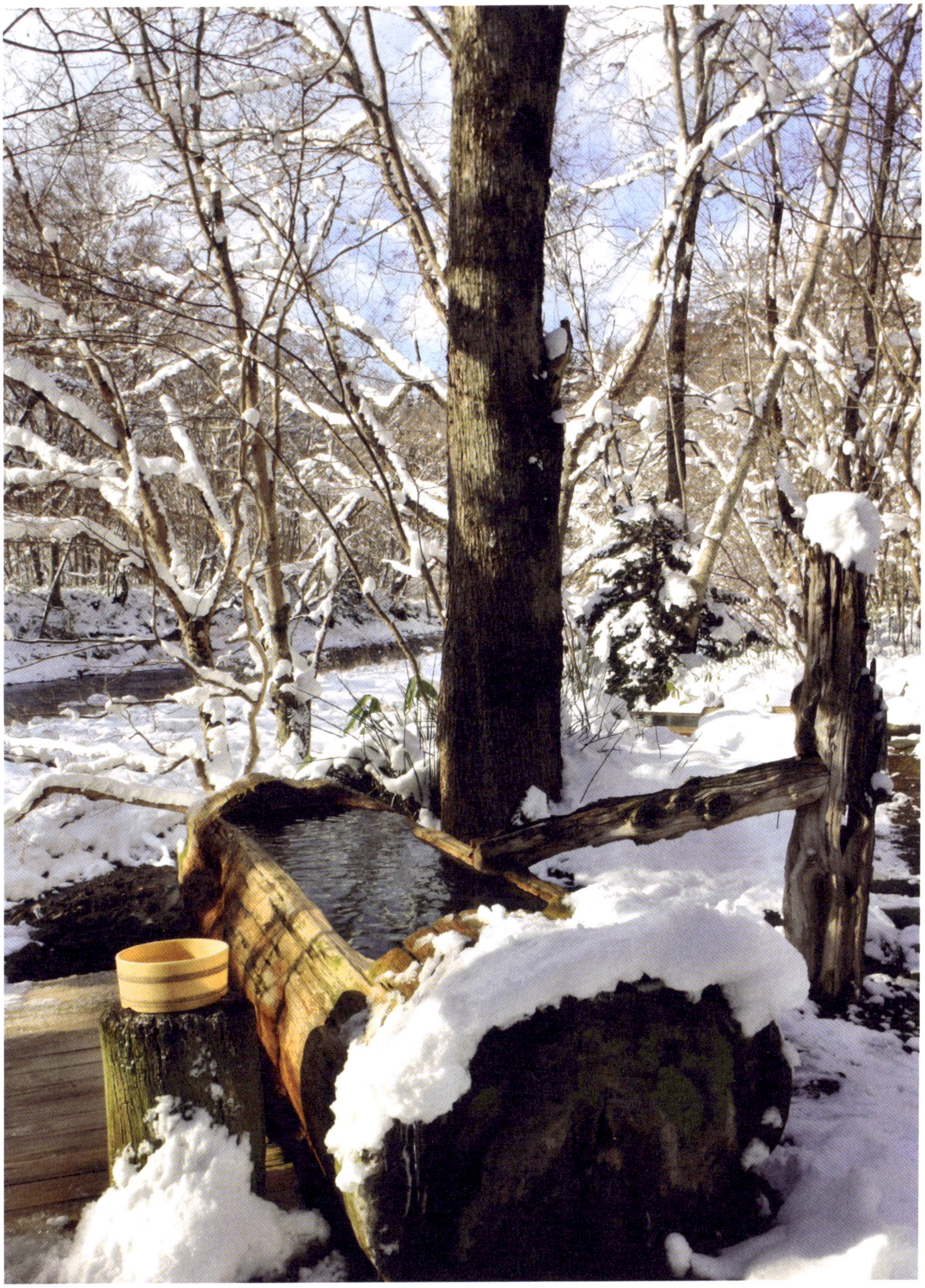

ABOVE The gorgeous tree trunk onsen bath at the private Tochi no Yu overlooks the river.

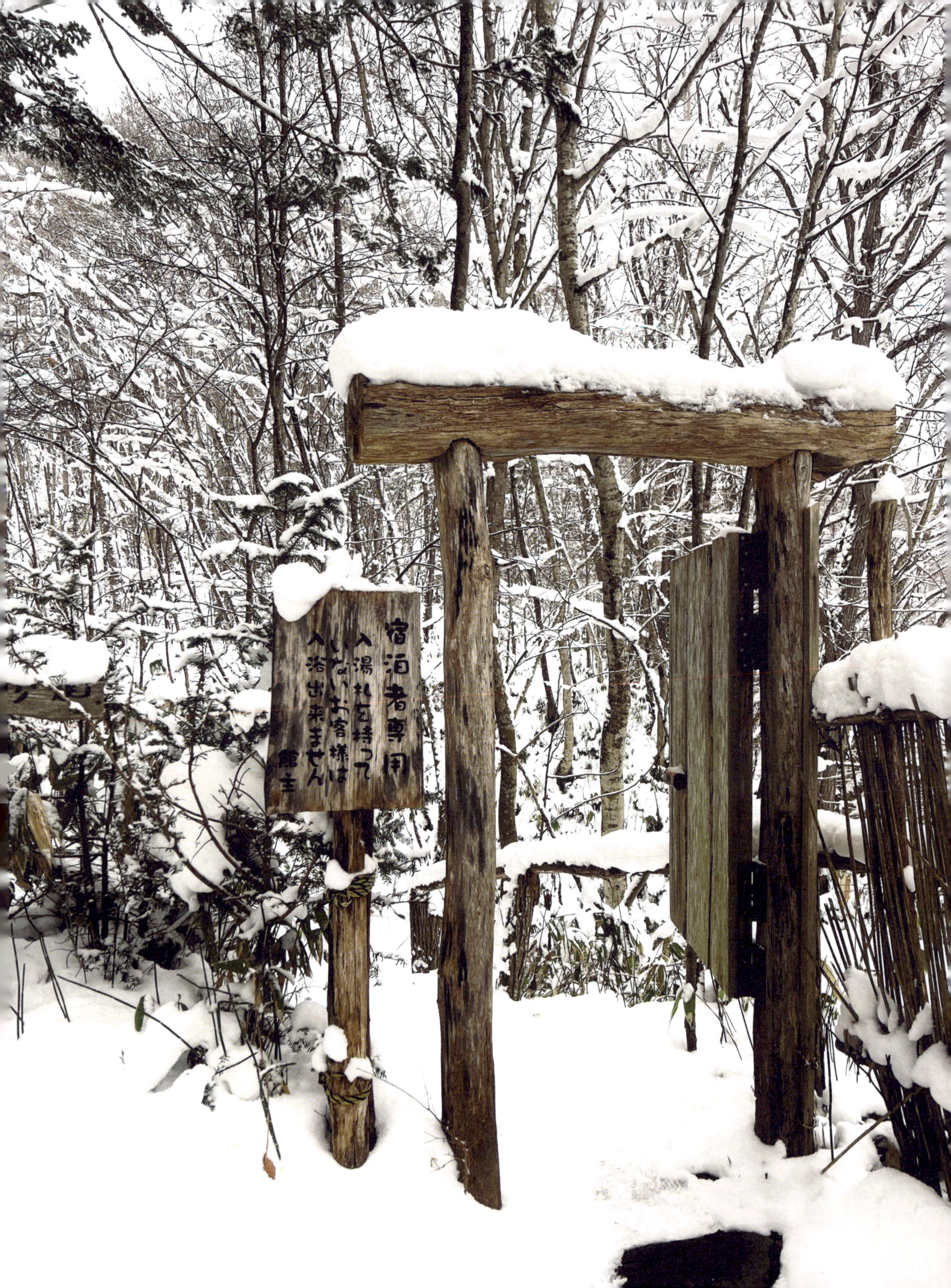
宿泊者専用
入湯札を持って
いないお客様は
入浴出来ません
館主

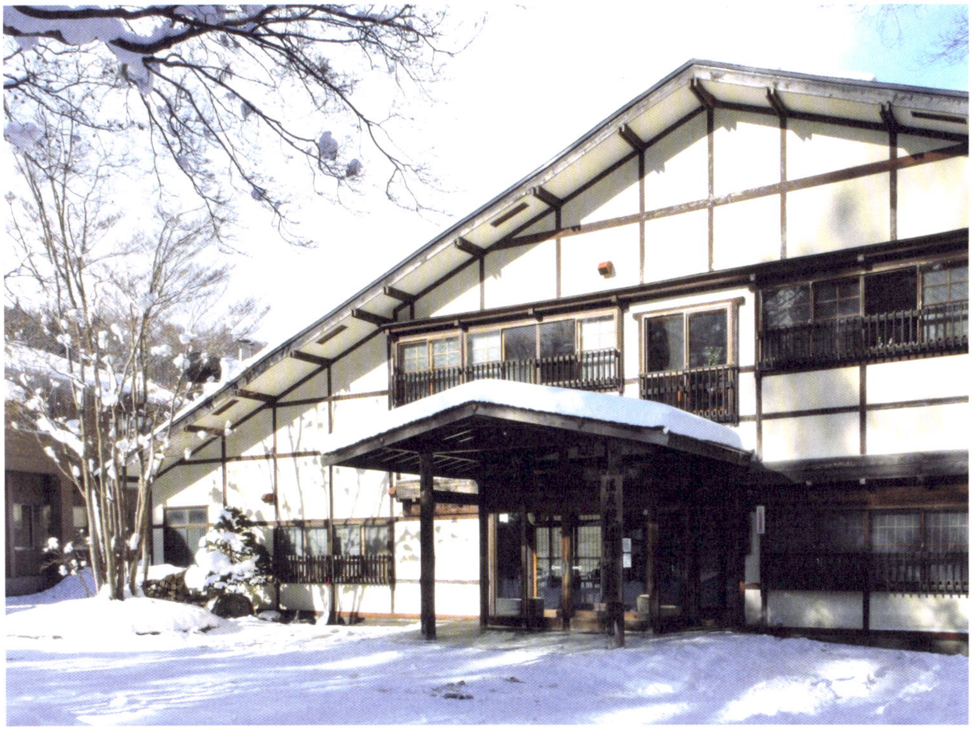

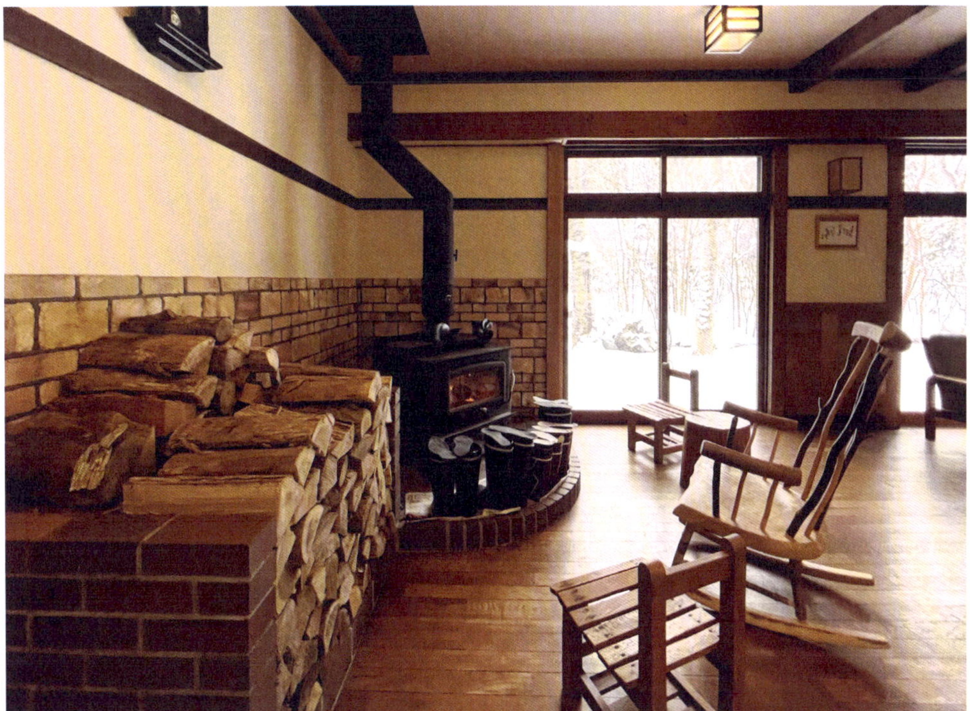

ABOVE Visitors can warm themselves by the fire in Ginkonyu's cozy wooden lounge.

Maruhon Ryokan
Takashima • Gunma Prefecture

AN ONSEN INN REVITALIZED BY ONE MAN'S VISION

Enjoy peaceful, relaxing moments in this stunning, award-winning hinoki onsen bath and serene rest area, draped in shadows and light.

Midway between the two famed onsen towns of Kusatsu and Shima lies the sleepy hamlet of Sawatari Onsen, where the modern era has not diminished its charming, retro Showa atmosphere. Known as the "finishing bath of Kusatsu Onsen," the silky, alkaline onsen waters of Sawatari soothe skin roughened by Kusatsu's highly acidic onsen. Devastated by a great fire in 1945, Sawatari was revitalized in 1959, and since then continues to protect the waters and increase awareness of its therapeutic, beautifying onsen.

Among the eight onsen ryokan in Sawatari, Maruhon Ryokan shares the inspiring story of a person who took a courageous leap of faith to start fresh. Around 20 years ago, Fukuda Satoshi was a banker who fell in love with the onsen waters of Maruhon Ryokan, and, hearing it was in danger of closing due to succession issues, decided to help the family find a buyer. However, due to the complexity of onsen ownership rights, no buyer was successful. Wanting to keep the legacy of this Edo-era ryokan alive, Fukuda-san decided, with the previous owner's blessing, to take ownership of the inn himself, even changing, for the sake of succession, his family register name. Leaving his banking job, Fukuda-san moved with his family to the mountains and embraced the onsen ryokan life.

Pure *gensen kakenagashi* onsen waters flow into the three baths available at Maruhon Ryokan; historically, the most well-known is the large *konyoku* mixed onsen decorated with a mosaic of tiles, which sits within an impressive Showa-era hinoki bathhouse and offers female-only bathing between certain hours. A freely reservable private open-air onsen, made of Aomori Hiba cypress wood, is a perfect choice for those who may be a bit shy.

Bringing Maruhon firmly into the present is the third onsen bath, the women's bath. Designed by Kubo Tsushima Architects, the aromatic hinoki bathhouse seamlessly connects the ryokan's two accommodation wings. The bathhouse offers both a resting and bathing space, with a gracefully curving hinoki wall acting as both a comfortable backrest and a diffuser for the sun's gentle rays streaming in from the skylight and open-air vent. Male bathers may also enjoy this space during specific hours of the day.

Many visitors, especially solo travelers, choose to stay multiple nights in Satawari in order to partake in the ancient practice of onsen *toji*.

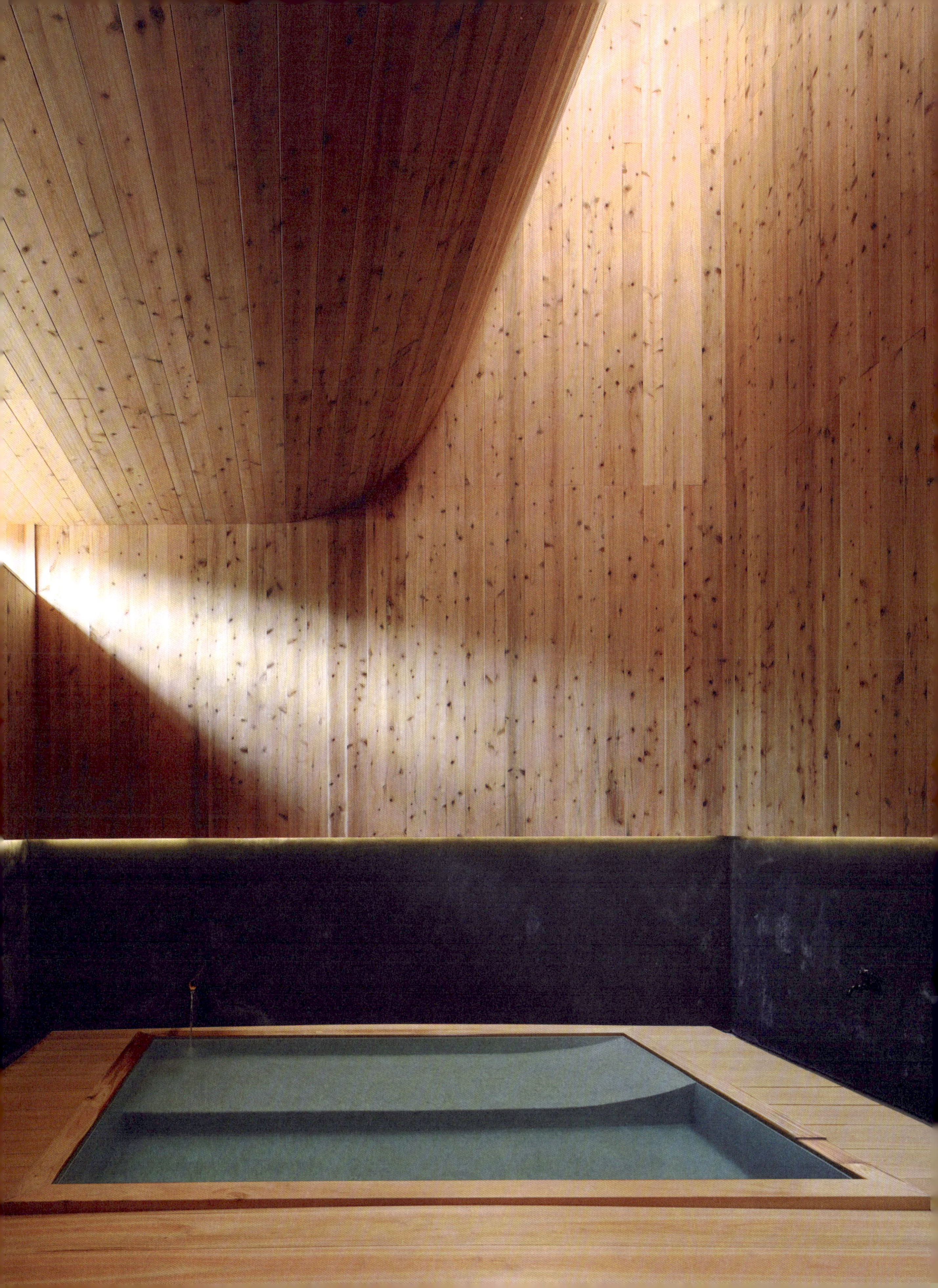

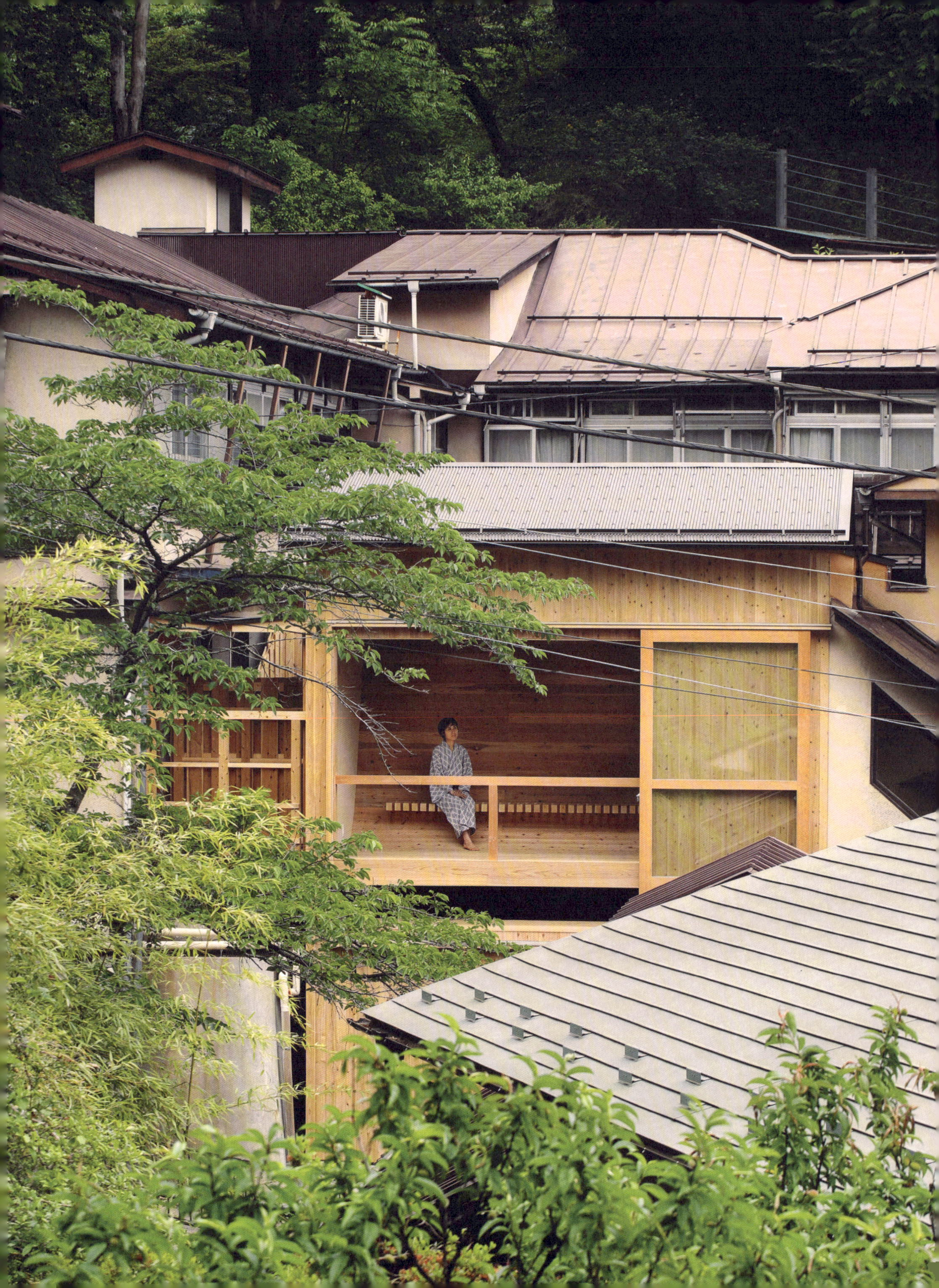

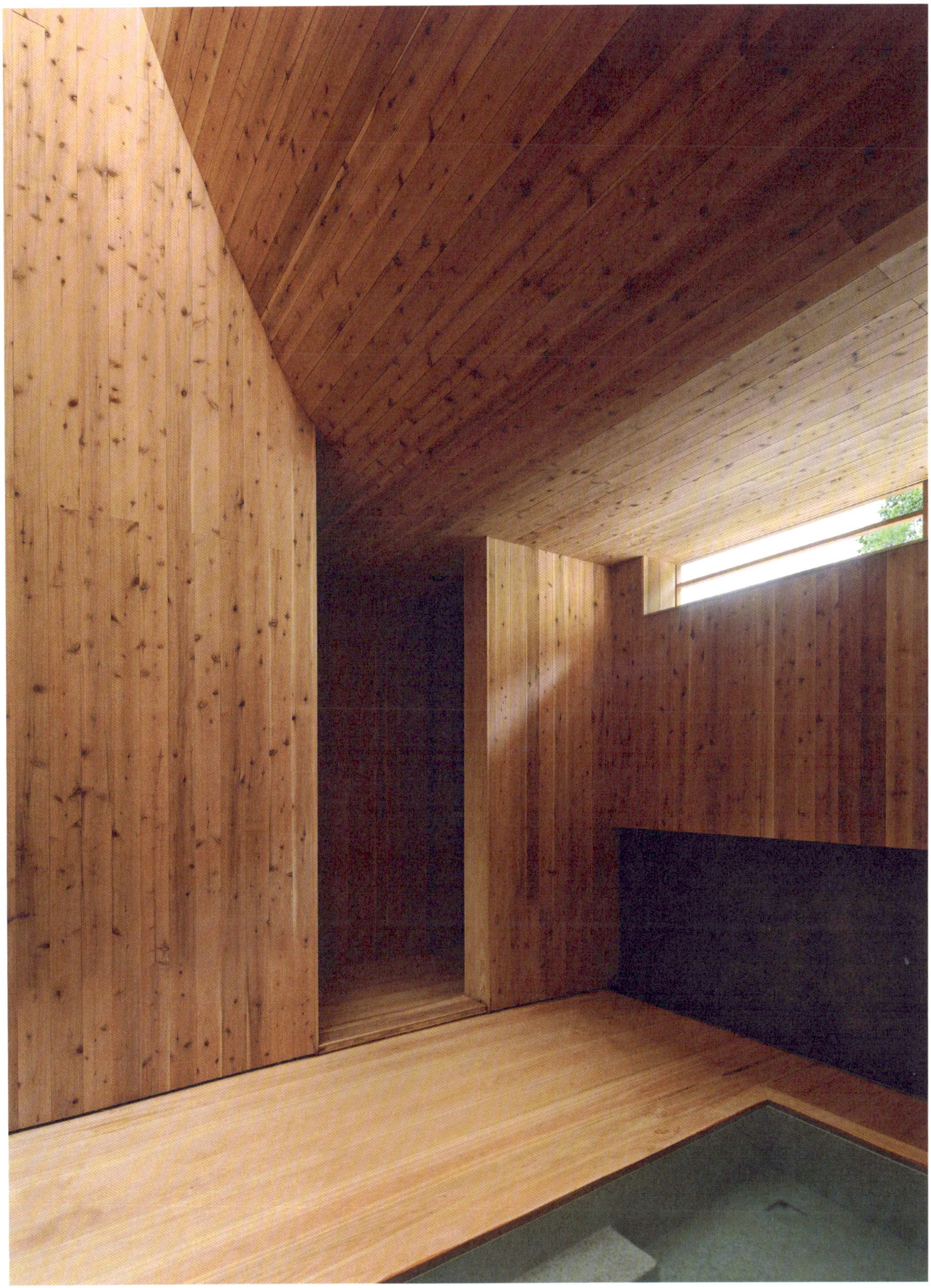

ABOVE The play of light and shadow mixed with the scent of hinoki wood creates a unique onsen-bathing experience.

Noboribetsu Onsen
Noboribetsu • Hokkaido Prefecture

WANDER THE MAJESTIC HELL OF JIGOKUNDANI

Soaring clouds of onsen vapors drift gently over the vast valley, creating an impressive, eerie environment for wandering exploration.

South of Sapporo lies Hokkaido's most famous onsen town: Noboribetsu. Renowned for its 10 plentiful onsen sources, each with its own unique characteristics to soothe, heal, and beautify, the town is located just below the extraordinary Jigokudani (Hell Valley), which supplies Noboribetsu with most of its onsen waters.

Created by the volcanic activity of Mt. Hiyori over 10,000 years ago, Jigokudani is a huge crater valley of 27 acres (11 hectares), where local lore states that the Yukijin (demon gods) guard the healing waters as penance for tormenting humanity. Rising clouds of onsen steam compliment the vivid hues of the mountain greenery and the various shades of earth and rock, creating an otherworldly, ethereal landscape that is eerily breathtaking. This geothermal wonderland, with its bubbling onsen and steaming fumaroles, is evocative of the country's historical depictions of the hellish realm, yet offers a bevy of delights for its visitors.

Several walking trails are found throughout Jigokudani and Noboribetsu, with the main trail taking one right through the heart of Hell Valley. One of the area's longer trails, perfect for the adventurous walker, gives way to spectacular views over the area and leads to Oyunuma Pond, a mesmerizing sulfuric pond with a distinct milky-blue hue. The steaming, mineral-rich onsen water that pours from the pond forms the Oyunuma River, which offers weary trekkers restful, therapeutic footbath pools set amid the lush natural surroundings.

Noboribetsu Onsen became popular as a destination to heal and recuperate during the Edo period, when, in the 1850s, the carpenter Takimoto Kinzo and his wife Sata moved to Hokkaido. Sata suffered from severe dermatosis and Kinzo sought desperately for a way to help ease her pain. One day, Kinzo decided to seek the truth behind all the stories he had heard about the healing properties of Noboribetsu's onsen springs, and he carved a path through the craggy mountains to reach the steaming valley of Jigokudani. Here, he built a small hut by the springs, hoping the waters would provide relief and cure Sata's ailment. Over time, after regularly bathing in the onsen, Sata's dermatosis was miraculously healed.

Once aware of the onsen's benefits, Kinzo eventually opened an inn so others could partake of the healing waters. This inn would later become today's Takimotokan, named after Kinzo by his descendants.

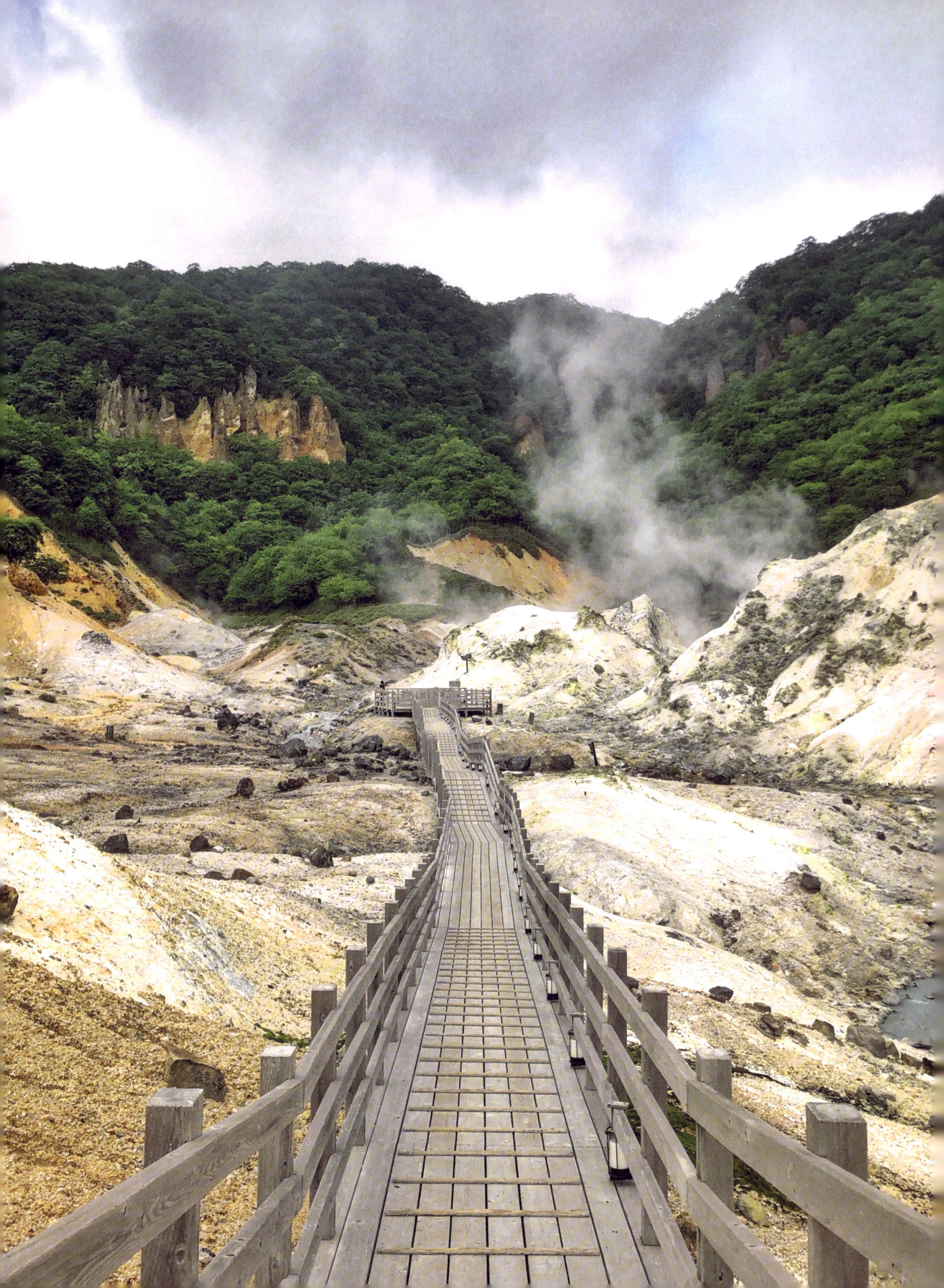

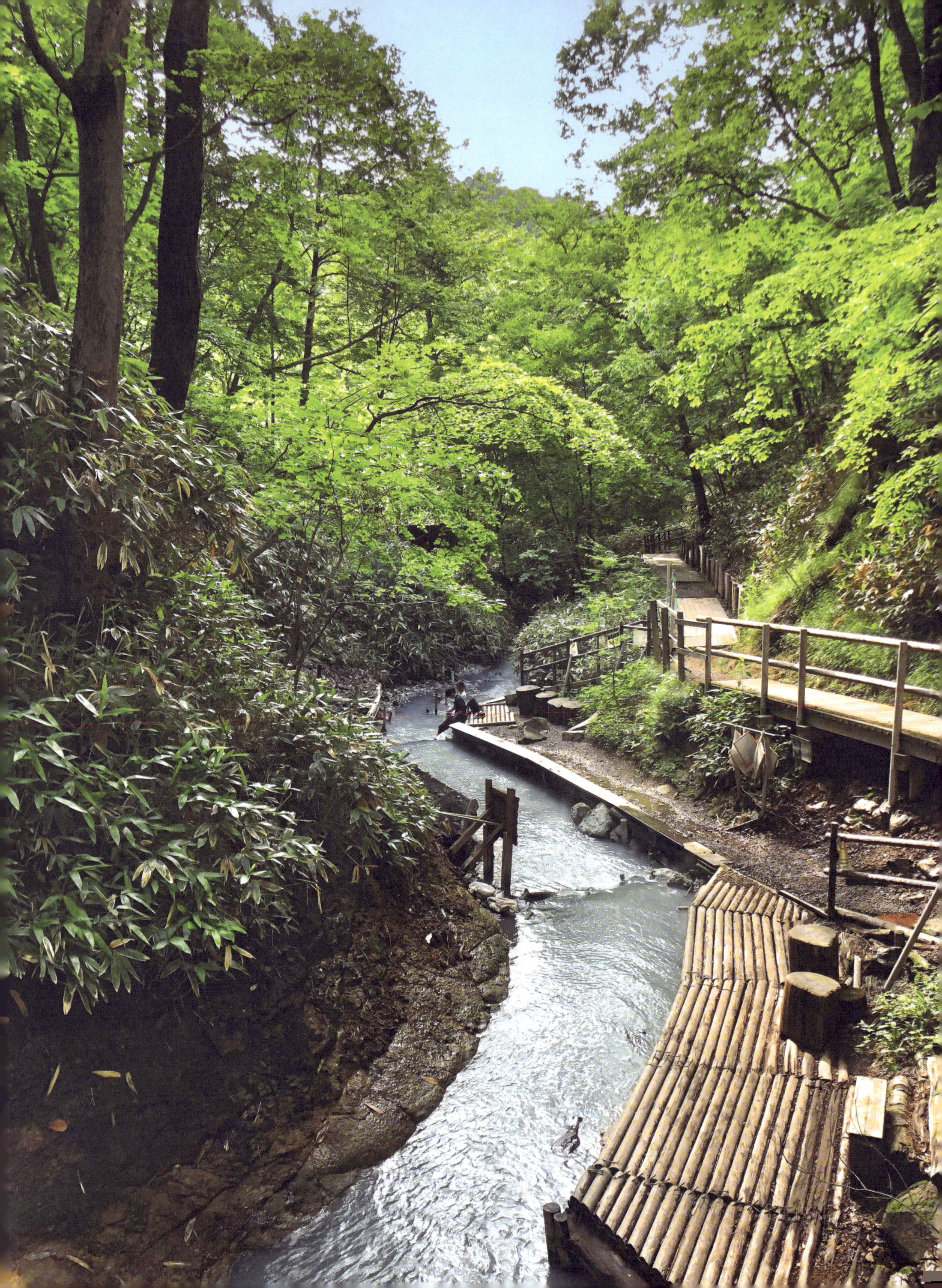

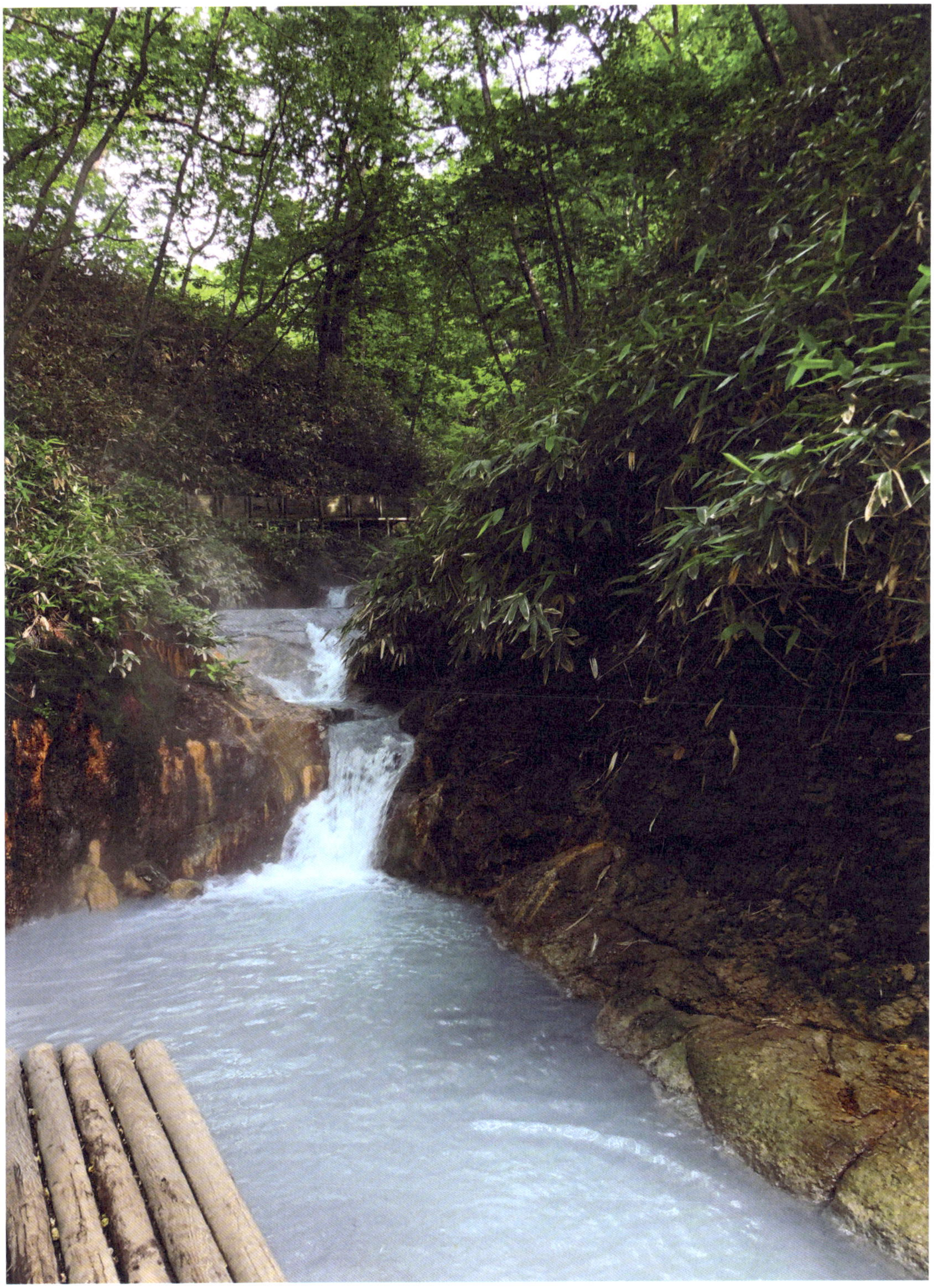

LEFT Visitors taking a moment to enjoy the natural onsen footbath flowing from the Oyunuma River.

Kurokawa Onsen
Minamioguni ● Kumamoto Prefecture

ONE OF THE COUNTRY'S MOST BELOVED ONSEN TOWNS

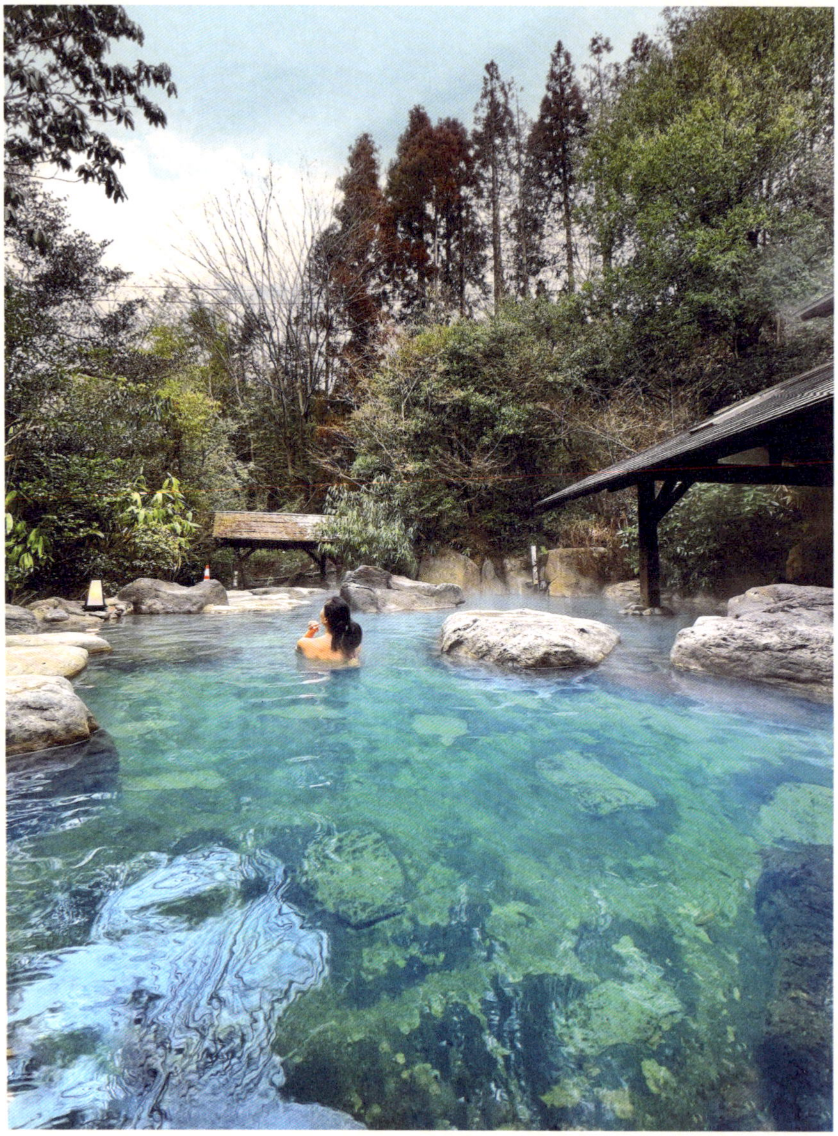

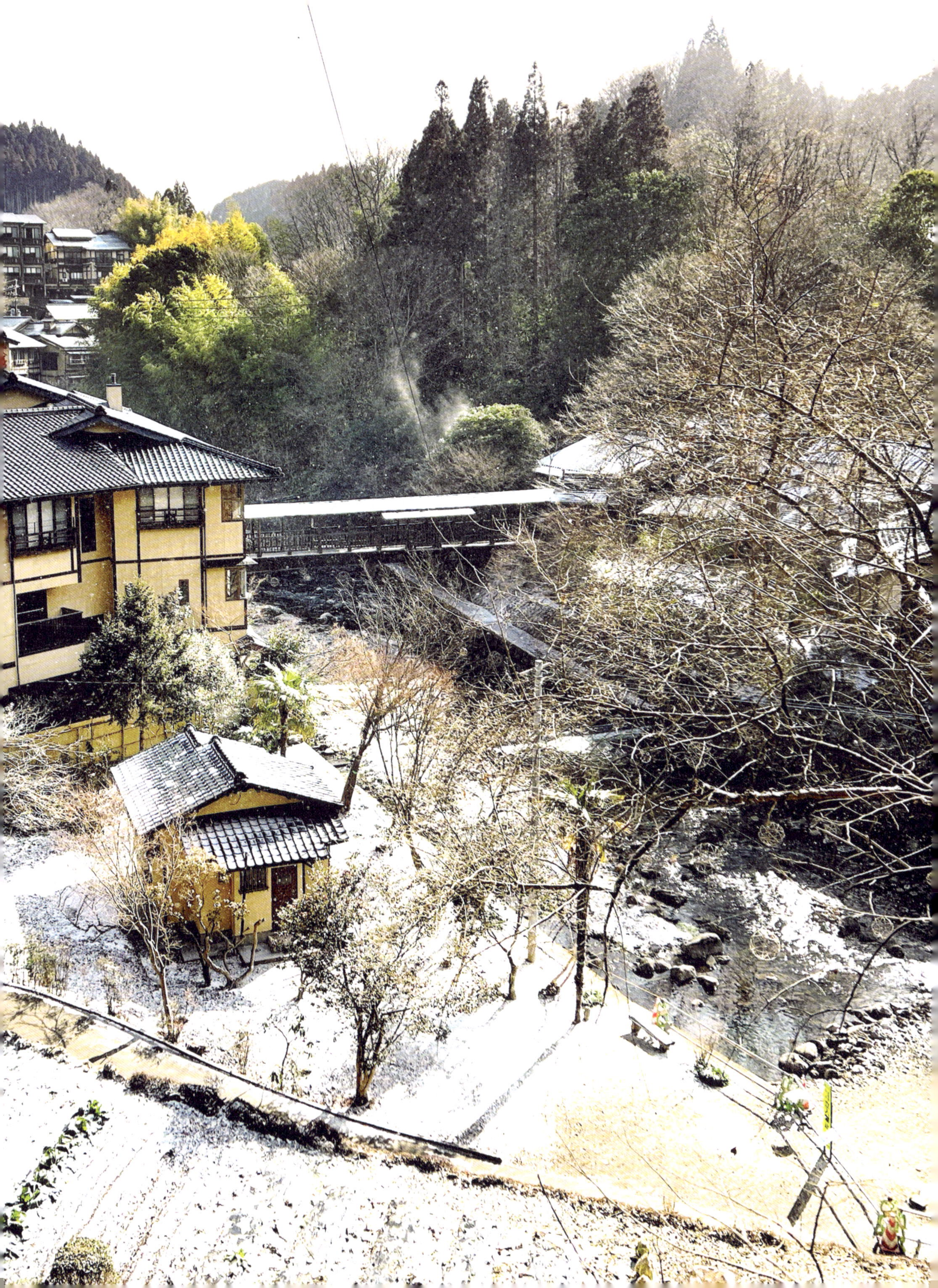

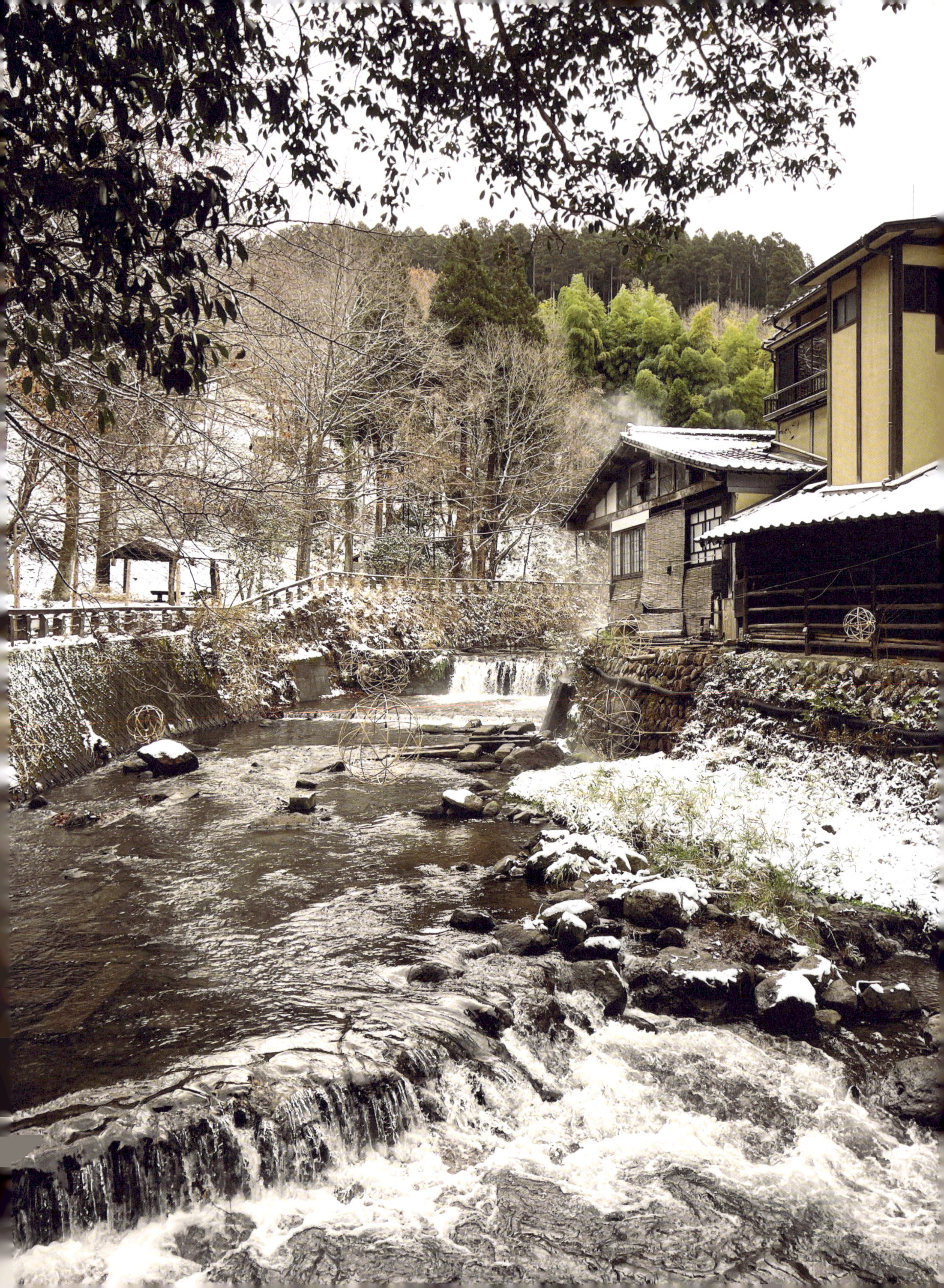

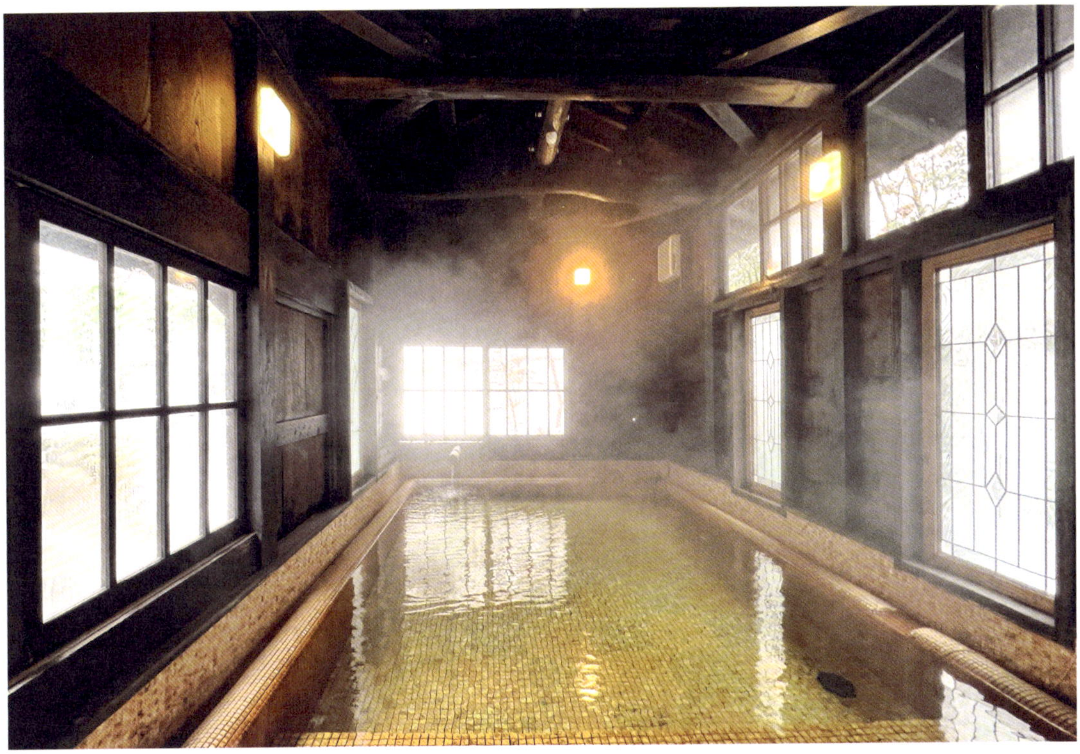

LEFT The Tanoharu River flows throughout Kurokawa Onsen.

In the lush mountains of Kyushu, stroll amid traditional, Sukiya-style onsen ryokan en route to a *rotenburo meguri.*

Known as a rest stop and recuperation point for daimyo and their vassals during the Edo period, Kurokawa Onsen's various springs are said to have been discovered when a poor young salt seller from the Eastern Bungo Province wanted to acquire a melon for his sickly father. Having no money, the son made an offering of salt to the local *jizo* statue and stole a melon from a nearby farm. Enraged, the farmer tried to cut off the boy's head, but the head of the statue fell instead, protecting the boy. A divine voice intervened in the fray and said that the head must be enshrined near Kurokawa; from then on, onsen springs were said to have gushed forth.

The town has retained its charming traditional atmosphere through the efforts of the locals, who have passed ordinances to keep the town free from neon signage, loud colors, and, most importantly, the towering concrete onsen hotels that were often constructed during the housing-bubble era. The townscape is characterized by the surrounding natural scenery, with wooden Sukiya-style onsen ryokan dotting the forest greenery, small boutiques and cafes, uneven stone streets, and a picturesque river weaving through the town. With the town generally accessible by foot, many visitors will choose to wear the traditional *yukata* (lightweight kimono) and *geta* (sandals) as they move between the baths.

With 28 onsen baths and roughly 30 small onsen ryokan lodgings, Kurokawa Onsen was built on the popular practice of onsen *meguri*, establishing itself as a place for *rotenburo meguri*, where travelers attempt to soak in as many of the breathtaking outdoor onsen as possible during their stay. Though many are

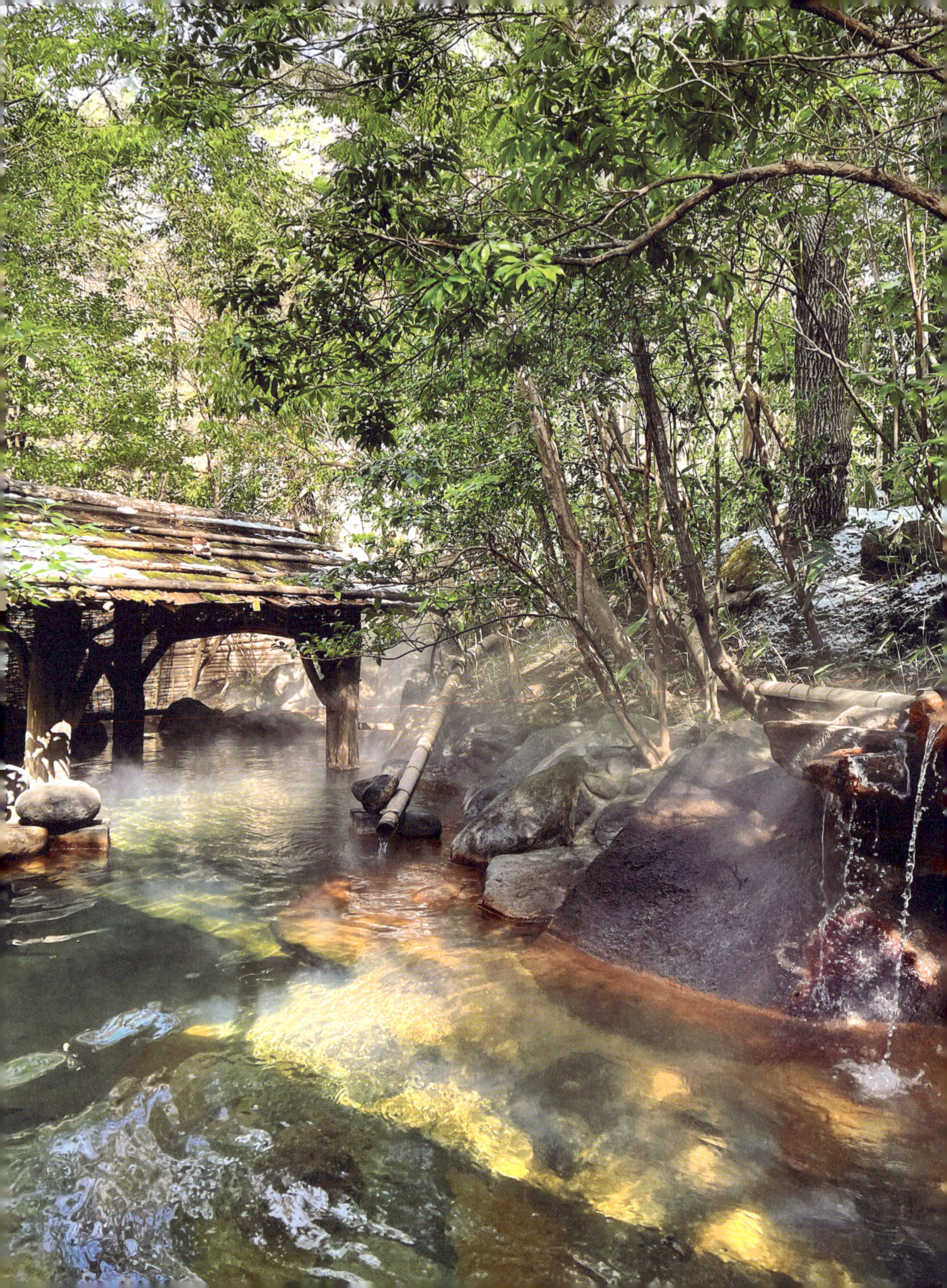

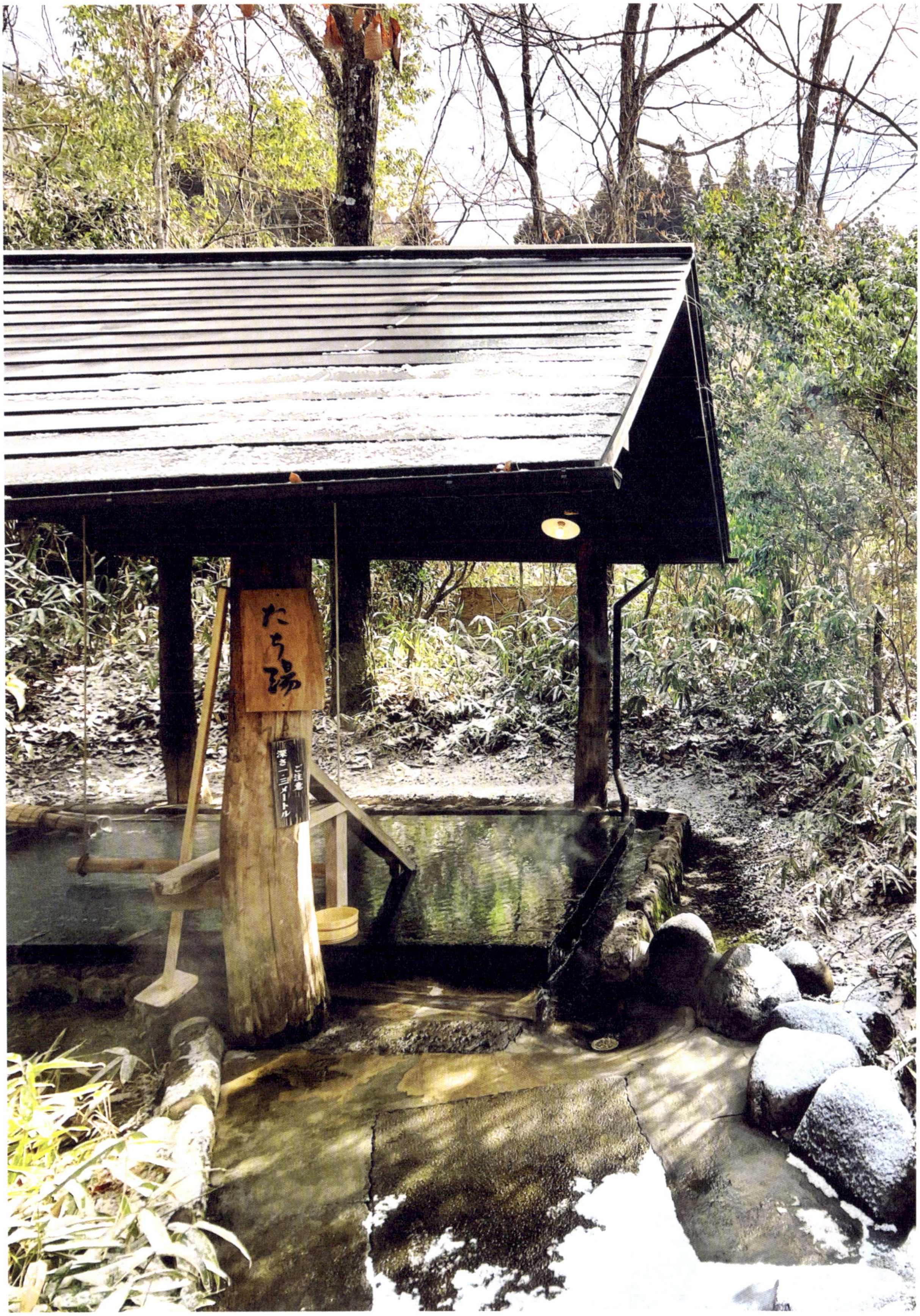
たち湯
ご注意
深さ一・三メートル

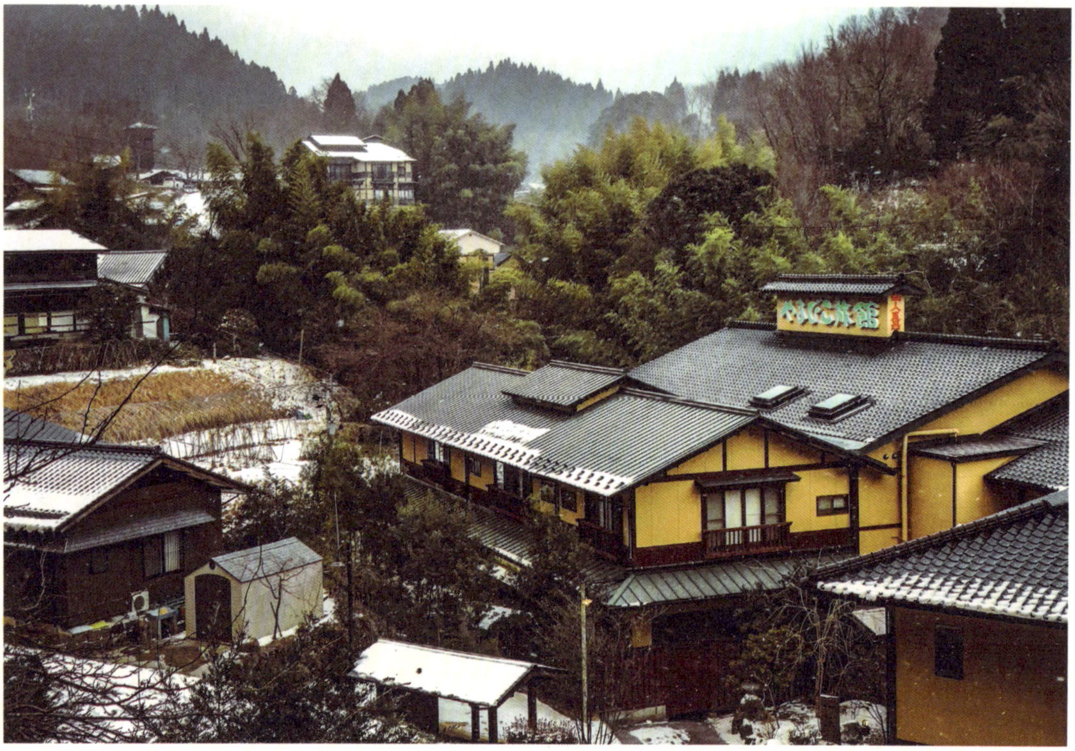

RIGHT One of the many onsen *rotenburo* for which Kurokawa is so well known.

located close to the heart of the town, the most spectacular *rotenburo* are found a little further along the mountain valley in either direction, where they are framed by the beautiful seasons and situated riverside.

A wooden cedar pass known as a *tegata* grants discounted admission to the onsen at three different ryokan of the visitor's choice. Passes can be purchased by both day visitors and overnight travelers, and are provided complimentary with stays at some onsen ryokan. The *tegata* also functions as a kind of decorative *ema*, a wooden plaque found in Shinto tradition, which travelers hang at the shrine after completing their *rotenburo meguri* to display the stamps of the ryokan visited along their journey.

In winter, visitors can walk down to the river after dinner or following the last onsen soak of the evening to view the pretty bamboo lantern illuminations floating in the water. Although memorable in every season, autumn brings out fiery colors in the maple trees, providing an striking backdrop to one's outdoor baths.

Though many visitors are more than welcome to visit Kurokawa as a day trip, as many of the ryokan's public onsen allow day trippers, to properly experience the multitude of *rotenburo* available, an overnight stay is essential, with many choosing to spend multiple nights to leisurely explore not only their ryokan's onsen but other neighboring ryokan too. Don't be surprised to encounter locals and returning patrons visiting their favorite onsen several times during the day.

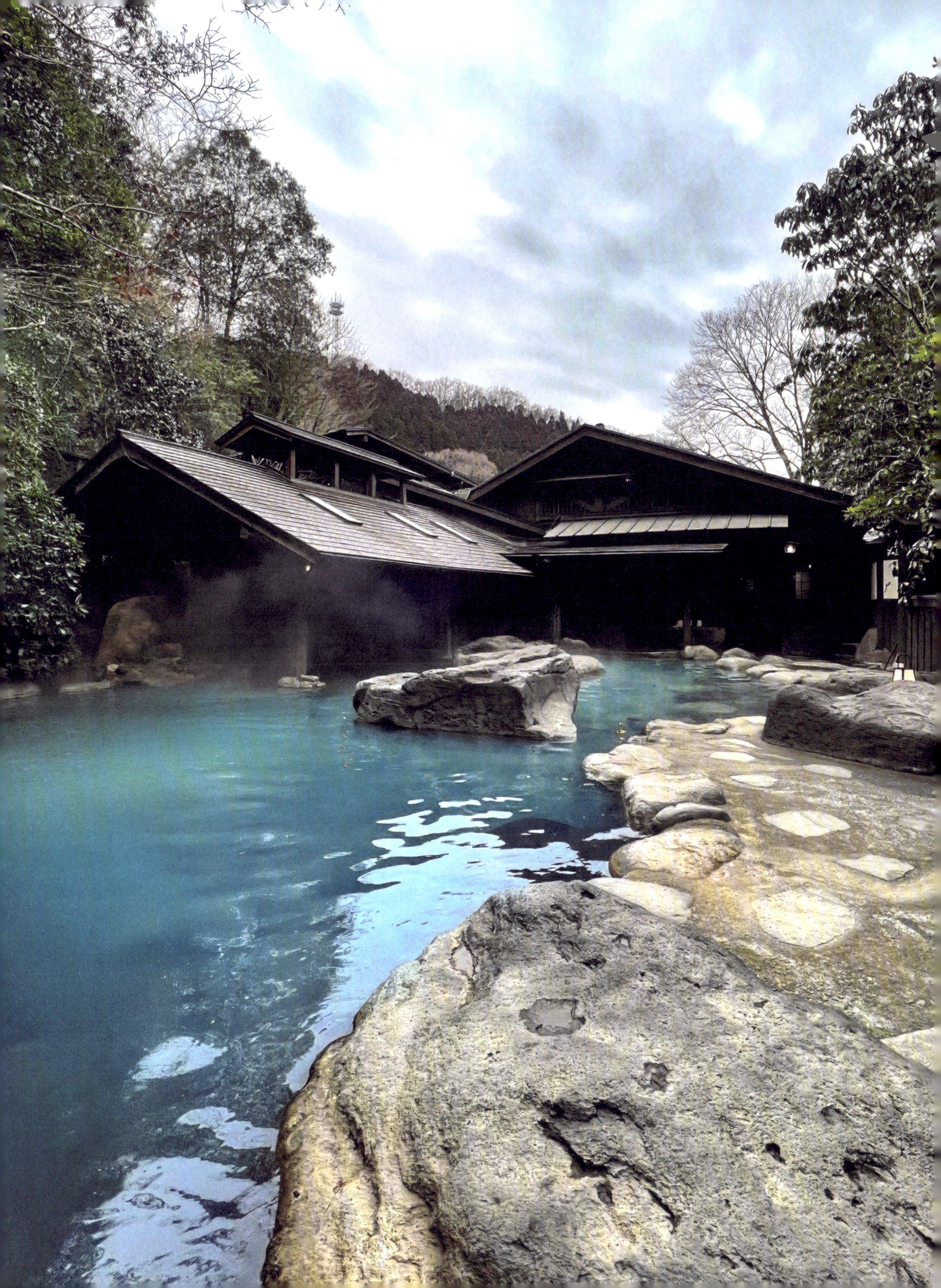

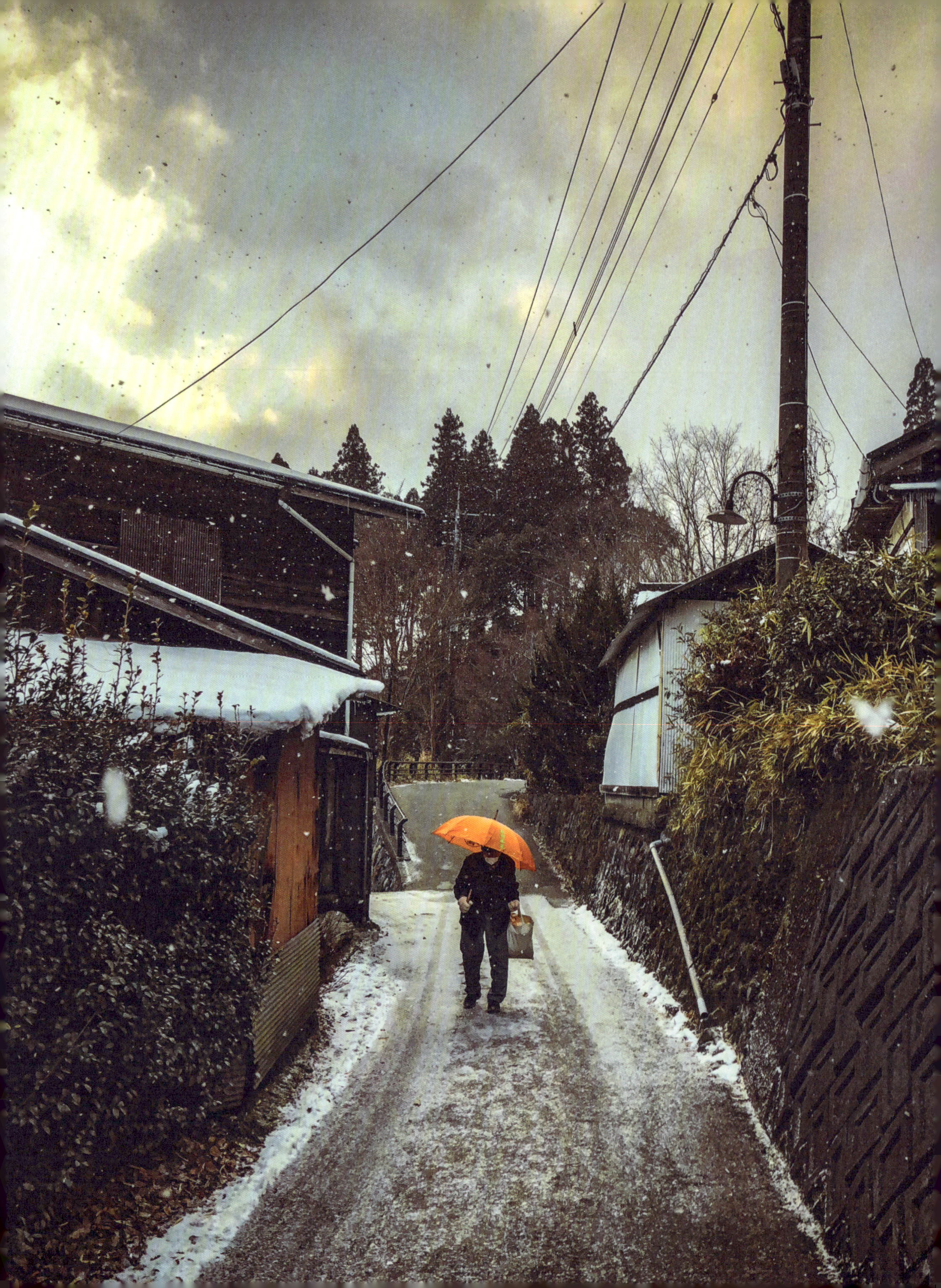

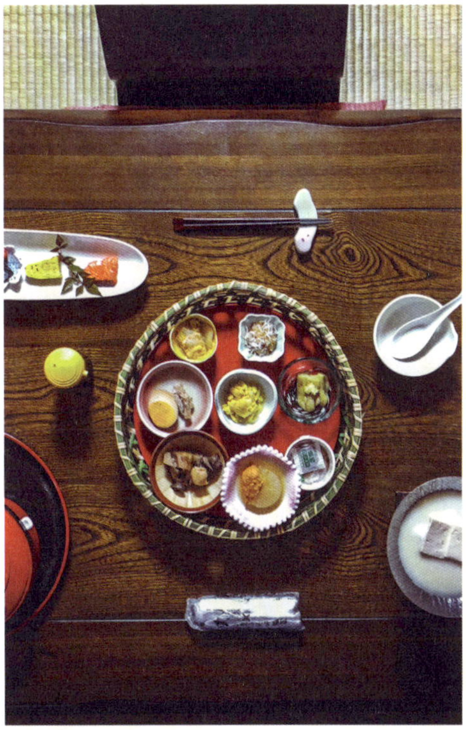

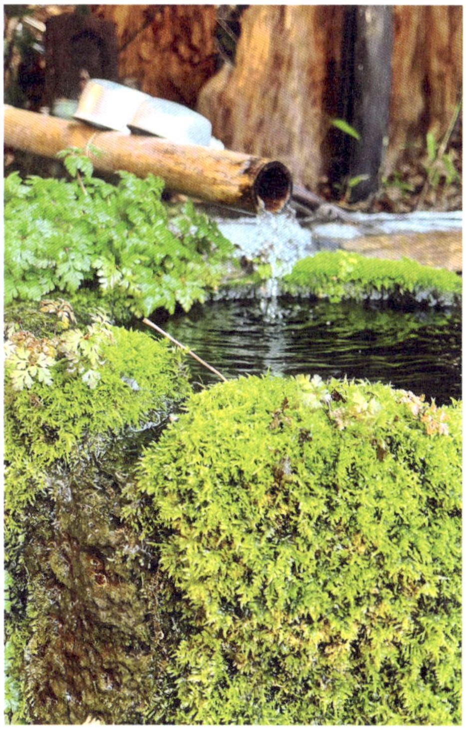

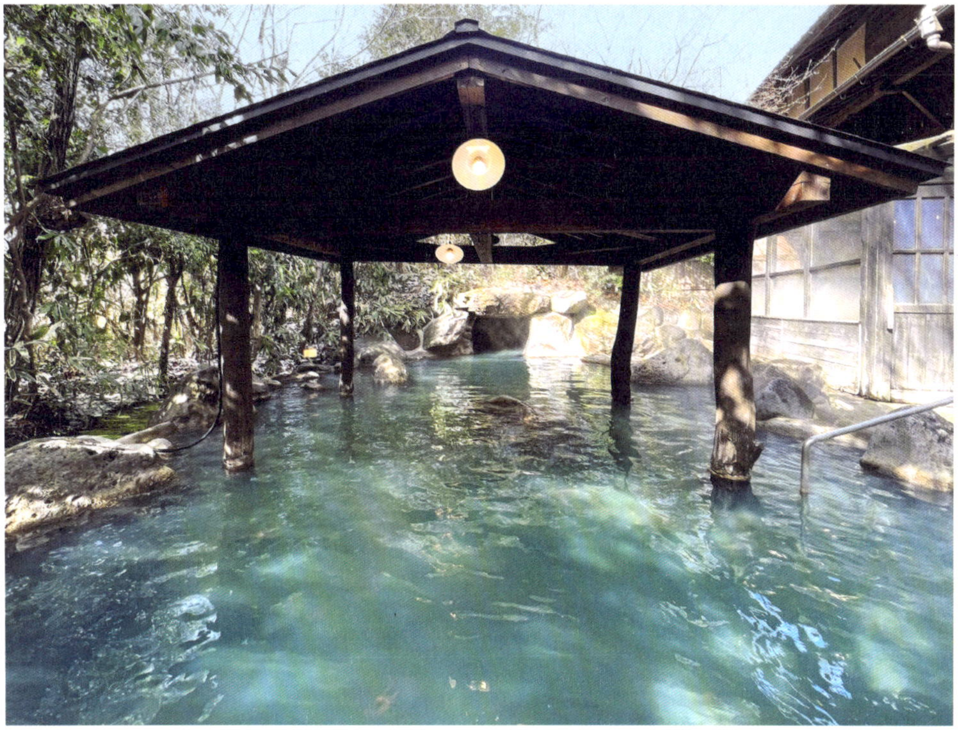

LEFT A local going about his day as the snow begins to fall.

FUFU Kyoto
Kyoto, Nanzenji Area • Kyoto Prefecture

A PLACE WHERE MODERN LUXURY AND TRADITIONAL JAPANESE *OMOTENASHI* MERGE

Treat yourself at this elegant onsen haven in the historic and culturally rich city of Kyoto.

Wandering through Kyoto's serene and meticulously preserved Higashiyama District, visitors stroll along narrow cobblestone streets lined with pottery shops, charming boutiques, traditional teahouses, exquisite *kaiseki* restaurants, and numerous ancient shrines and temples. It is in this peaceful locale that one finds the resplendent FUFU Kyoto, one of ten FUFU properties renowned for their contemporary, luxurious, and sophisticated resort aesthetics celebrating the richness and beauty of Japanese culture.

Perched on the shores of the Lake Biwa Canal and a stone's throw from the important cultural heritage sites of Nanzenji Temple and Heian Jingu Shrine, FUFU Kyoto is located near some of Kyoto's best sightseeing destinations. The beautifully landscaped modern garden Murin-an can be found next door, offering tranquil walks to begin each day.

FUFU Kyoto itself is peacefully set within a former Japanese garden, and some of its original maple and pine trees remain on the grounds today, enhancing the serene setting. Within the grounds lies Yae-Hitoe, a detached villa overlooking the garden where guests can slowly savor the changing seasons or partake in cultural activities like traditional tea ceremonies or ikebana—the art of flower arranging.

Each of the 40 rooms at FUFU Kyoto has its own private onsen bath, found in either circular, square, or rectangular designs and constructed from aromatic and therapeutic Japanese hinoki wood, which add to the sanctuary-like ambiance of the spaces. A simple alkaline onsen sourced from Nose Art Lake flows into every bath, allowing guests to fully enjoy the water's soothing, healing qualities in complete privacy. There is no communal public onsen bath at FUFU Kyoto, giving each stay an enticingly exclusive vibe.

Neutral tones, wooden accents, and earthy colors set the backdrop of the rooms, where sliding shoji doors reveal windows filled with seasonal landscapes. Subtle ikebana decorations are housed in artisanal vases, which grace little alcoves or adorn the walls, enhancing the beauty of FUFU's elegant Japanese minimalism. Wonderfully spacious, all rooms contain restful lounging areas, whose warm and homey feeling promises a relaxing retreat after the day's adventures and where the carefully prepared *kaiseki* banquets can be enjoyed.

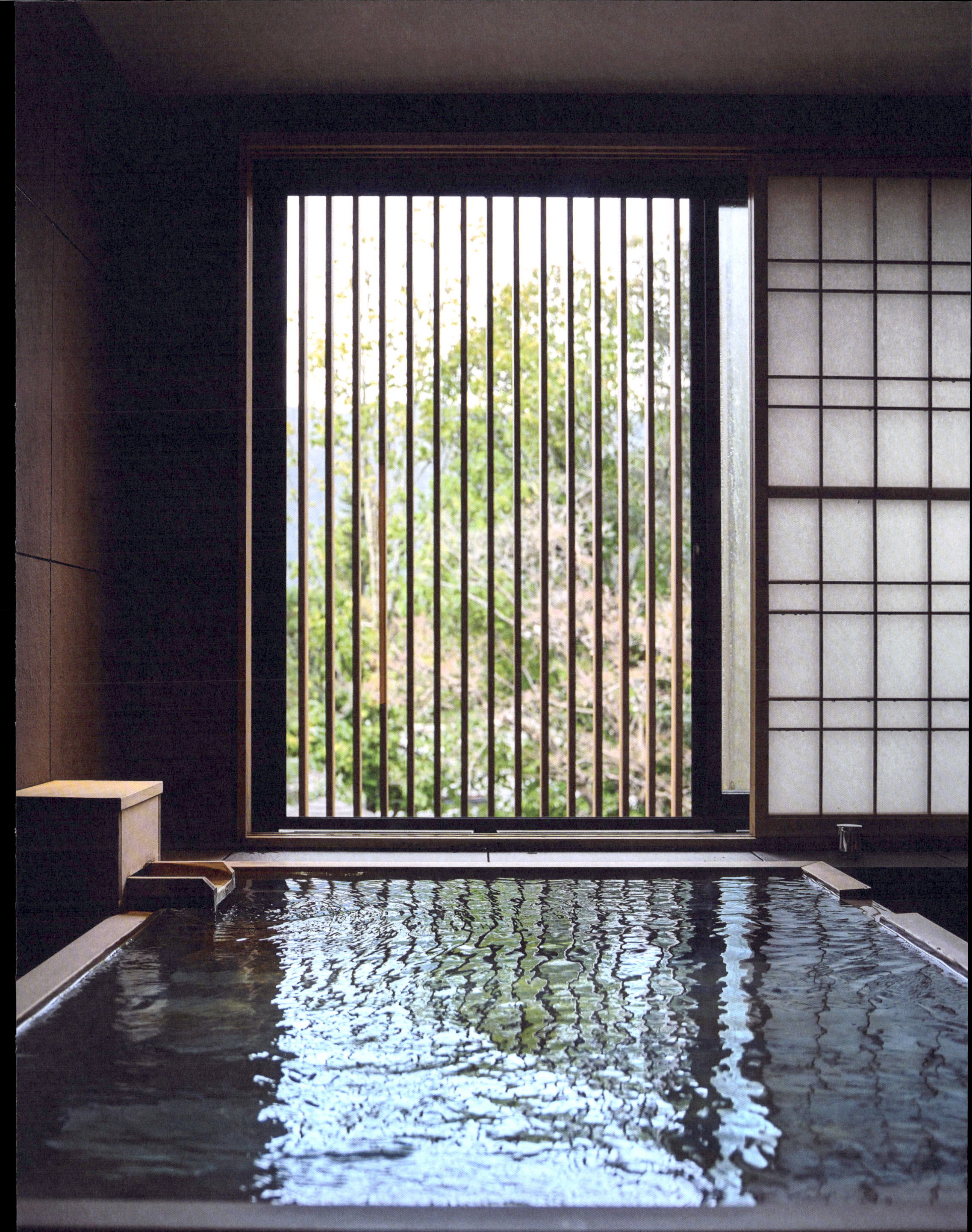

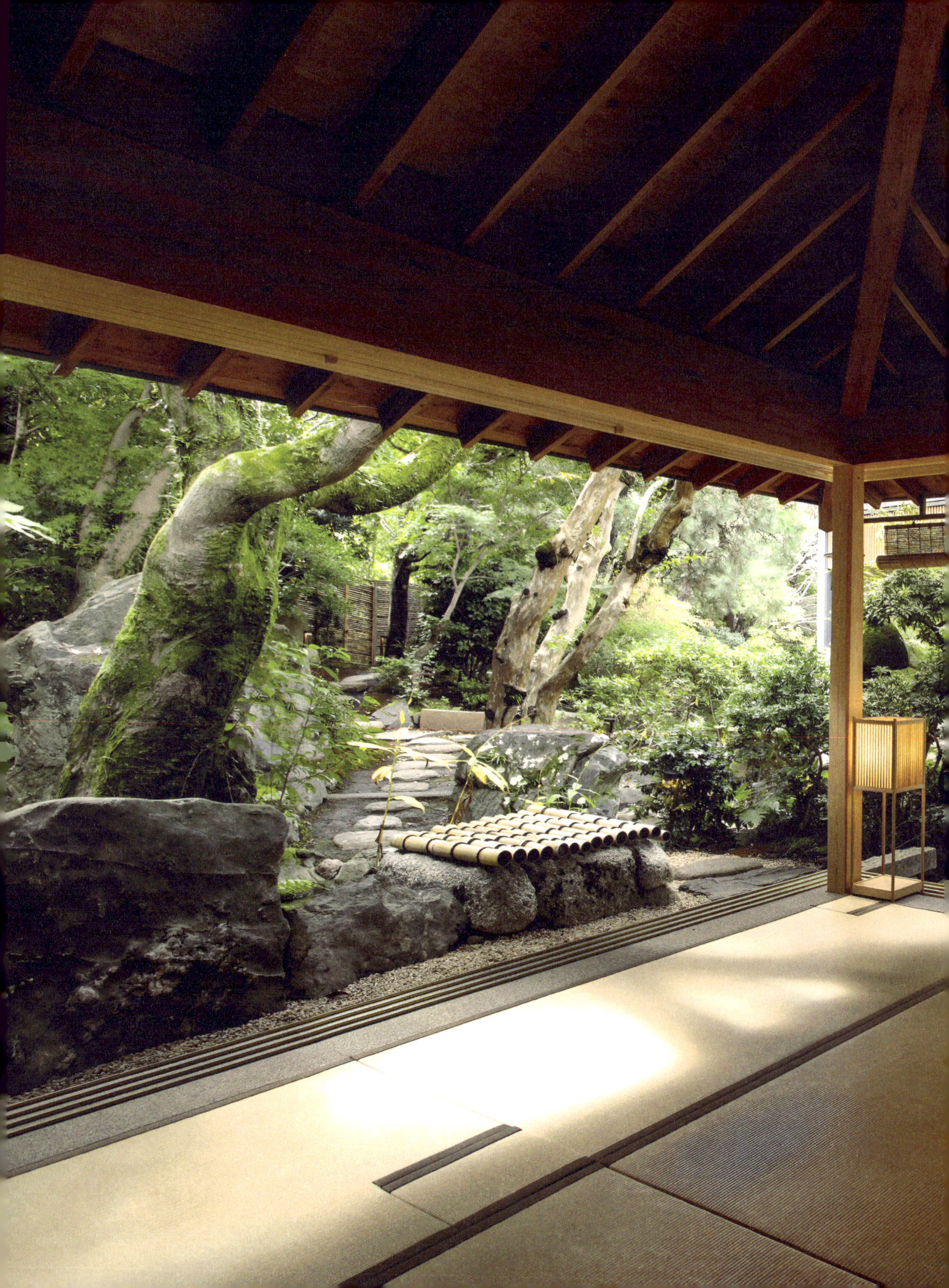

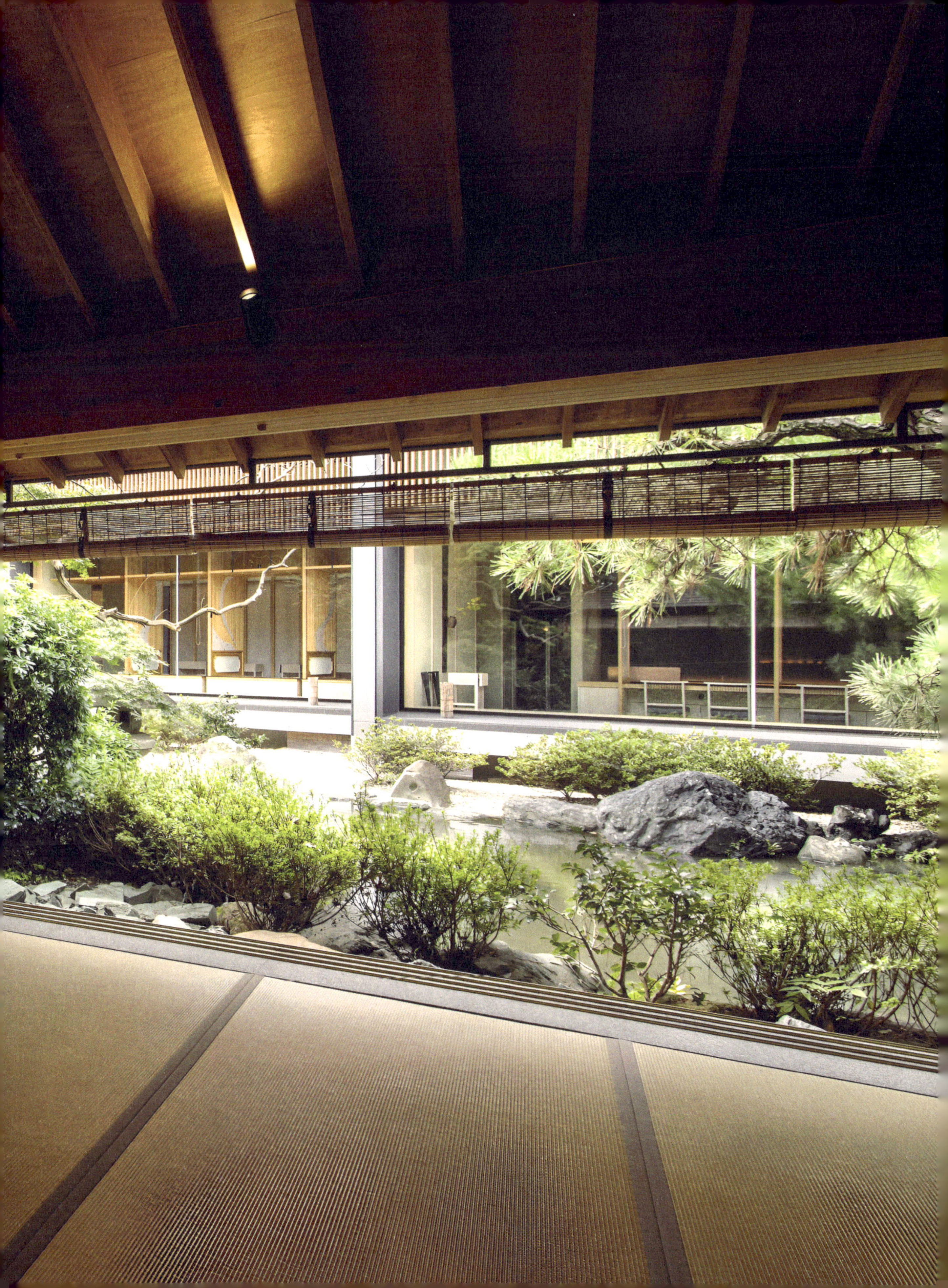

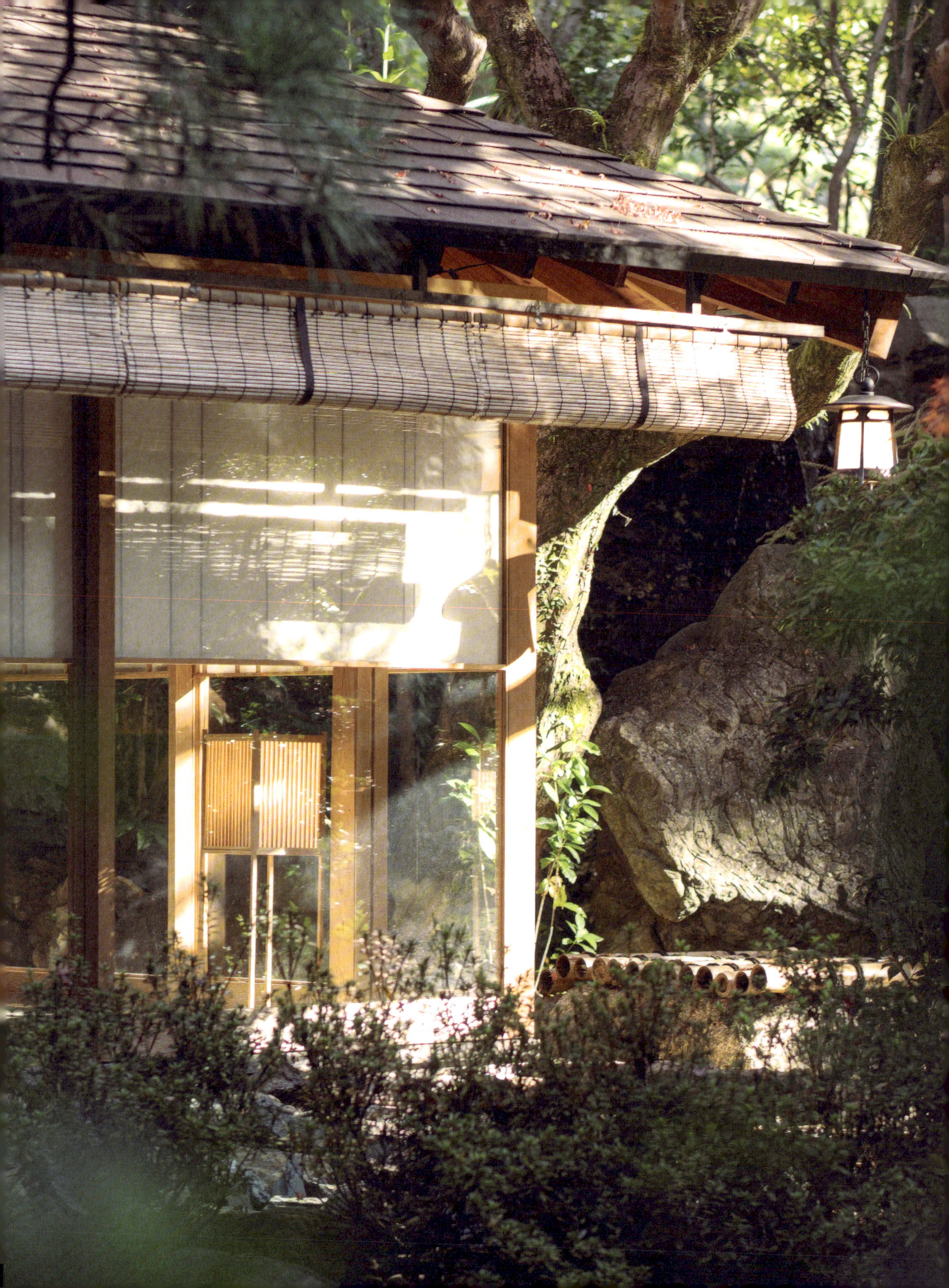

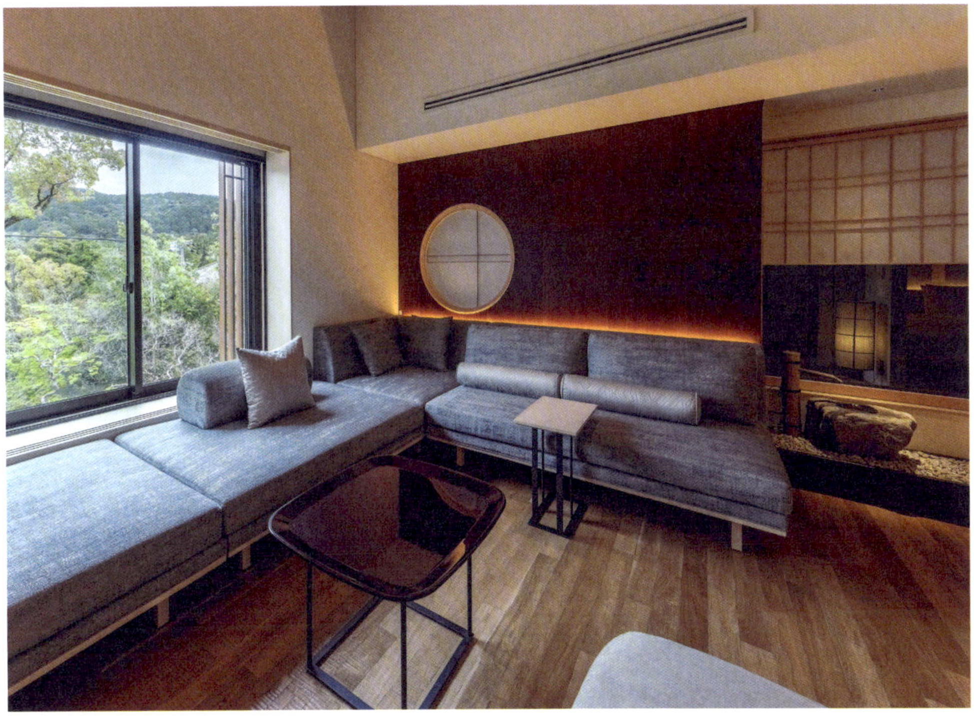

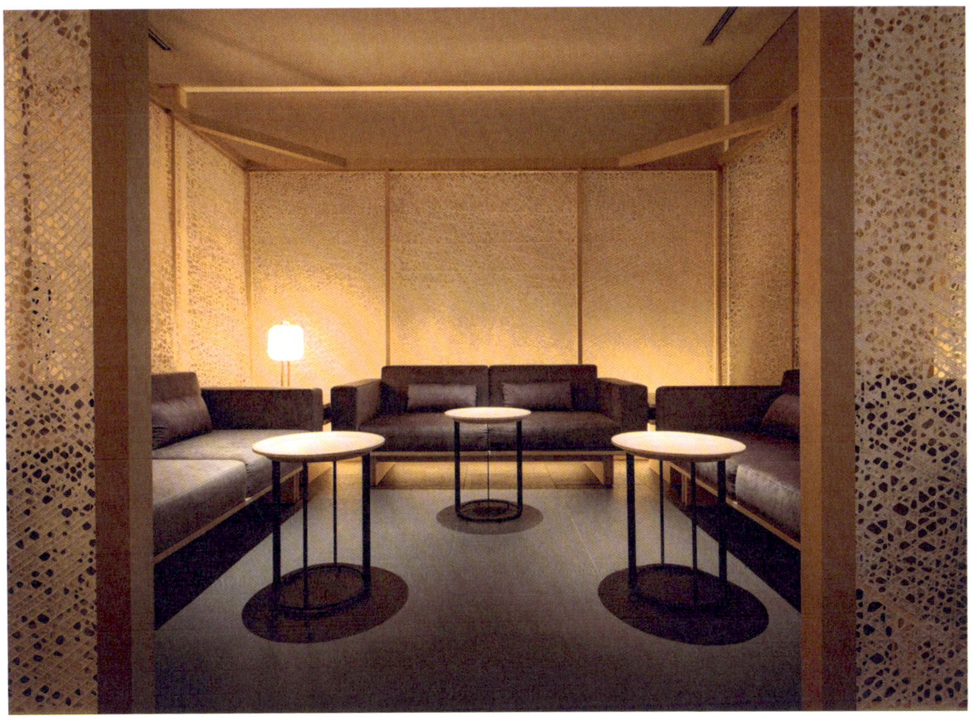

ABOVE, TOP, AND RIGHT Blending modern design elements with traditional Japanese aesthetics, FUFU Kyoto puts luxury first and foremost.

Asan Kotonami
Manno-cho • Kagawa Prefecture

INDULGE IN A LUXURY TREEHOUSE VILLA ESCAPE

Soothe the soul amid the majestic trees in the peaceful Satoyama Hutte cottages, where sounds of the mountain landscape inspire deep appreciation.

Although Japan's smallest prefecture, Kagawa holds an abundance of charms, including a delightfully retro onsen town located at the base of the Shinto shrine Kotohira-gū (or Konpira-san to the locals). Kotohira-gū is the head shrine in a tessellation of 683 others, each dedicated to the guardian god of the sea, fertility, and medicine, Omononushi. The picturesque Kotohira-gū requires an impressive 785 ascending steps in order to reach the main shrine, and a further 583 steps to arrive at its inner shrine. After spending time exploring Kotohira-gū, visitors often descend to the onsen town of Kotohira to rest their feet in the town's footbath and to meander through the many small boutiques and local restaurants.

Venturing out from Kotohira to the scenic Asan Mountains offers travelers the opportunity to enjoy the natural surroundings of Asan Kotonami, a peaceful onsen retreat. Here one can appreciate the slowness of time, feel the gentle mountain breeze, and listen to the sounds of the flowing river and waterfall.

The cozy *auberge* ambiance of Asan Kotonami carries through not only in the warm, wooden interiors of the main building but also to the village of nine Satoyama Hutte villas dotting the mountain landscape above. Rooms in the main building are finished with calming wooden walls, sliding shoji doors, and modern Japanese design aesthetics. Many also have their own private onsen. The standalone villas are furnished with similar design elements and contain spacious balconies replete with lounging hammocks and day beds offering majestic mountain views. Here, one really feels as though they are living in their own private treehouse. Guests at the Satoyama Hutte villas also enjoy a complimentary session at the private open-air onsen.

Regardless of where one stays, one will likely spend an inordinate amount of time enjoying all of the retreat's many open-air onsen, whose waters flow from a private onsen source called Migo Onsen. The riverside onsen, Sesaragi, is nestled amid lush forests and offers waterfall views, while even the indoor onsen are semi-open-air, encouraging bathers to embrace the practice of *shinrin-yoku*, or forest bathing. Here, one might also take time to peacefully recline in the sleeping onsen bath or enjoy standing in the deep bath to further enjoy this tranquil and deeply contemplative environment.

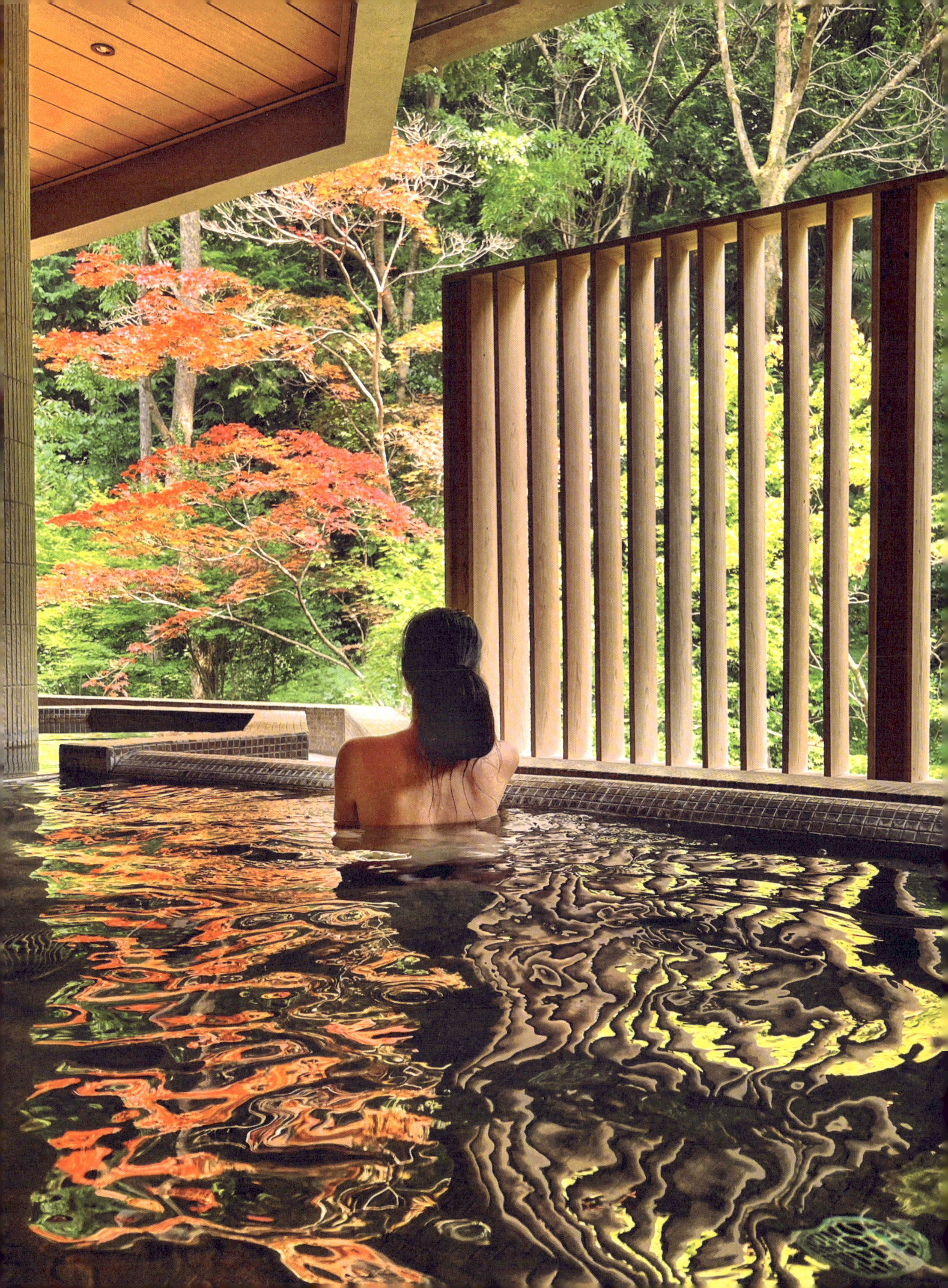

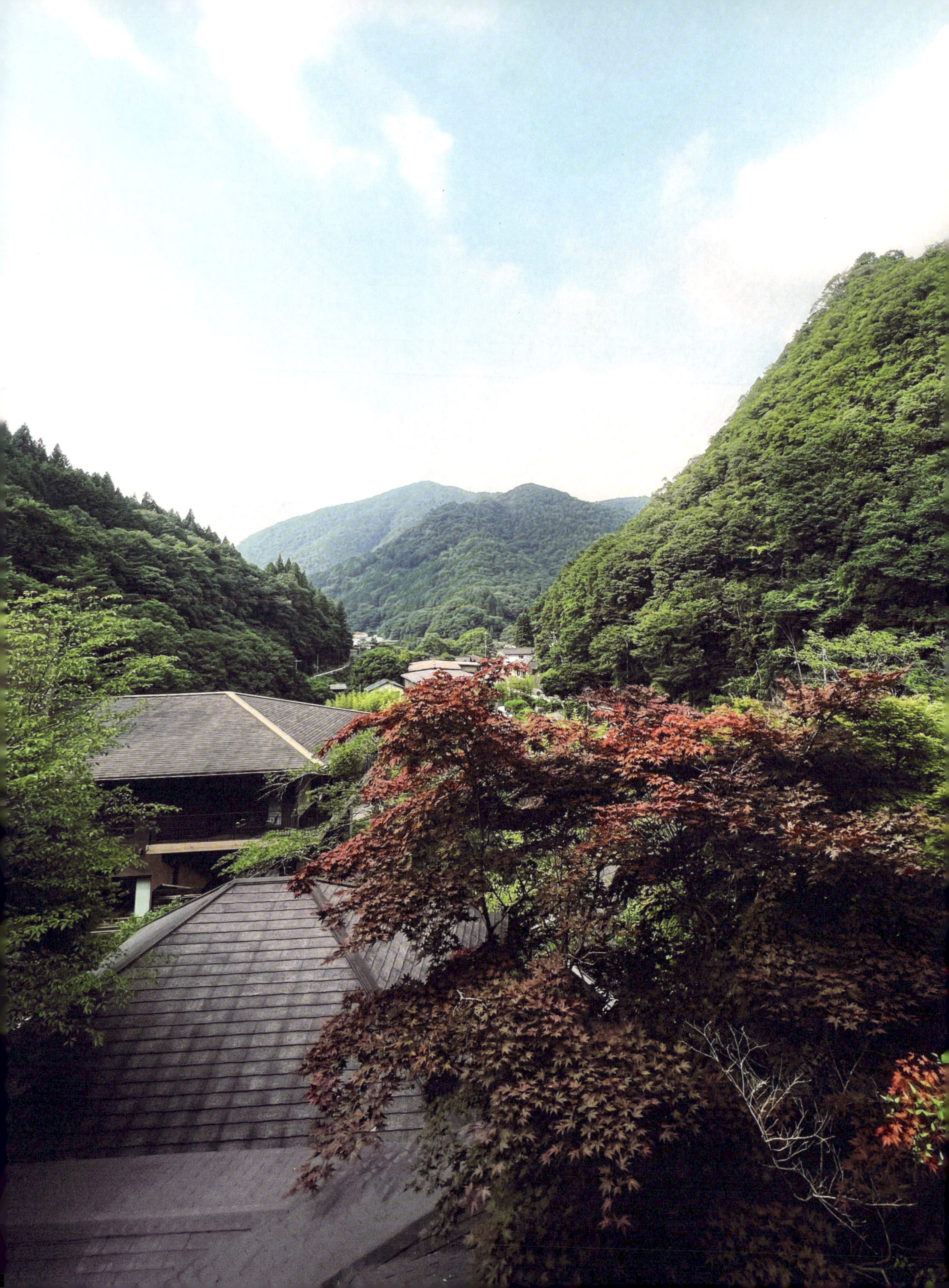

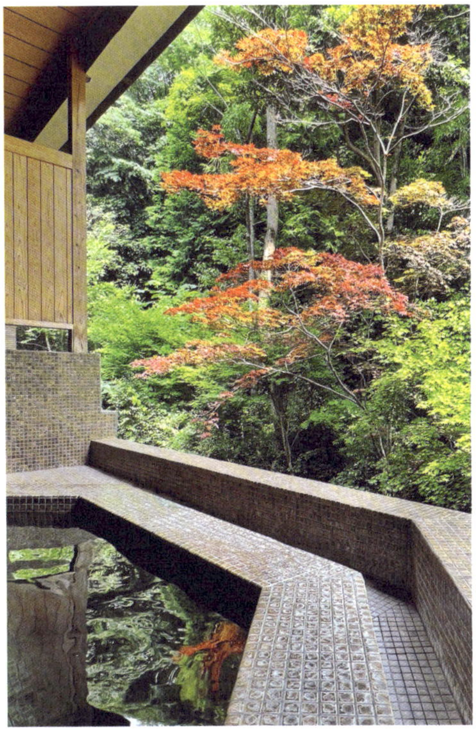

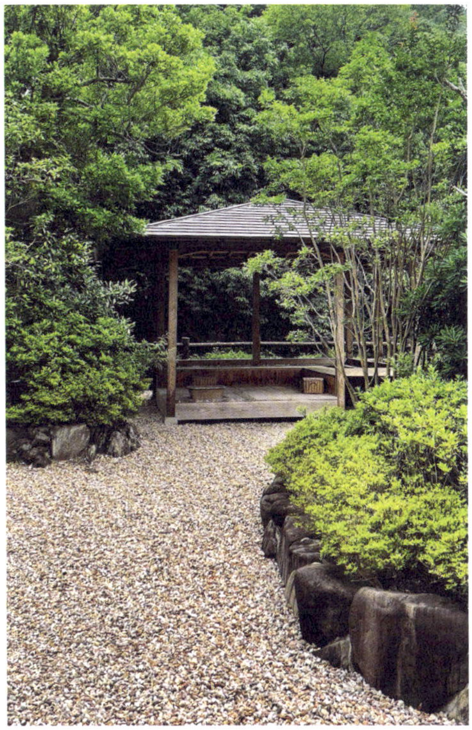

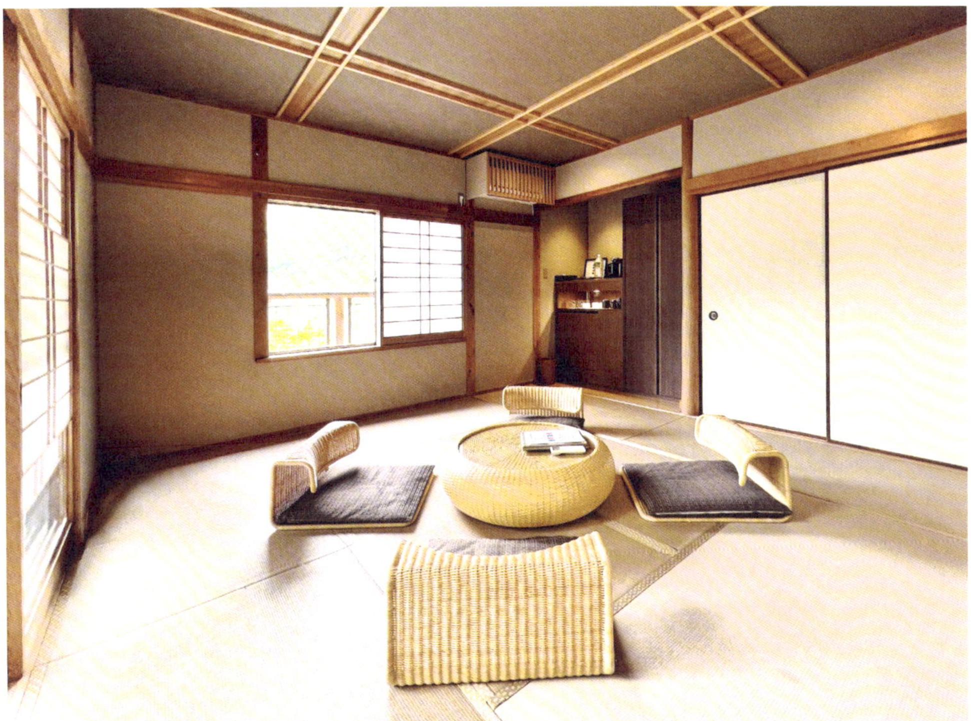

LEFT A stay at the Satoyama Hutte of Asan Kotonami offers stunning views of the Asan Mountains.

Aoni Onsen
Kuroishi • Aomori Prefecture

TIME STOPS FOR TRAVELERS AT THIS HIDDEN HAVEN

Journey to this sheltered ryokan offering multiple onsen baths, a favorite of those who delight in the charms of *hitou.*

One finds the remote Aoni Onsen deep within a forested valley in Aomori Prefecture, between Lake Towada and Hirosaki. As you enter the valley, watch as the signal bars on your phone disappear, leaving you without distraction and fully present in the moment.

Also called Lamp-no-yado (Lamp Inn), Aoni Onsen was established in 1929, and is spread out along the Aoni Valley's mountain stream. It features a main building, three annexes, and four different onsen baths. Previously inaccessible during the snowy winter months, the onsen ryokan began opening all year round in 2001.

Its rustic, traditional atmosphere, Sukiya-style architecture, and secluded location make Aoni Onsen one of the most beautiful *hitou*, or secret, onsen in Japan. Simple Japanese tatami rooms are available in the main building, while slightly bigger tatami rooms are found in the annexes. Bathrooms are communal and all rooms are without televisions and electrical outlets—here, one may practice onsen *toji* in its true form.

Hearty meals sourced from the local area are prepared for guests in the large dining hall, where a traditional *irori* hearth often slow-cooks delicious *ayu*, a river fish. One can enter the hall wearing the ryokan's homey *yukata* (cotton kimono) and *haori* (jacket), sit cross-legged amid the low tables, and feast on the wholesome and nourishing food.

As dusk falls, the glimmering, soft light cast by the oil lamps creates a relaxing ambiance within the wooden interiors, allowing guests to retire fully relaxed to their rooms and be well-rested for the following day.

Visitors can easily experience a miniature onsen *meguri* without ever leaving the ryokan, as a small indoor hinoki (Japanese cypress) onsen is housed within the main building—this also enables an easy late-night soak. Nearby one finds Kenroku-no-Yu, a large hinoki semi-open-air onsen within a separate bathhouse, whose floor-to-ceiling windows afford views of the seasonal scenery. Filled with onsen steam in winter when the windows are shut, the bathhouse has an almost mystical appearance. While the men's and women's baths are essentially mirror images of each other, the women's bath also contains two small outdoor onsen.

Also on-site, Takimi-no-Yu has a small indoor rock onsen as well as an open-air *rotenburo* for soaking. Many visitors also love the larger, open-air *konyoku* (mixed gender) onsen opposite Takimi-no-Yu, which also features a small barrel onsen that is best appreciated when the snow falls.

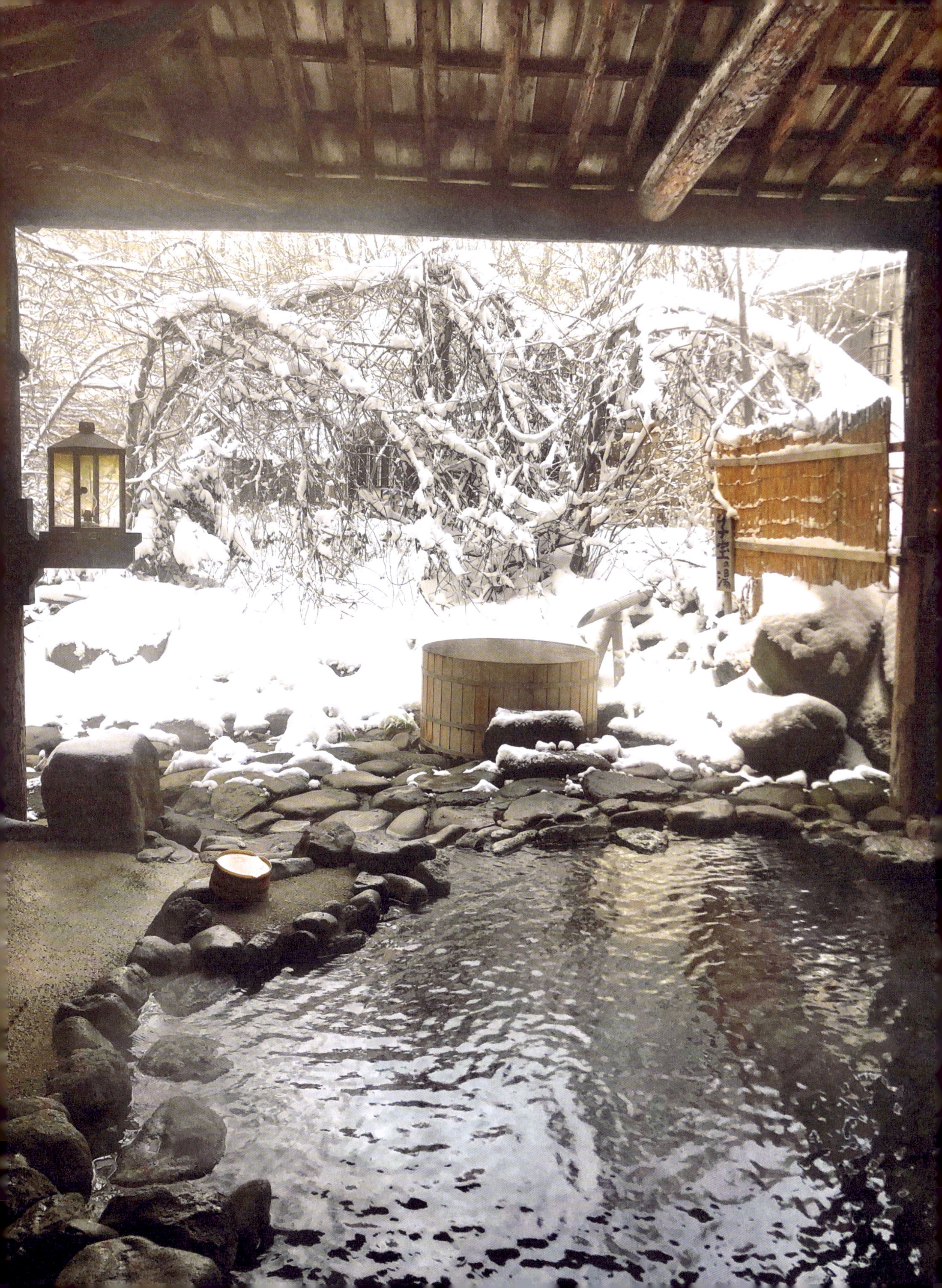

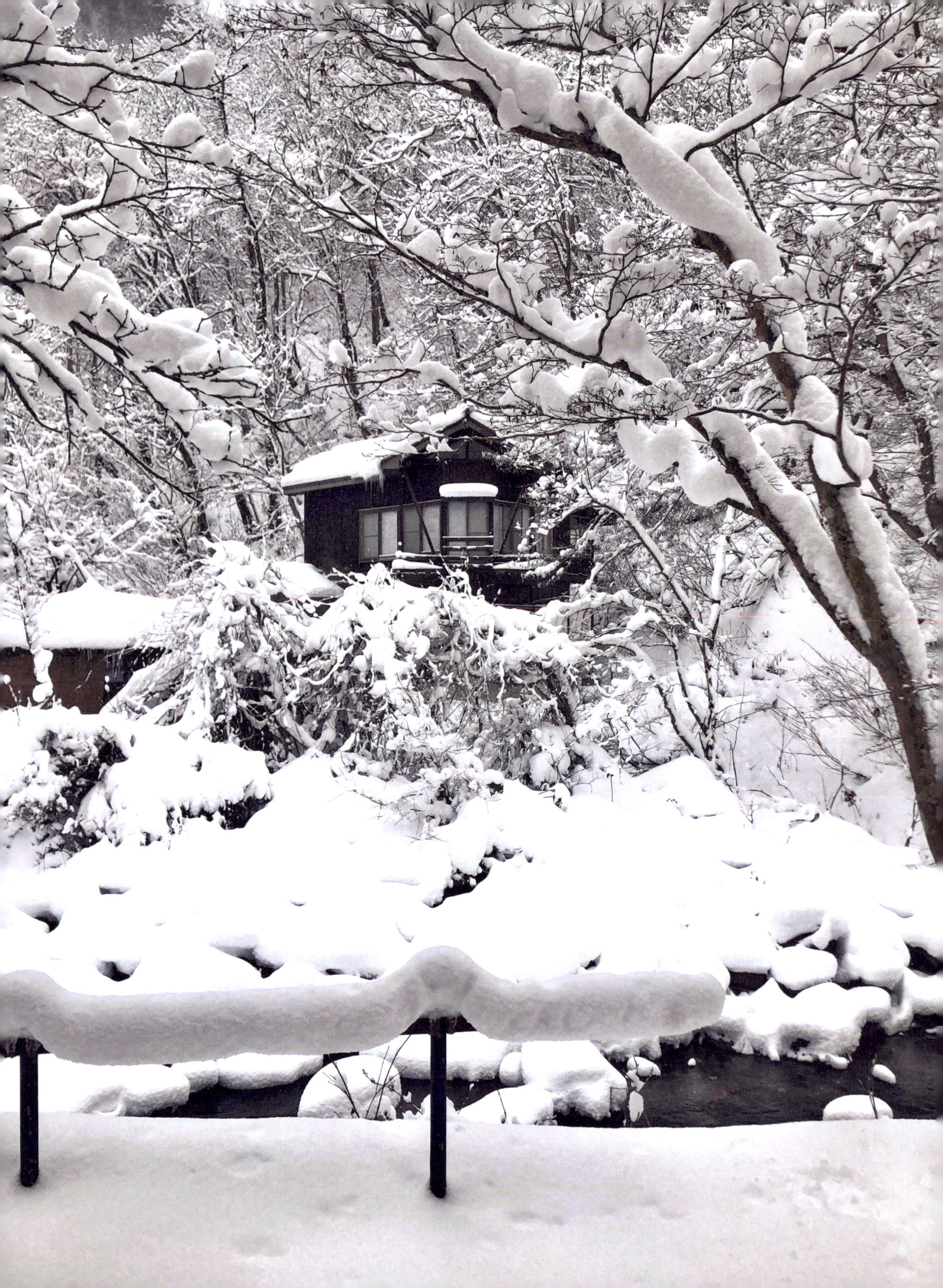

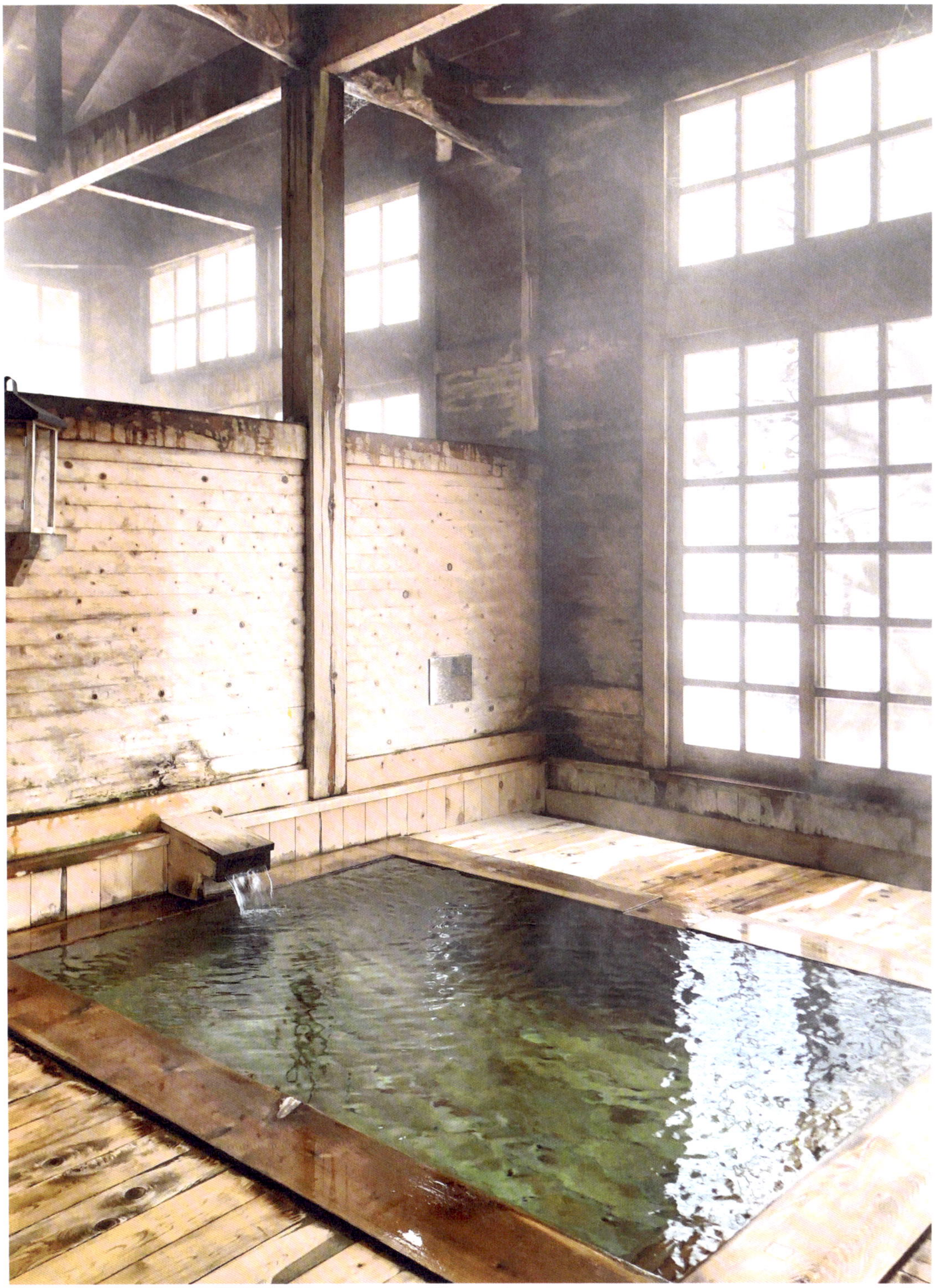

ABOVE The public onsen bathhouse of Kenroku-no-Yu, where the hinoki aroma fills the atmosphere.

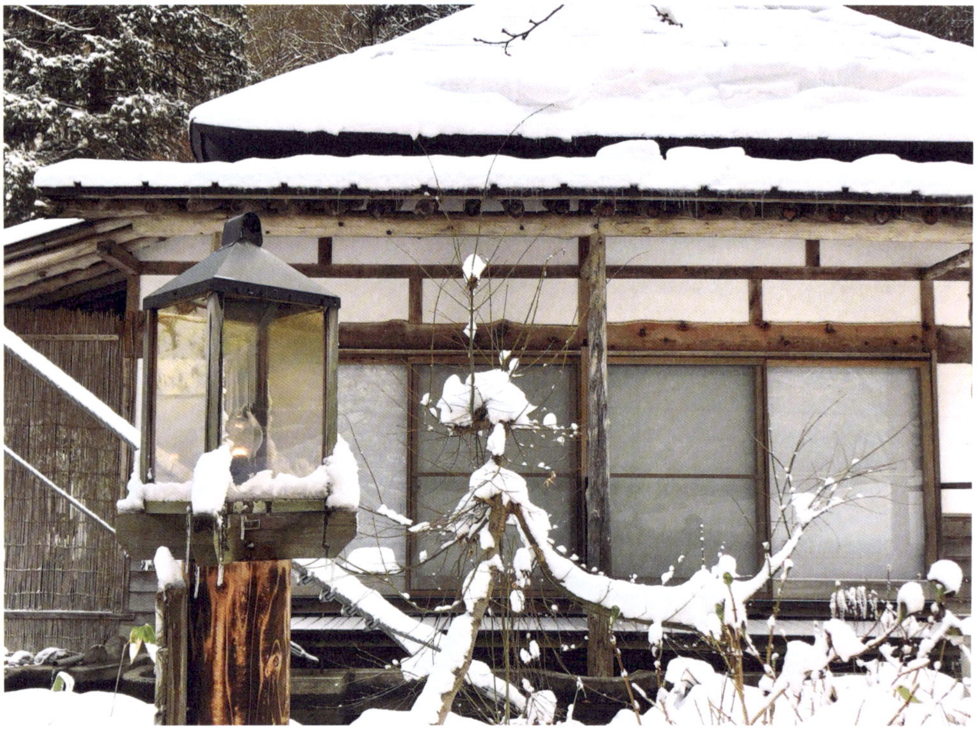

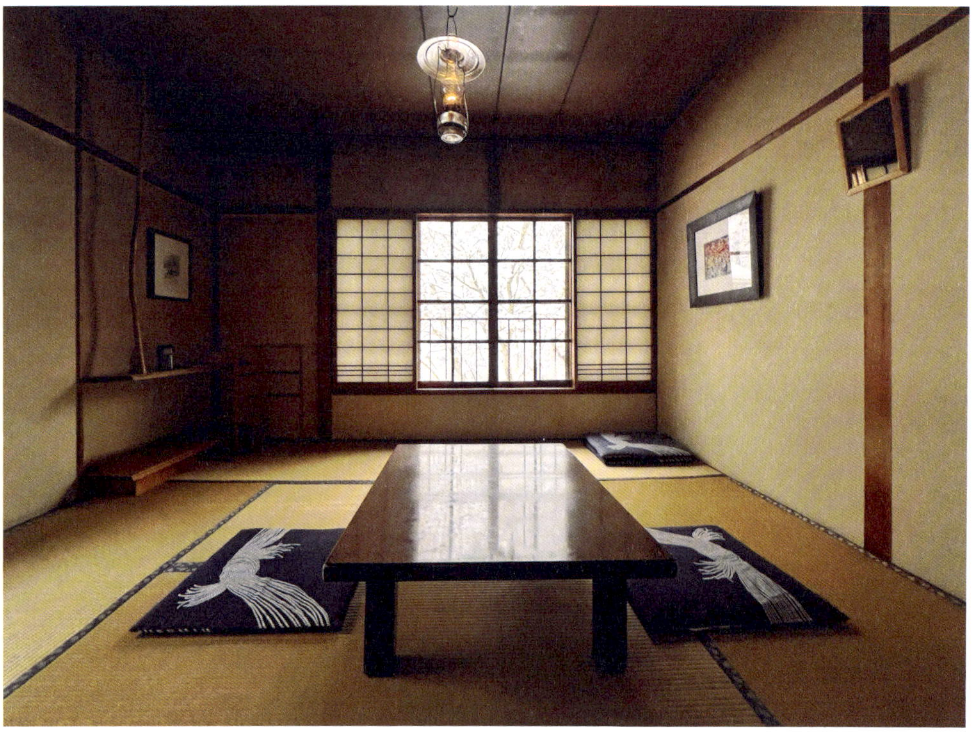

RIGHT The barrel bath of the popular *konyoku* (mixed) onsen.

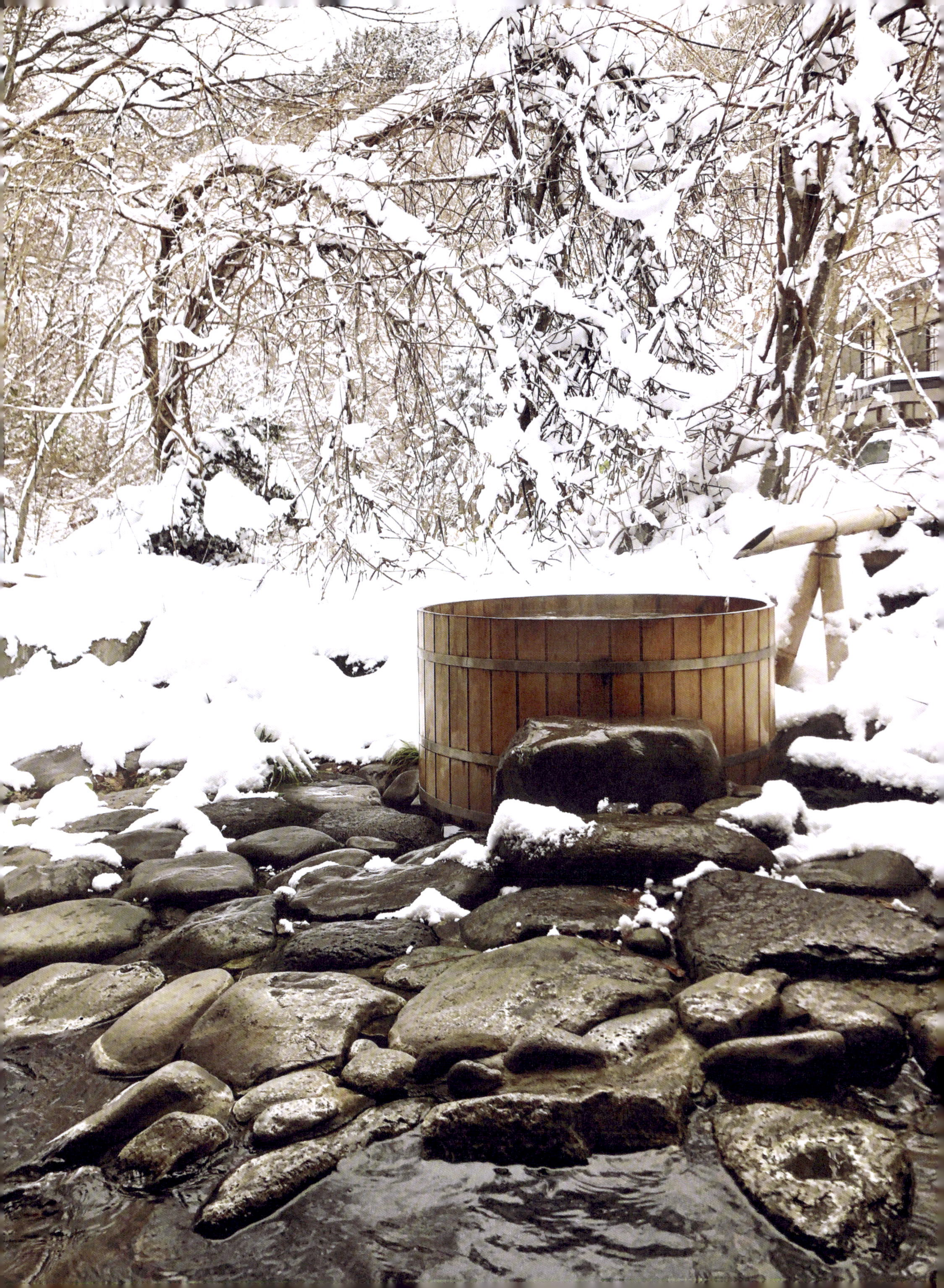

Kosenkaku Yoshinoya
Totsukawa Village • Nara Prefecture

AN IDYLLIC, REMOTE MOUNTAIN GETAWAY IN JAPAN'S LARGEST VILLAGE

Take in the sounds of the river and surrounding nature at this rare, "free-flowing" town.

A winding drive along narrow mountain roads brings one to Totsukawa Village, set deep in the mountains of Nara Prefecture. The village is home to Japan's oldest shrine, Tamaki-jinja (built in 37 BCE), which once guarded against fire and served to ward off evil spirits.

A true rarity, Totsukawa is known as a "free-flowing onsen village" due to the copious amounts of pure *gensen kakenagashi* onsen water rushing through it. Three onsen towns are found along the banks of the beautiful, teal-hued Totsukawa River, each offering slightly different experiences. Tosenji Onsen is the oldest of the three and possesses a simple sulfur spring, while Kamiyu Onsen is a hidden public bath located on the river and Totsukawa Onsen is beloved for its skin-beautifying *bijin-no-yu*, its drinkable onsen water, and its magnificent scenic vistas.

In the heart of Totsukawa Onsen, Kosenkaku Yoshinoya is a delightfully cozy, family-run onsen inn whose history dates back some 100 years. Warm and welcoming, every room is a spacious, simple 10-tatami affair, each with a comfortable *engawa* sitting area that leads to a balcony with stunning mountain views mirrored back on the lake's surface. All the rooms are named after local mountain ranges, trees, and rivers.

The indoor onsen is spacious with wide windows and lake views. The onsen water flows freely and its silky texture is wonderfully luxurious against the skin, while its steam gives off even more cleansing moisture. However, the onsen temperature can be quite high, so one should make sure to acclimate by using the traditional *yu-oke* bucket to pour the onsen water over the body a few times after showering.

After a long soak, walk down to the open-air onsen set on the high precipice of the river bank and immerse yourself in its waters and the sounds of nature. Framed with greenery, both the men's and women's *rotenburo* offer lush views of the richly hued lake, although the women's bath has let the greenery grow a bit more to ensure privacy. Each outdoor onsen also features a small onsen bath carved from an ancient tree trunk—perfect for solo bathers. The setting is so beautiful that no matter the weather, whether it be pouring rain, mist-enshrouded, or glistening with sunlight, the bathing experience here is magical.

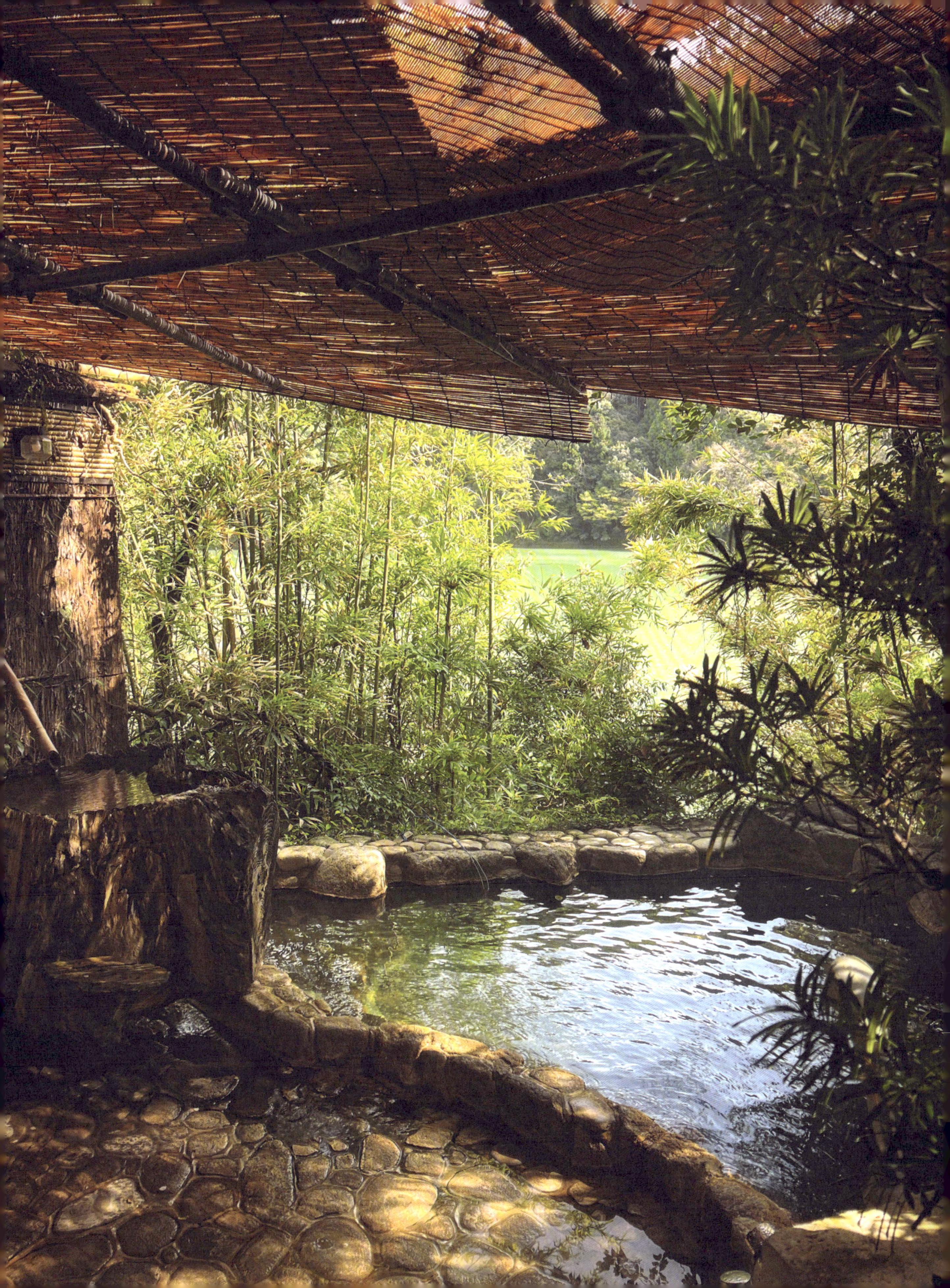

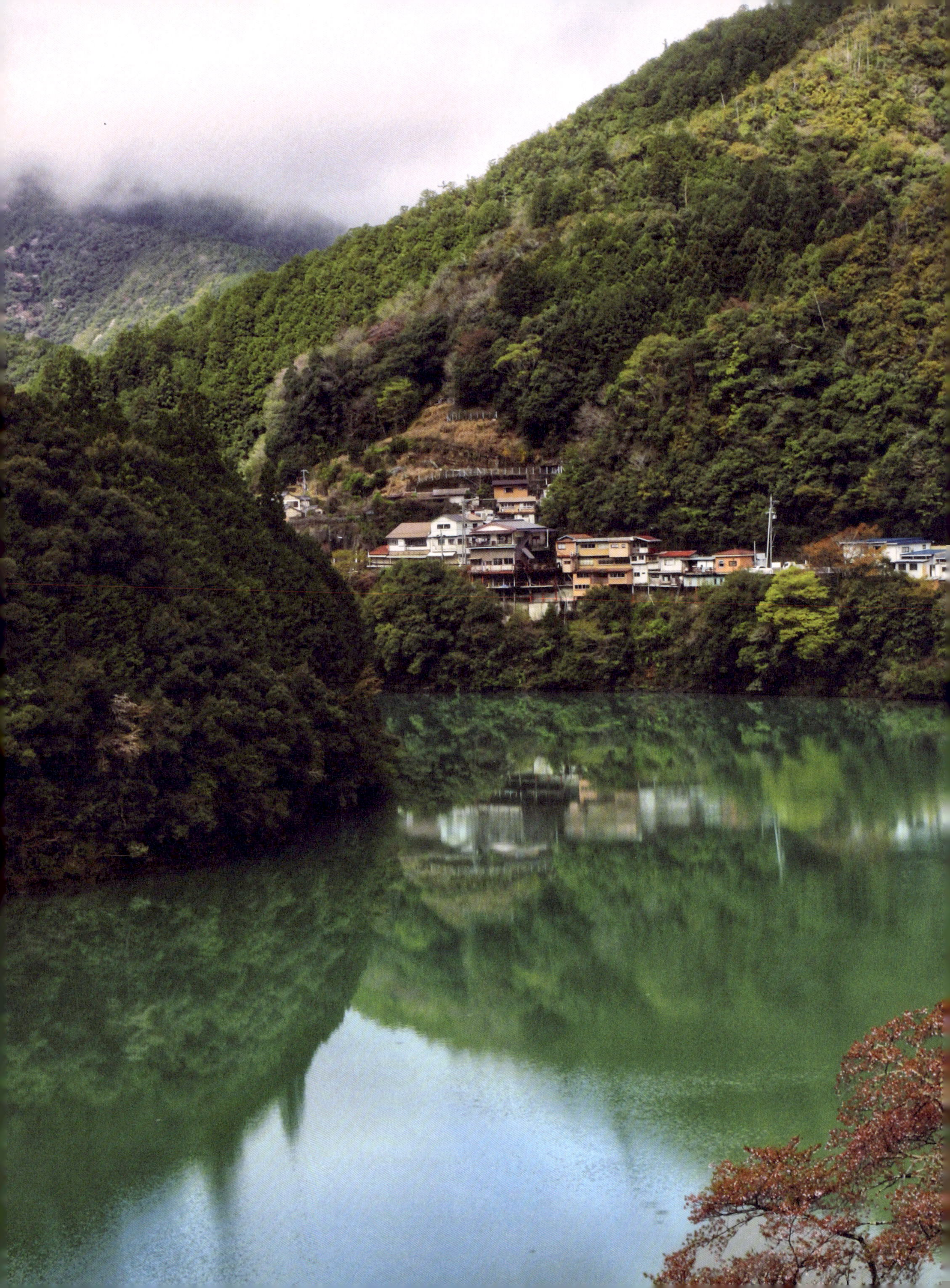

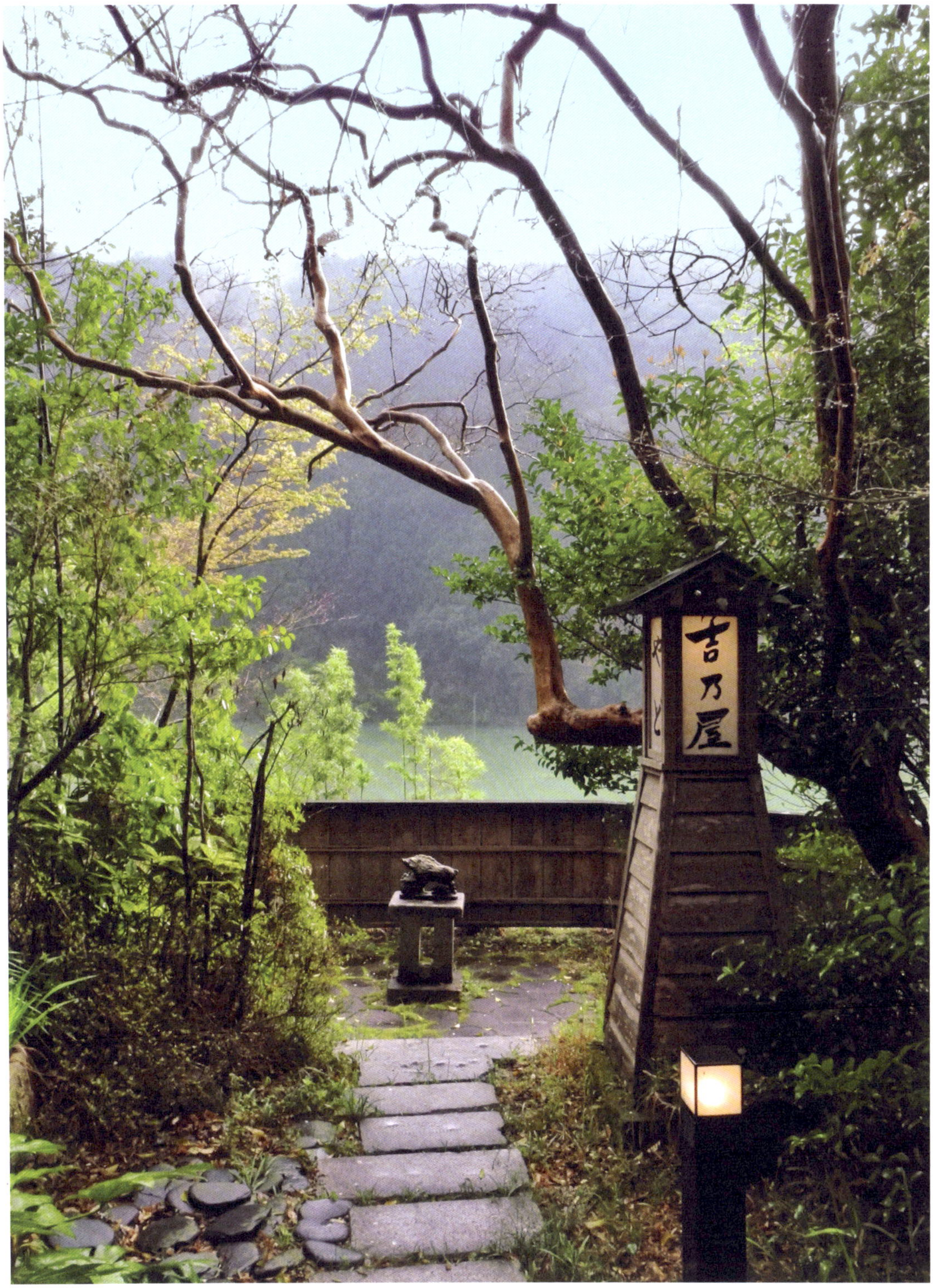

LEFT Reflections of the local scenery are mirrored in the rich, emerald waters of the Furusato Dam Lake.

Shimogoten: Ryujin Onsen
Tanabe • Wakayama Prefecture

EXPERIENCE ONE OF JAPAN'S TOP THREE *BIJIN-NO-YU*

This timeless ryokan, set beside the Hidaka-gawa River in a quiet mountain village, incorporates parts of the historic original inn.

On the Kii Peninsula, along the upper reaches of the rich, turquoise-hued Hidaka-gawa River, lies a small, secluded, and historic mountain hamlet renowned for its silky, beautifying onsen waters. Ryujin Onsen, named for a dragon god, is found at the southern midway point linking the sacred sites of Koyasan and the Kumano Kodō pilgrimage region. Ancient lore tells that the onsen source was originally discovered by religious pilgrims, and was later developed after the famed Buddhist monk, Kobo Daishi, had a prophetic dream that led him to the spot.

The Edo period saw the daimyo Tokugawa Yorinobu, feudal warlord of the Kishu Tokugawa clan, establish Ryujin Onsen in 1639 as a personal retreat, constructing two inns, Kamigoten (Royal Palace) and Shimogoten (Lower Lodgings), for his immediate family and vassals. Elements of these historic inns remain today, offering visitors a fascinating glimpse of the old feudal system.

Shimogoten's present structure is built around parts of the original inn, which currently function as the lobby, communal lounge, and dining areas, each decorated with lovely antiques and historic ephemera. The inn's simple yet spacious tatami rooms look out over the Hidaka-gawa River, with some featuring cozy, sunken *kotatsu* tables and private, open-air onsen baths to ensure a restful time.

Guests can spend their stay soaking in the comfortable public indoor onsen, whose Ozashiki bath is one of the few remaining tatami onsen baths in Japan, or enjoying the aromatic scent and benefits of the hinoki onsen. However, the indisputable highlight of Shimogoten is the splendid, open-air *rotenburo* onsen, overlooking the turquoise waters of the river and its rocky banks. This onsen is also a rarity, as it's one of the few traditional *konyoku* left in the country, and, as such, all bathers must wear towels.

The sleek, velvety, lotion-like quality of the onsen feels luxurious against the skin; one can easily stay immersed in its waters for long stretches while listening to the healing sounds of the river. Time can also be devoted to wandering the lovely riverbank, dipping one's toes into the crisp, clear waters, climbing the steps to the local onsen temple, and traversing the many historic suspension bridges over the river.

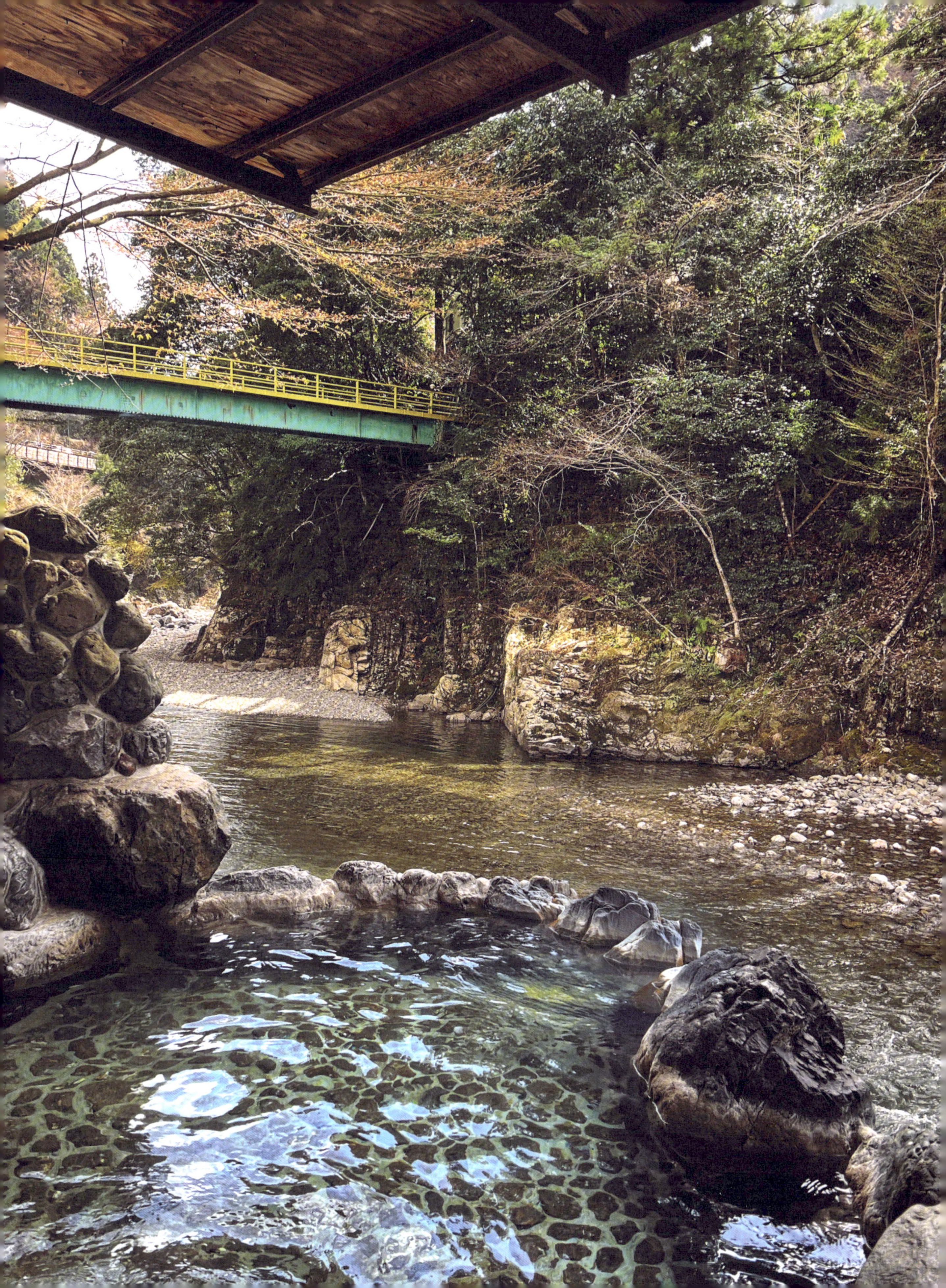

Rankeisou
Sanjo • Niigata Prefecture

ESCAPE TO THIS PEACEFUL ONSEN RETREAT IN THE COUNTRYSIDE

Reset and heal the body, mind, and soul in this secluded destination, where life moves leisurely and time seems to stop.

Nestled in a grove of oak and cedar trees in the remote reaches of Niigata Prefecture, Rankeisou is a countryside mountain inn renowned for its onsen *toji* sojourns. Standing alone in the river valley, the ryokan melds seamlessly with its breathtaking surroundings, with its aged, warm wooden exterior appearing as one with the trees. Built in the traditional Japanese architectural style, Rankeisou might give the impression of a feudal lord's countryside manor, yet its origins are much humbler.

Roughly 100 years ago, at the end of the Taisho era, a man named Otake Yasukichi decided to leave the hectic city behind and returned to his hometown to start digging a well by means of his own *kazusa-bori* (a unique, deep-well-digging contraption traditionally made from bamboo). Yasukichi was a quiet man by nature and his neighbors, friends, and family were unsure of what he aimed to achieve. For two years, he used the *kazusa-bori* and his own bare hands, digging until he struck bedrock from which flowed a lukewarm, saline water that effortlessly cleaned and healed wounds.

Around this discovery, he built a simple, communal lodging to which people traveled from far and wide to bathe in the therapeutic waters and heal in the natural environment. Those who could afford it paid with money or food, while those who could not assisted in helping around the premises.

Currently, Rankeisou's 17 rooms are distributed among three annexes that together form one expansive, three-story inn. Each of the three structures offers a different experience: Ryokufukan is a nationally registered cultural property from the early Showa period, a former traditional inn and restaurant that was relocated to Rankeisou. The Keiryukan annex offers rooms with picturesque scenes of the valley and a spacious communal onsen on the first floor, while Suiyukan is a single-story house decorated with art pieces and designed with refined modern simplicity.

Besides the large communal onsen, where both men and women have separate baths, visitors can also enjoy a sizable indoor onsen and an outdoor rock *rotenburo;* there are additionally three scenic open-air onsen found higher up on the hillside along the Sumon River. Iwayu has both a semi-open-air hinoki onsen and a splendid, spacious rock *rotenburo,* while Fukayu offers two more onsen to try: another semi-open-air hinoki onsen and a deep outdoor hinoki onsen. Both beautifully showcase the attractiveness of each season and are available for overnight guests between the hours of 16:00 and 22:00, after which they open to the public again.

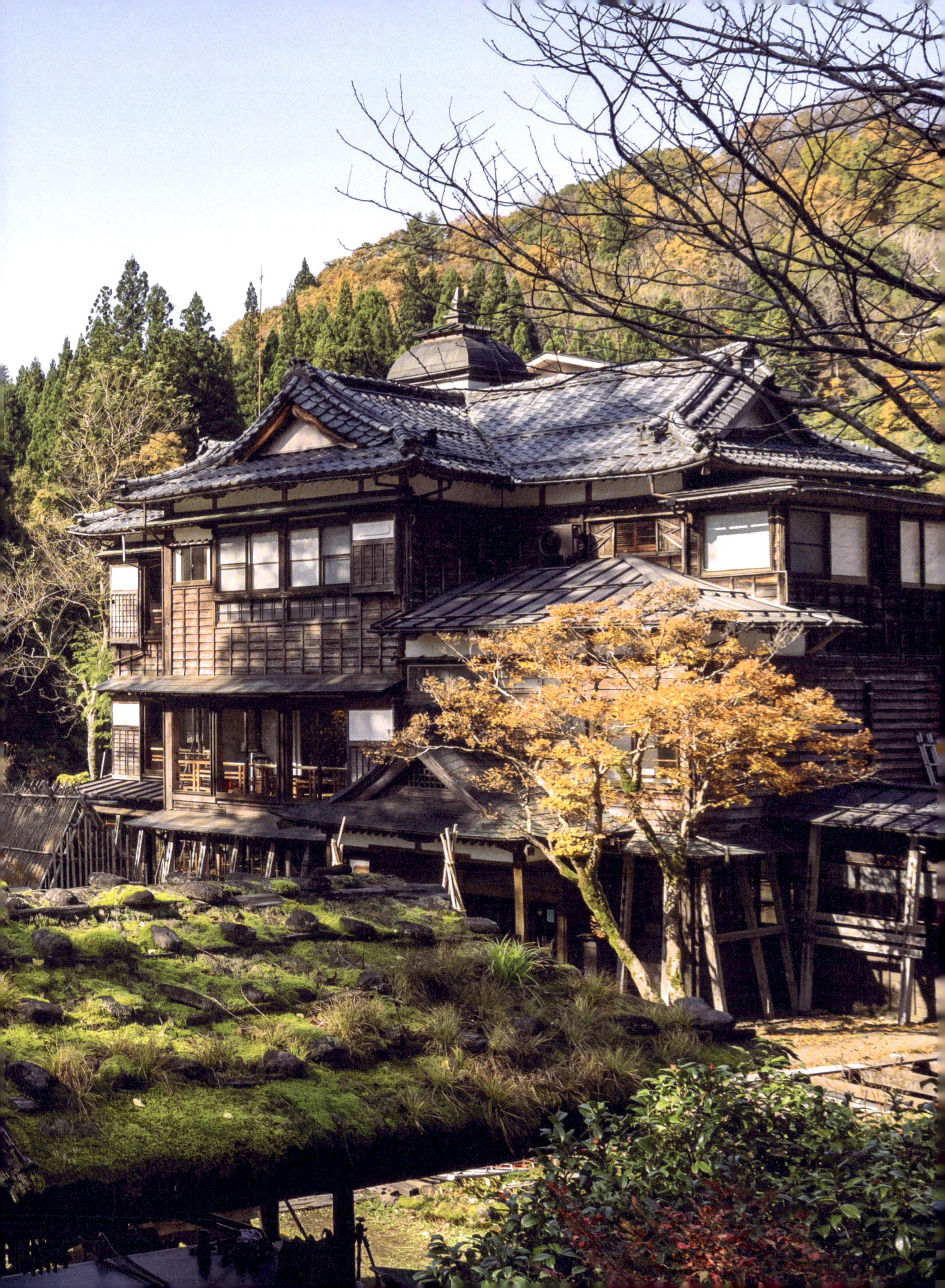

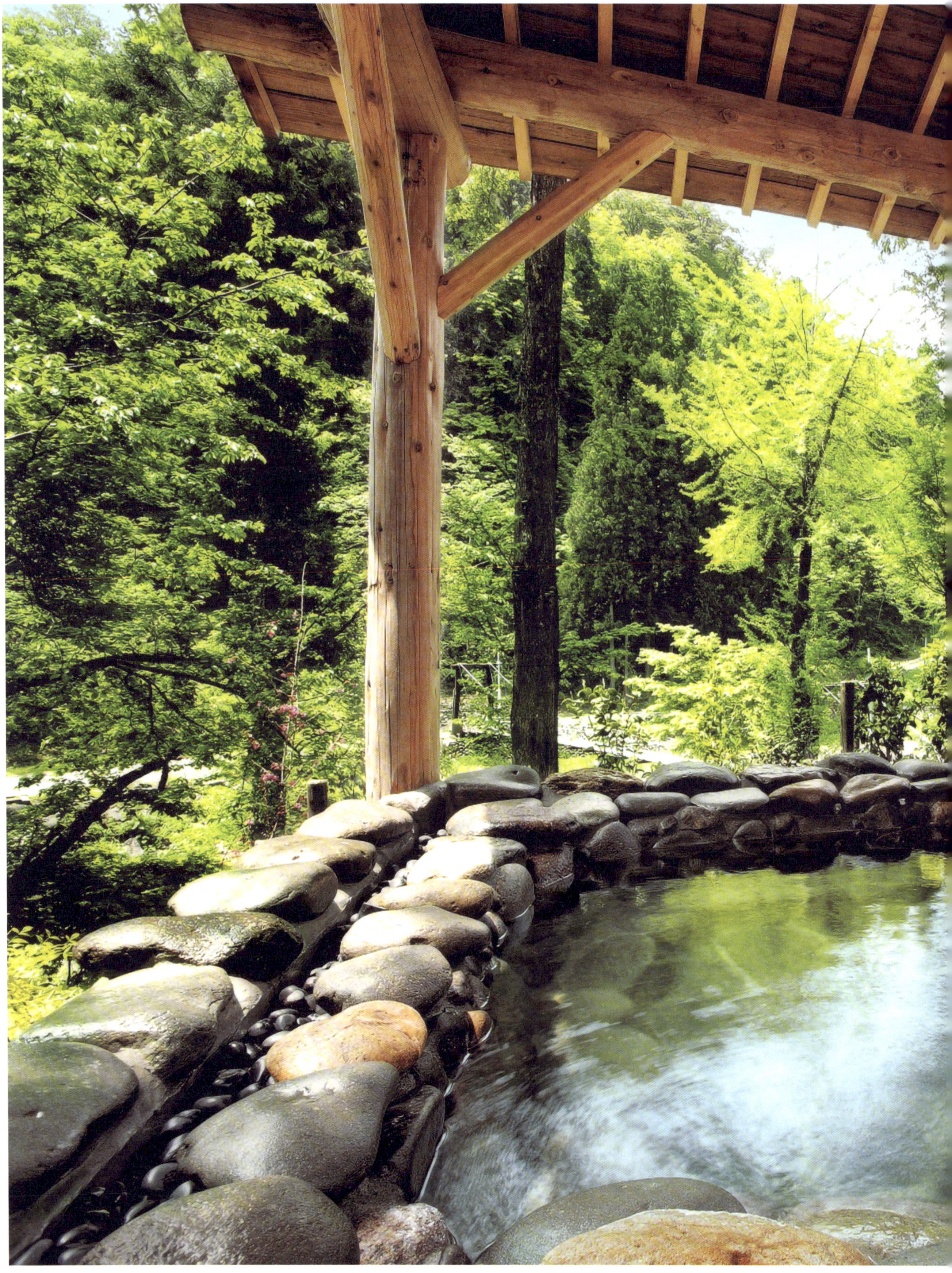

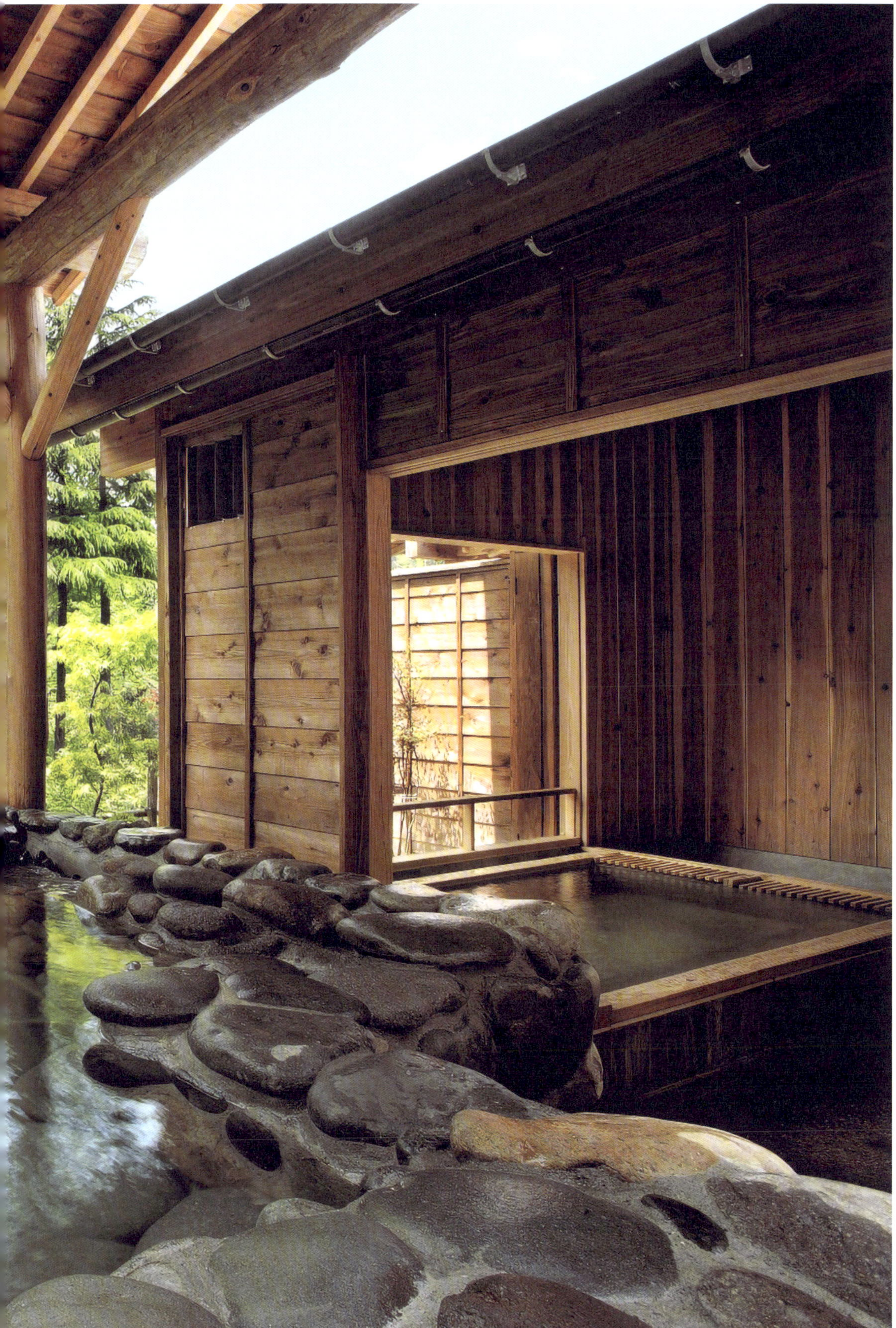

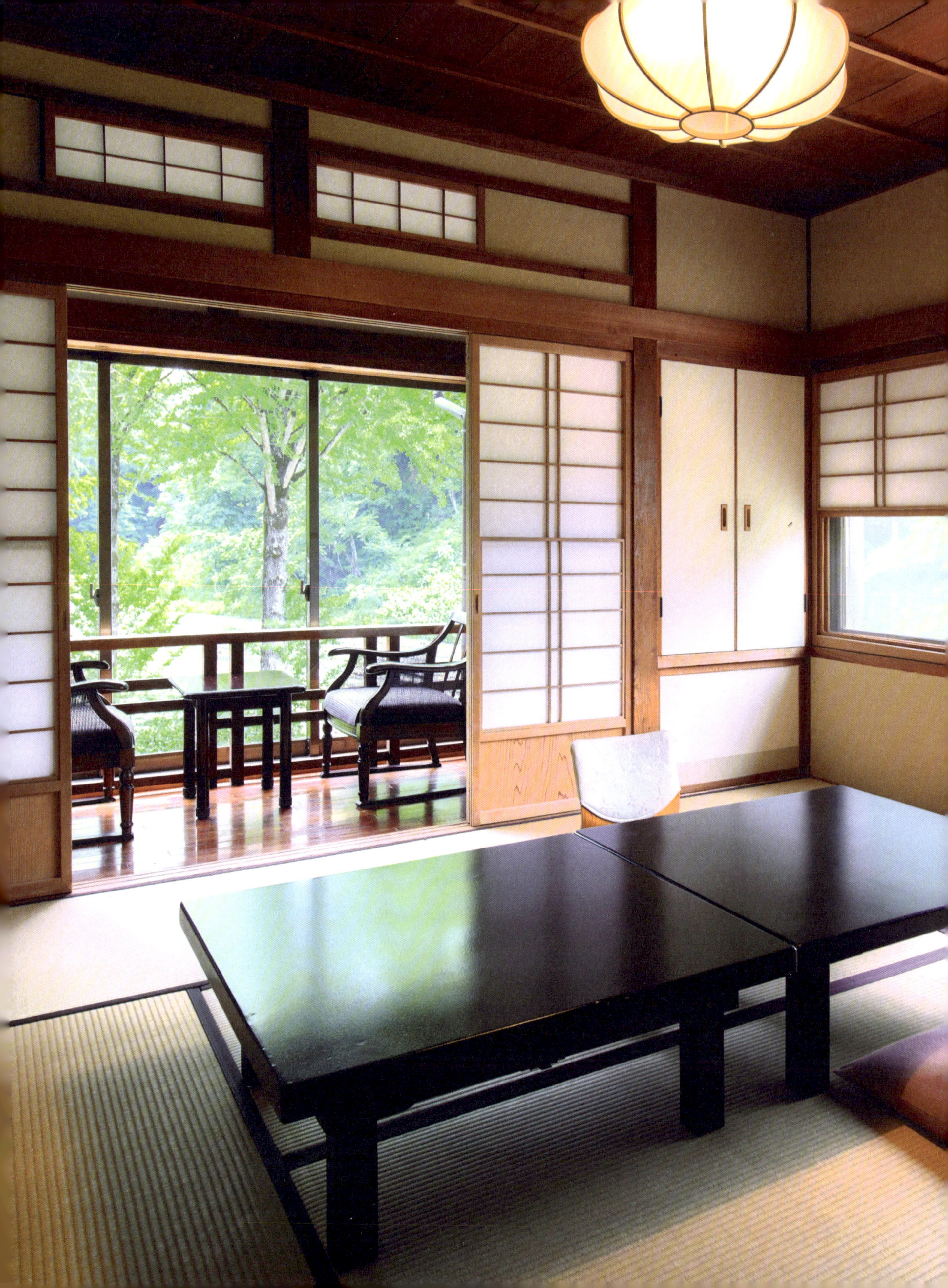

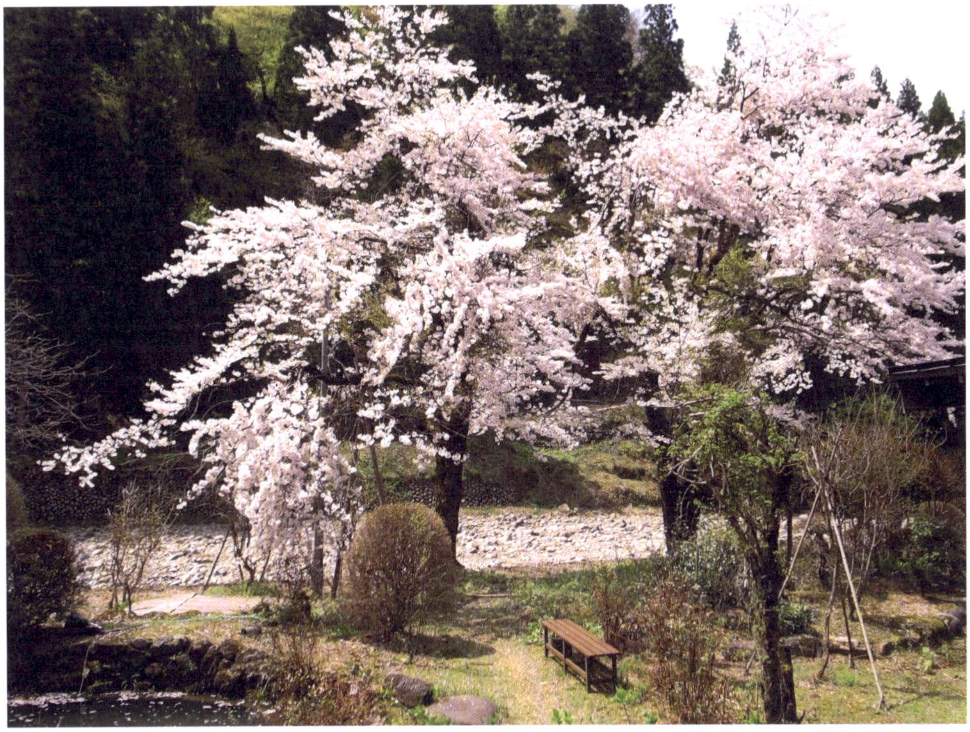

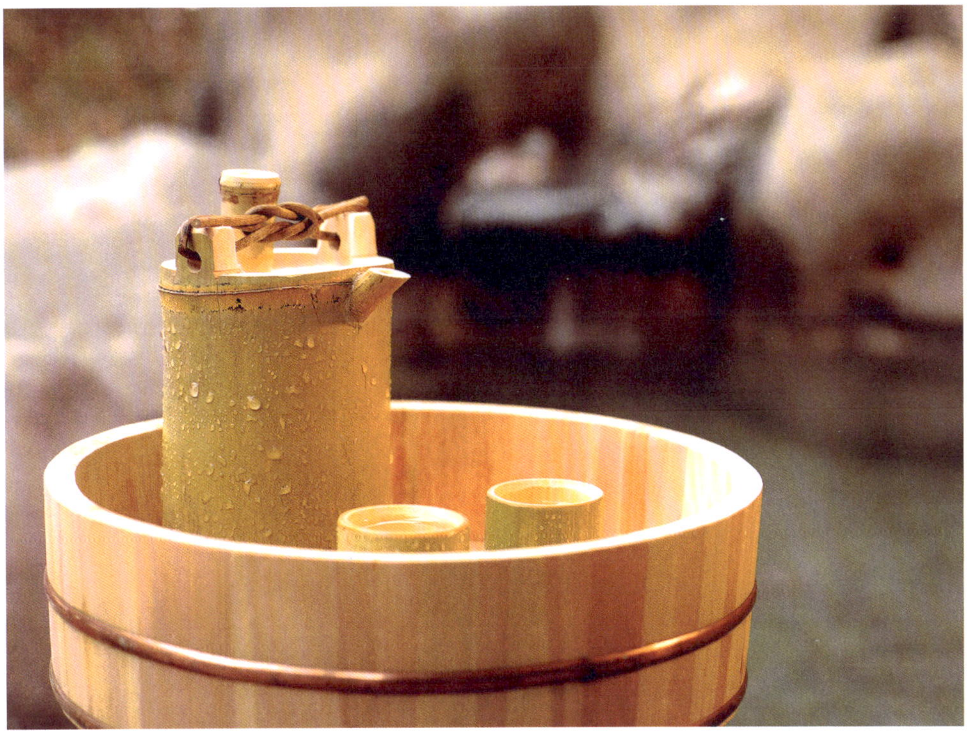

LEFT Wide *engawa* terraces offer restful views of the changing scenery around Rankeisou.

Yufuin Onsen
Yufuin • Oita Prefecture

WANDER THIS PICTURESQUE ONSEN TOWN WITH MT. YUFU IN THE DISTANCE

One of Japan's loveliest onsen towns is quietly nestled in the peaceful countryside amid a setting of rice paddies, rising onsen steam, nearby mountains, and leisurely walking trails.

Surrounded by mountains, with the majestic twin peaks of Mt. Yufu featuring prominently in the scenic backdrop, Yufuin Onsen lies within a flat river basin surrounded by picturesque rice paddies and countryside farmhouses. A much-loved onsen town in Oita Prefecture, Yufuin offers a simpler, more down-to-earth experience in comparison to neighboring Beppu—no large concrete structures or rising onsen hotels are found here. Yufuin's low wooden buildings, encircled by lush green areas, rising onsen steam, and misty morning fog shrouding Mt. Yufu, create an ethereal atmosphere.

The town is spread out around the basin, with a main shopping street lined with sweet cafes, small restaurants, boutiques, and museums. The charming Yufuin Floral Village is a popular stopover. Constructed to resemble the English Cotswolds, it draws many visitors for its special charm, with miniature thatched houses containing numerous shops and eateries that lend it a Studio Ghibli-like atmosphere.

Though the main street can sometimes become crowded, as soon as one ventures off into the little side streets, the crowds disappear and one is left with peaceful countryside pathways and scenery. Yufuin is popular among day-trippers, who come for the shops and pretty setting; however, by late afternoon once they have departed, the quiet charm of the town becomes even more apparent. Yufuin's onsen ryokan and hotels—sprawling, single-story villas—are dispersed throughout the town away from the main street, but most are still easily walkable from the center. Staying overnight in Yufuin allows one to appreciate the serenity of the rural area without the crowds, while day visitors can bathe in several of the ryokan's public onsen for a fee.

During one's stay in Yufuin, a leisurely stroll around Lake Kinrinko—a small, scenic body of water found at the end of the main street where wild koi fish swim and white egrets stalk across the placid waters—is a definite must. Wooden walking paths encircle the lake, along which visitors will discover a small local shrine and a stone torii gate in the water on the lake's southern side. Early mornings and late afternoons are exceptionally lovely for such rambles, as the dawn mist or golden afternoon light casts its magic on the waters.

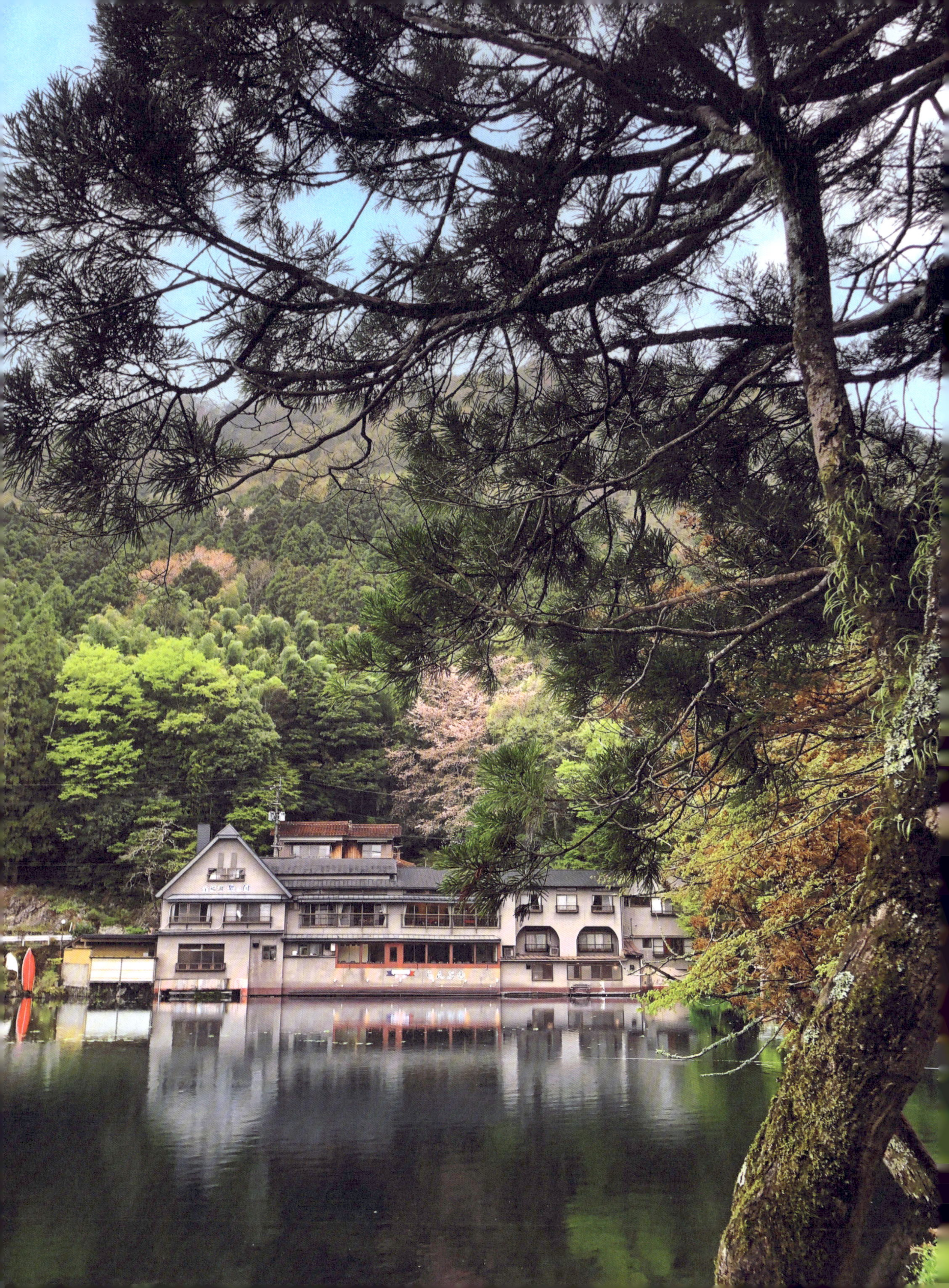

Ginzan Onsen
Obanazawa • Yamagata Prefecture

AN ICONIC AND BEAUTIFUL WINTER ONSEN GETAWAY

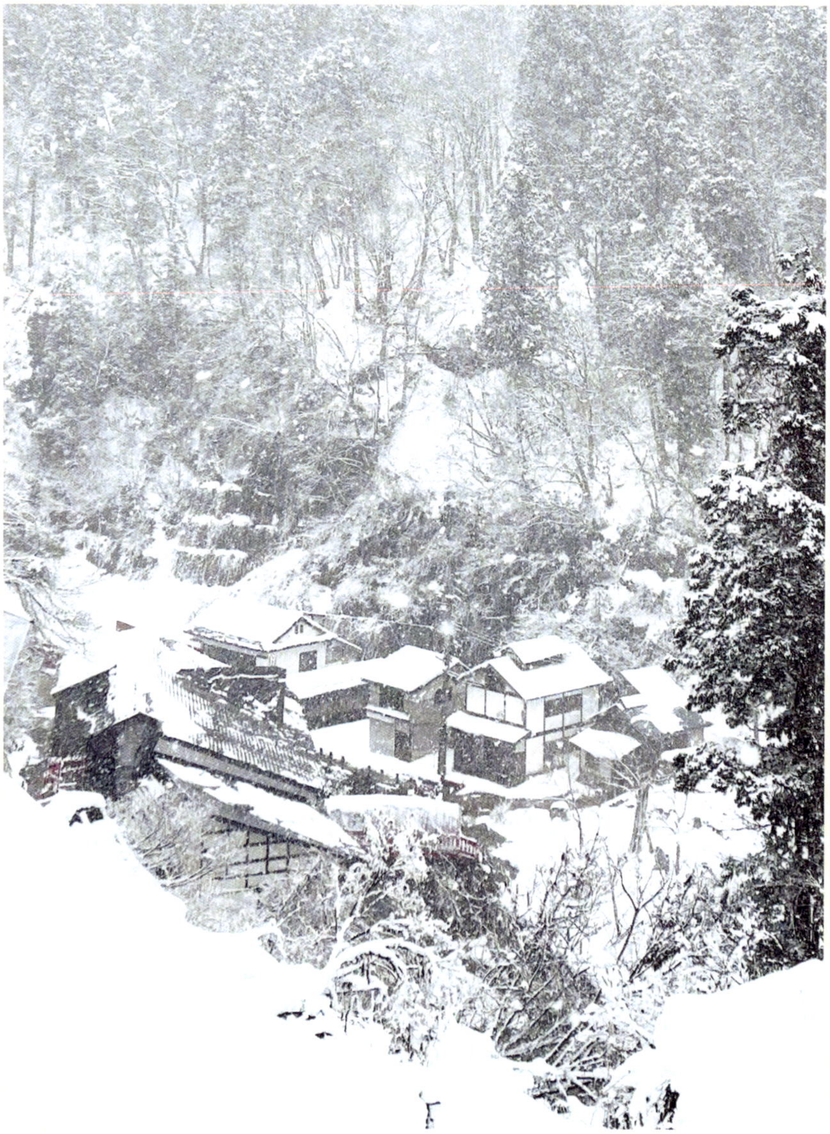

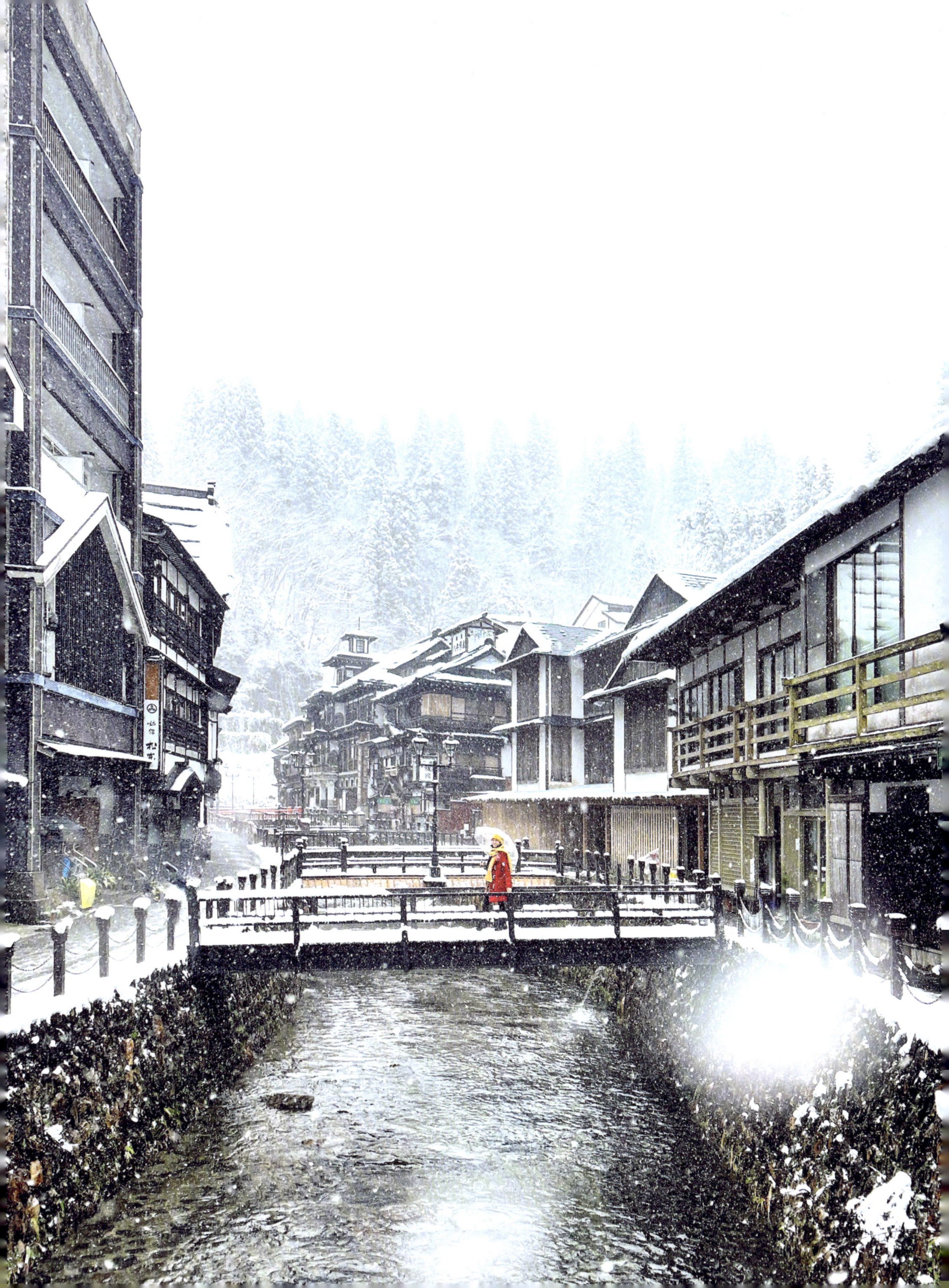

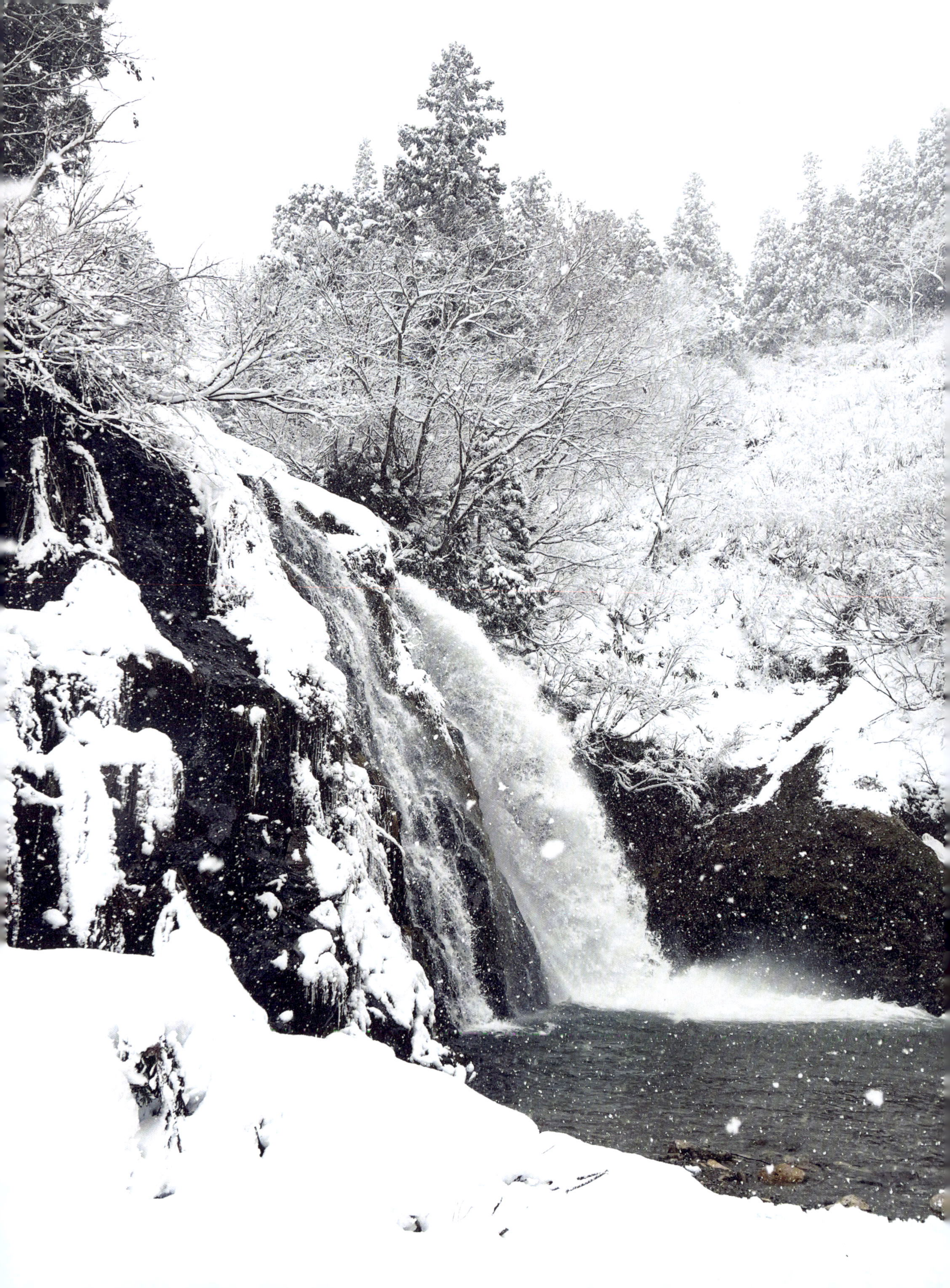

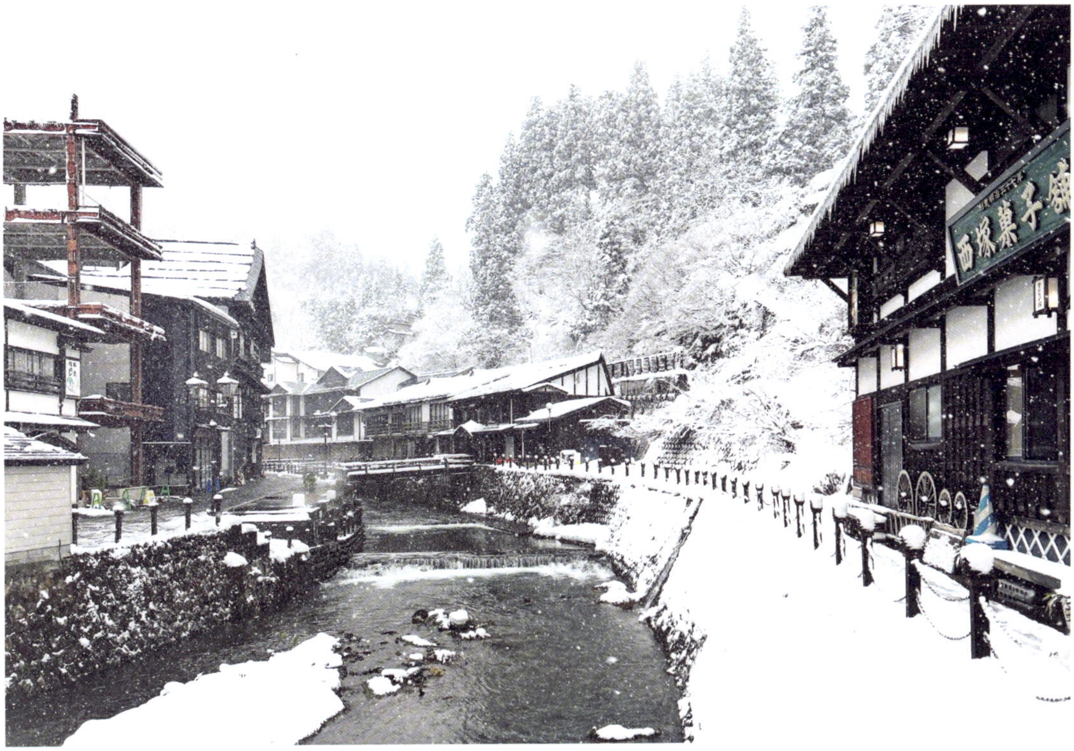

LEFT Shirogane-taki waterfall is striking in all seasons.

Beloved for its snowy scenery and the many glowing antique lamps dotting its streets, this picturesque onsen town is truly enchanting.

Deep in the mountains of Yamagata Prefecture lies the remote and renowned Ginzan Onsen. While beautiful in every season, it is perhaps the most magical in winter, when snowfall covers the town and creates a crisp, hushed winter wonderland. Traditional gas lamps cast their soft glow on the gentle snow flurries, creating a bewitching, old-world atmosphere set against a dramatic backdrop of giant, snow-capped pines.

Once the site of the Nobezawa silver mine, the town decided to rebuild itself as a premier onsen destination after it was closed. Named in honor of its industrial past, Ginzan Onsen loosely translates to "silver mountain hot springs." The mine, whose remnants remain behind the town, can be visited during the spring, summer, and fall seasons.

Along with the mine, one of the town's other main sightseeing spots is Shirogane-taki, an impressive 72-foot (22-meter) waterfall that cascades down powerfully in Shirogane Park. Located at the far end of the onsen town, Shirogane offers walking trails to Senshin Gorge and Choda Gorge, where visitors can view the gorgeous natural scenery and listen to the sounds of the mountain stream. It is particularly beautiful in fall when the crisp autumnal air arrives and the forest leaves lose their green, but inaccessible in winter due to the heavy snowfall.

The town's traditional wooden timber frame ryokan, with their white-plaster walls and intricate craftsmanship, were built using strict construction standards in order to preserve the beauty and elegance of the Taisho Roman architecture. For many travelers, Ginzan Onsen is also especially beloved for its cinematic associations, as it is believed to be another one

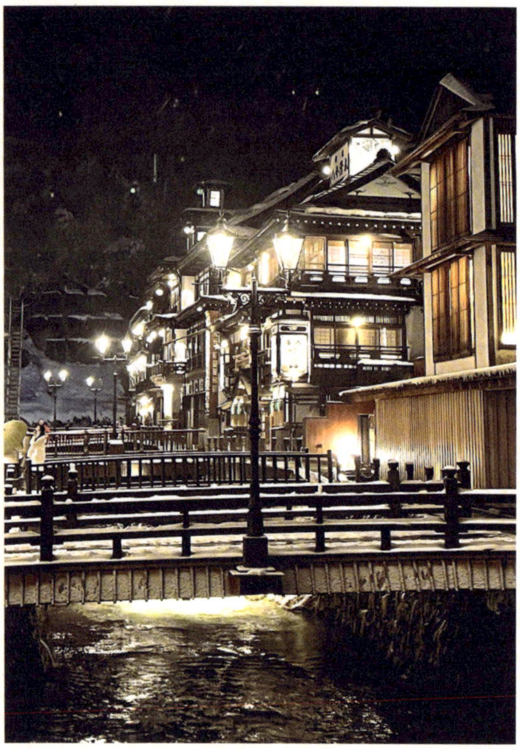

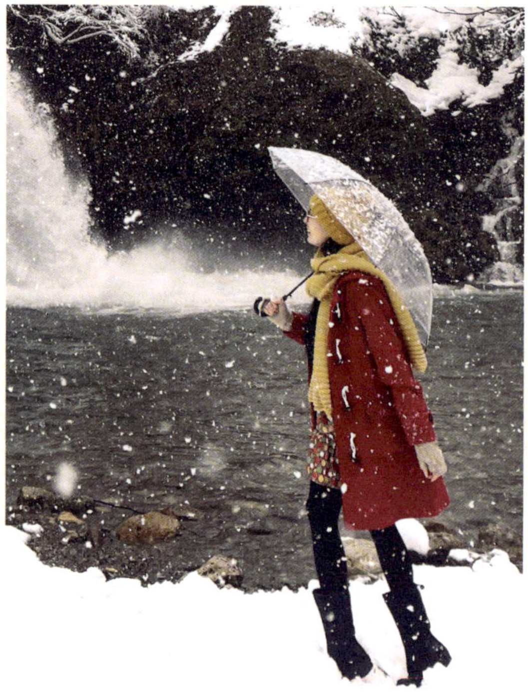

ABOVE LEFT At night, Ginzan Onsen glows with the light of traditional oil lamps.

of the inspirations for Miyazaki Hayao's most famous and critically-acclaimed movie *Spirited Away.*

Boasting 13 onsen ryokan along its quaint, pedestrian-friendly streets, complemented by a few shops and restaurants, Ginzan Onsen feels wonderfully untouched by modern life—making an overnight stay the perfect way to fully experience its exquisite historical charm. To preserve and protect the town, and to allow overnight onsen guests a more intimate experience, the town has recently implemented a ticketing system that limits day visitors. From the hours of 17:00 to 20:00, only 100 day visitors are allowed entry—during the evening hours, the town is open only to locals and guests staying at the town's ryokan.

Staying at one of these ryokan is also the best way to luxuriate in Ginzan's hot springs, as there is only one public bathhouse, Shirogane-no-yu, and two onsen footbaths for day visitors to use. Roughly half the onsen ryokan in town have less than 10 rooms in each of their properties. Ginzanso, with its 40 rooms, is the largest, while the remaining six have less than 20 rooms each. Overnighting in this mountain village is the best way to truly unwind. Its warm, restorative waters, historic architecture, and lack of evening crowds make for a truly transportative experience.

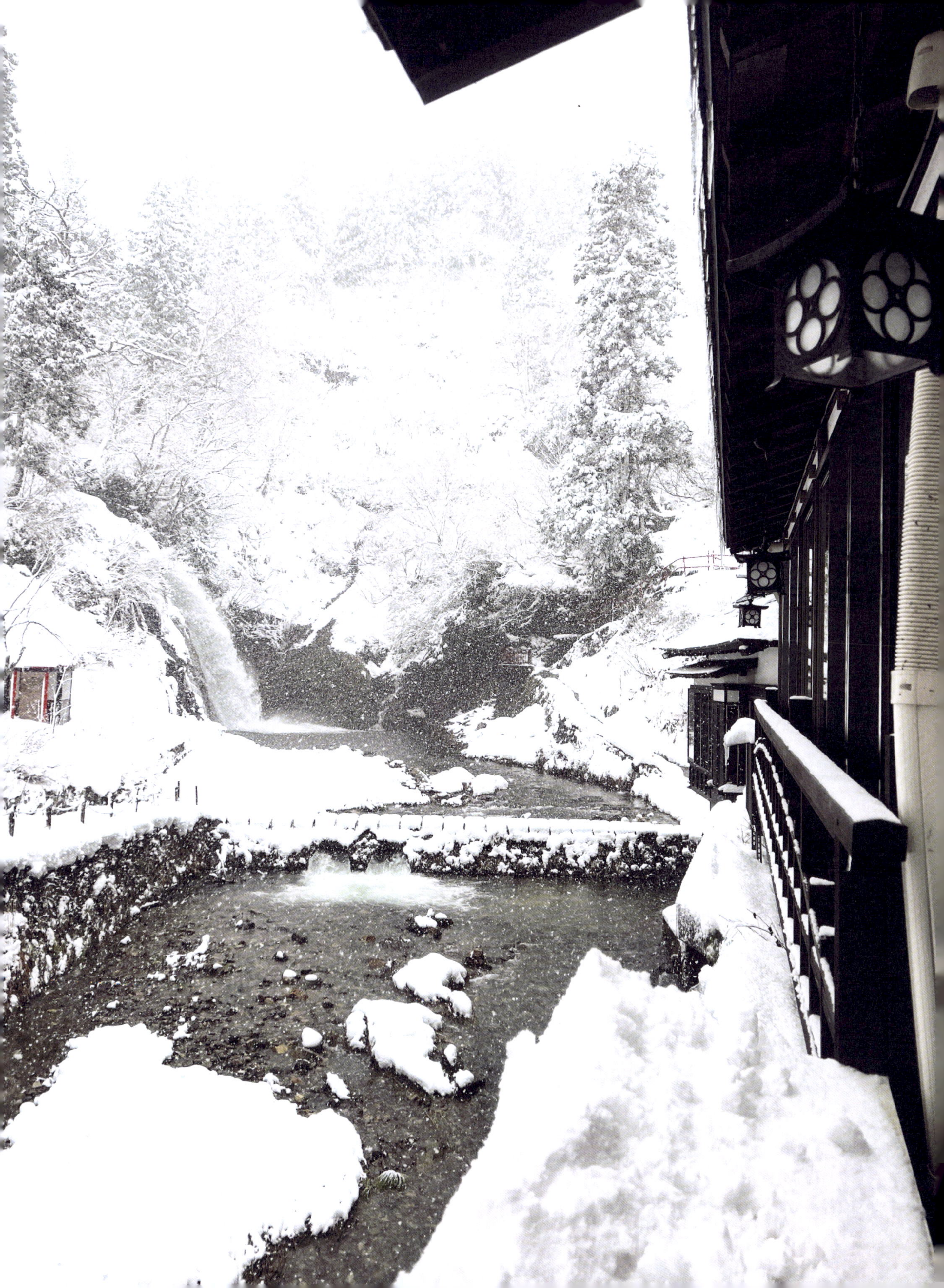

Takimikan, "the soba & waterfall inn"
Obanazawa • Yamagata Prefecture

REST PEACEFULLY AT THIS QUAINT ONSEN RYOKAN

Be sure to take time to fully relax in the magnificent rock *rotenburo*, where breathtaking views of the surrounding mountains greet you.

Nestled on a hilltop with sweeping views of the historic Ginzan Onsen and the cascading waterfall Shirogane-taki lies the charming Takimikan, a "soba and waterfall" ryokan evocative of Japan's Taisho Roman style. A curving white entrance, elegantly decorated with a traditional *kamon* symbol and a large wooden sign, greets guests as they enter the atmospheric interiors, whose high ceilings complement the large, exposed beams made from tree trunks. Travelers can relax and sip their welcome tea in a lobby finished with warm wood paneling and decorated with multiple antique *tansu* chests.

Formerly a beloved traditional soba restaurant, Takimikan still produces delicious, handmade Obanazawa soba from a recipe that has been passed down for generations. The noodles are featured in meals showcasing the regional Satoyama cuisine and can be enjoyed by overnight guests.

From the open windows of the main building's 14 cozy guest rooms, views of the impressive Ginzan mountain range create a relaxing, calming atmosphere. Unwind in the comfortable, cozy vintage chairs by the window as you watch the seasons pass, or doze on the plush, cushioned beds. Spacious tatami rooms, where vintage and antique furnishings contrast with bold primary colors painted on the tokonoma walls, speak to the influence of both traditional Japanese and Western design.

An easy walk down the hill leads guests to the heart of Ginzan Onsen, bypassing the Shirogane-taki waterfall where, at the waterfall's bridge, Takimikan's sister building, Bettei Takimikan, can be found. Four rooms are available in the annex, with both Yukihare and Shoryo offering elegant encounters with contemporary Japanese style, living areas furnished with traditional *chabudai* low tables, and incredible views of the waterfall. A private indoor onsen bath is also available for guests at Bettei Takimikan.

Some of the loveliest features of Takimikan are its public onsen baths, including a large communal indoor onsen with wonderfully scenic views. Its open-air *rotenburo* has panoramic views of the mountain ranges, and is the only rock *rotenburo* in the town. Every season is splendid, from the fragrant air of spring, to the vibrant fall foliage and the white snow of winter.

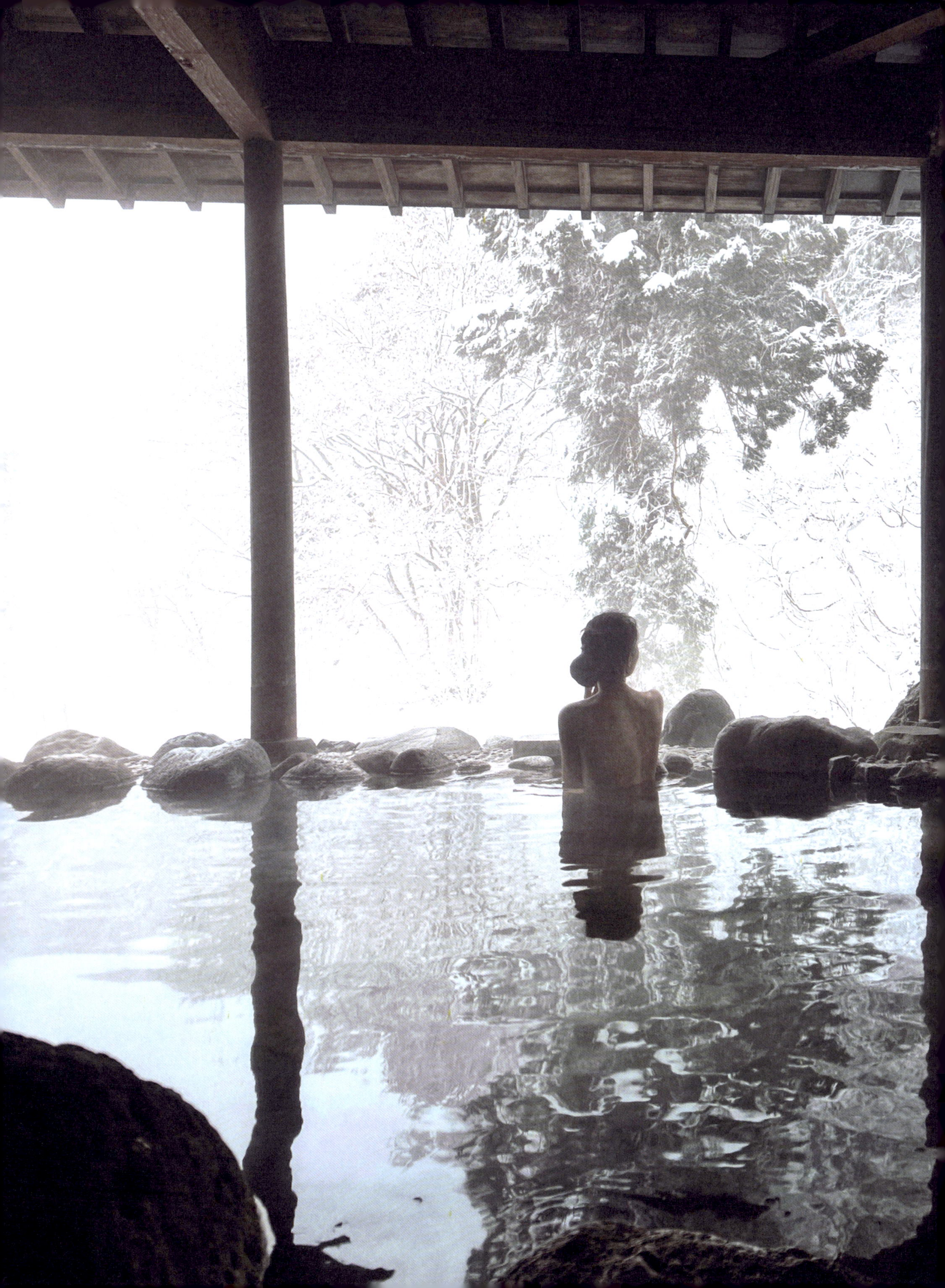

Satoyama Jujo
Minami-Uonuma • Niigata Prefecture

A HISTORIC *KOMINKA*, NOW A RELAXING ONSEN RYOKAN

Embrace the Japanese *satoyama* philosophy, where one experiences life in harmony with the environment, its ecosystems, and its natural resources.

Ensconced in the heart of Niigata's mountainous snow country, Satoyama Jujo is a 150-year-old *kominka* (traditional Japanese house) made entirely of strong hardwood *zelkova* and protected with layers of lacquer. Crafted from strong wooden posts and beams, the *kominka* stands as a beautifully restored and preserved example of Sukiya-zukuri architecture.

Inspired by *The Tale of Genji,* a classic work of literature from the Heian period, Satoyama Jujo literally translates to "10 stories of the mountain village," and it is through this philosophy of storytelling that they have chosen to redefine the luxury onsen ryokan experience, honoring the tradition of onsen culture while encouraging new experiences and discoveries. Their 10 carefully curated stories celebrate the themes of food, architecture, textiles, agriculture, the environment, art, the outdoors, relaxation, health, and gathering, allowing for a complete immersion in the region's rich culture and cuisine, and the magnificent scenic beauty of the Minami-uonuma region.

The traditional interiors of Satoyama Jujo are seamlessly furnished with modern, designer furniture and contemporary artworks. Guests are invited to dine at the onsen's restaurant, Sanaburi, where the menu has been built around local foraged seasonal produce and the deliciousness of Niigata's rice. Remarkably, while Niigata's rice is considered the best in the country, it is the rice from the Osawa district in Minami-uonuma—exactly where Satoyama Jujo is found—that is considered the best of the best.

Beyond the traditional *kominka* lies its modern extension, which houses guest rooms that are designed to blend the best of Japanese design with modern Western aesthetics. With their earthen tones and expansive windows, roughly half the rooms have their own private open-air onsen, showcasing excellent views of the lush and majestic surroundings.

One of the most impressive and memorable features of Satoyama Jujo is the open-air *rotenburo,* Amanogawa (Heaven's River), which is also the name for the Milky Way galaxy. Inspired by the concept of the popular infinity pool, the elegant *rotenburo* has been designed to provide bathers with stunning panoramic views of Mt. Makihata and the peaks running along the Gunma-Niigata border. Special care has been taken to ensure that no manmade structures obstruct the views as one unwinds. Regardless of the season or time of day, the experience soaking in the therapeutic, soft water of the onsen while admiring such views will never cease to disappoint. Be sure to bathe not only in the day but also after dark for glimpses of the starry sky.

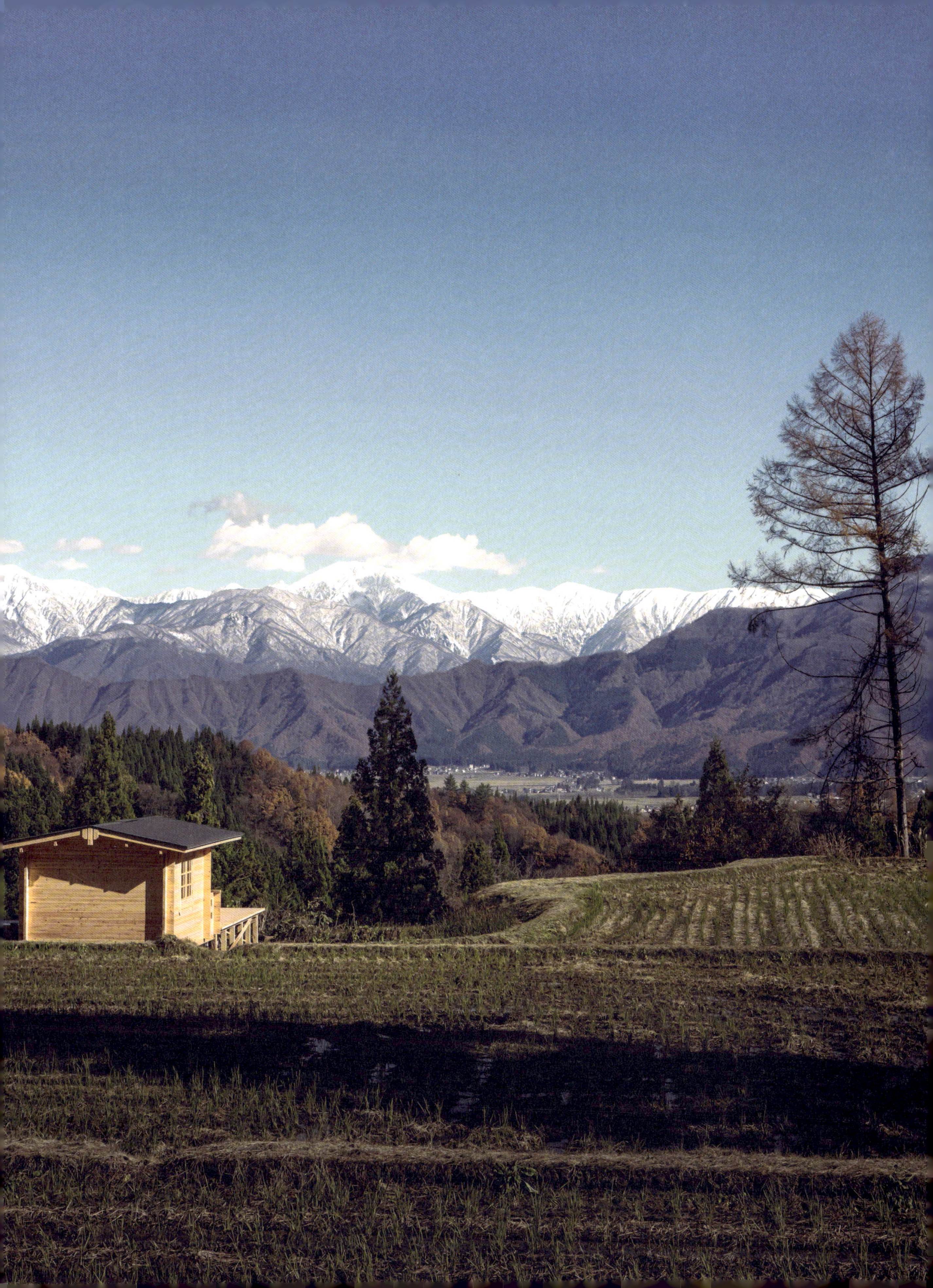

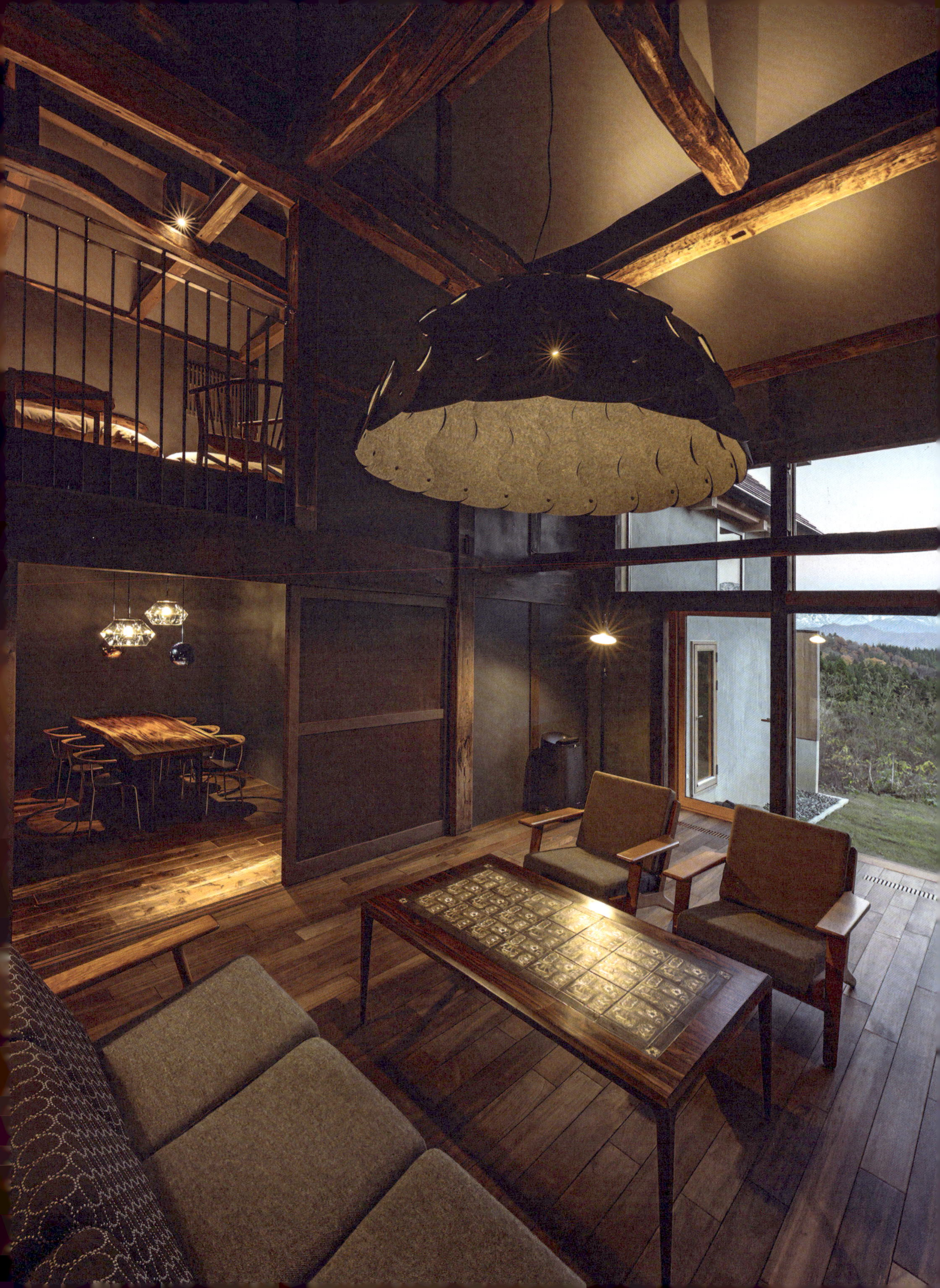

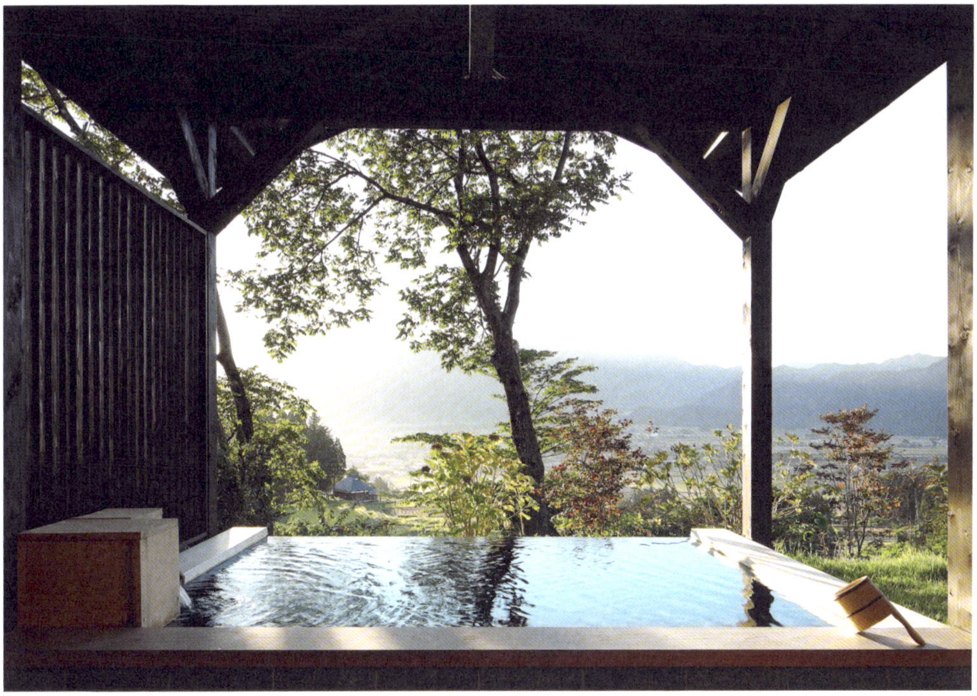

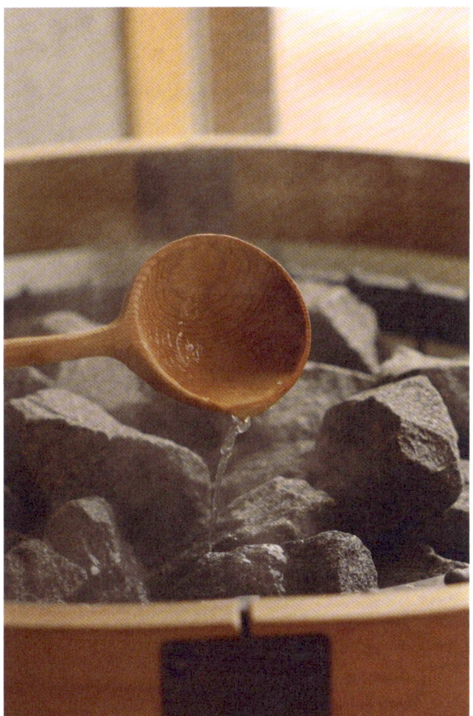

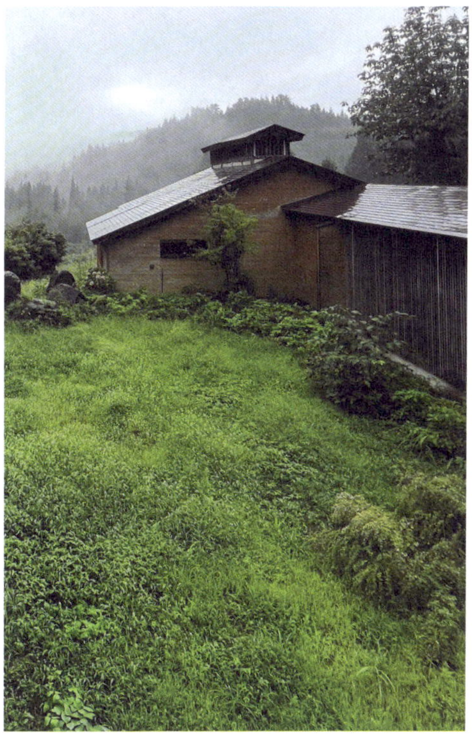

LEFT The luxurious interiors of Satoyama Jujo's standalone villas (Satoyama Jujo The House: Sen, Kiroku & Izumi) make for an impressively intimate stay.

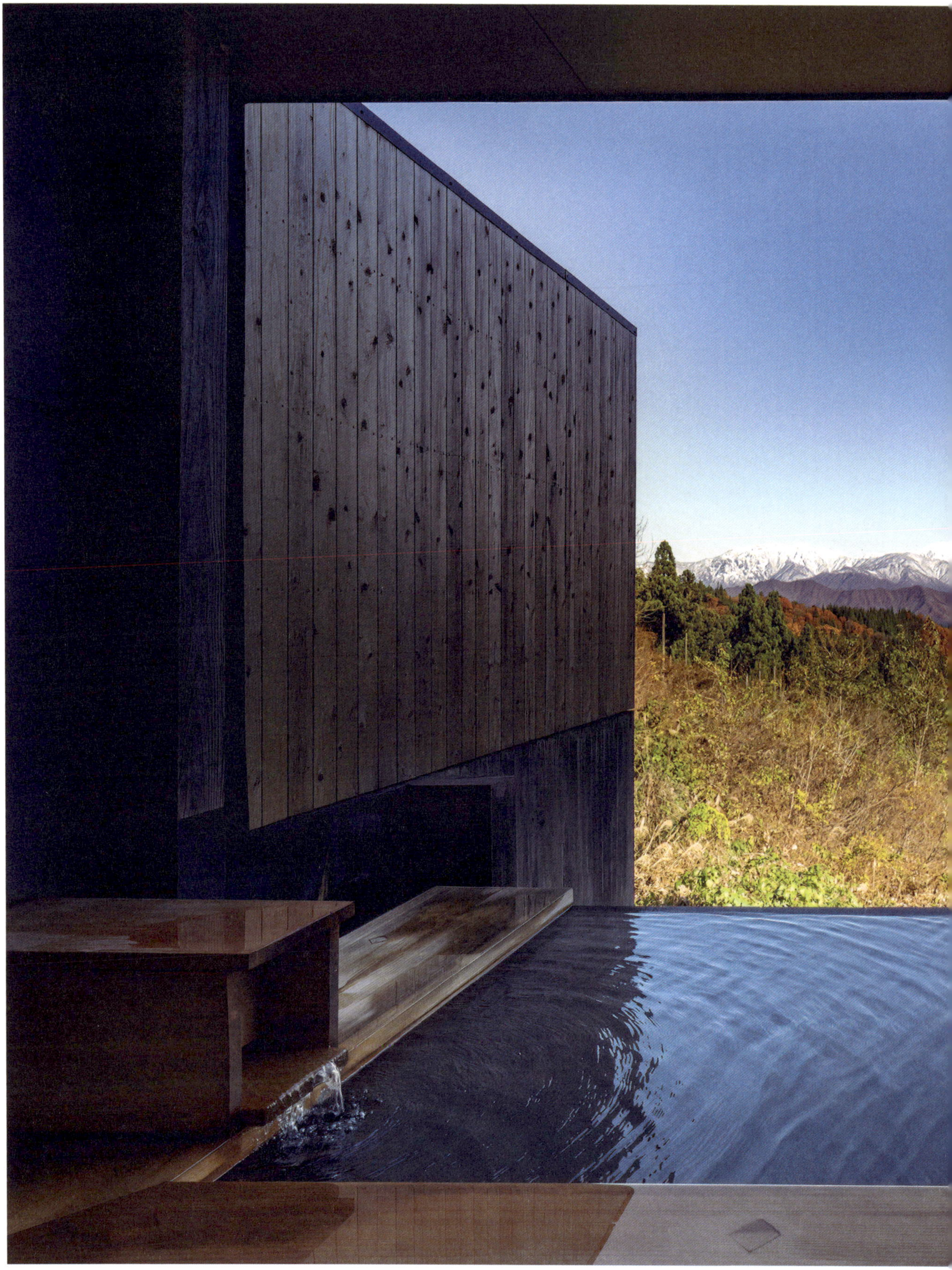

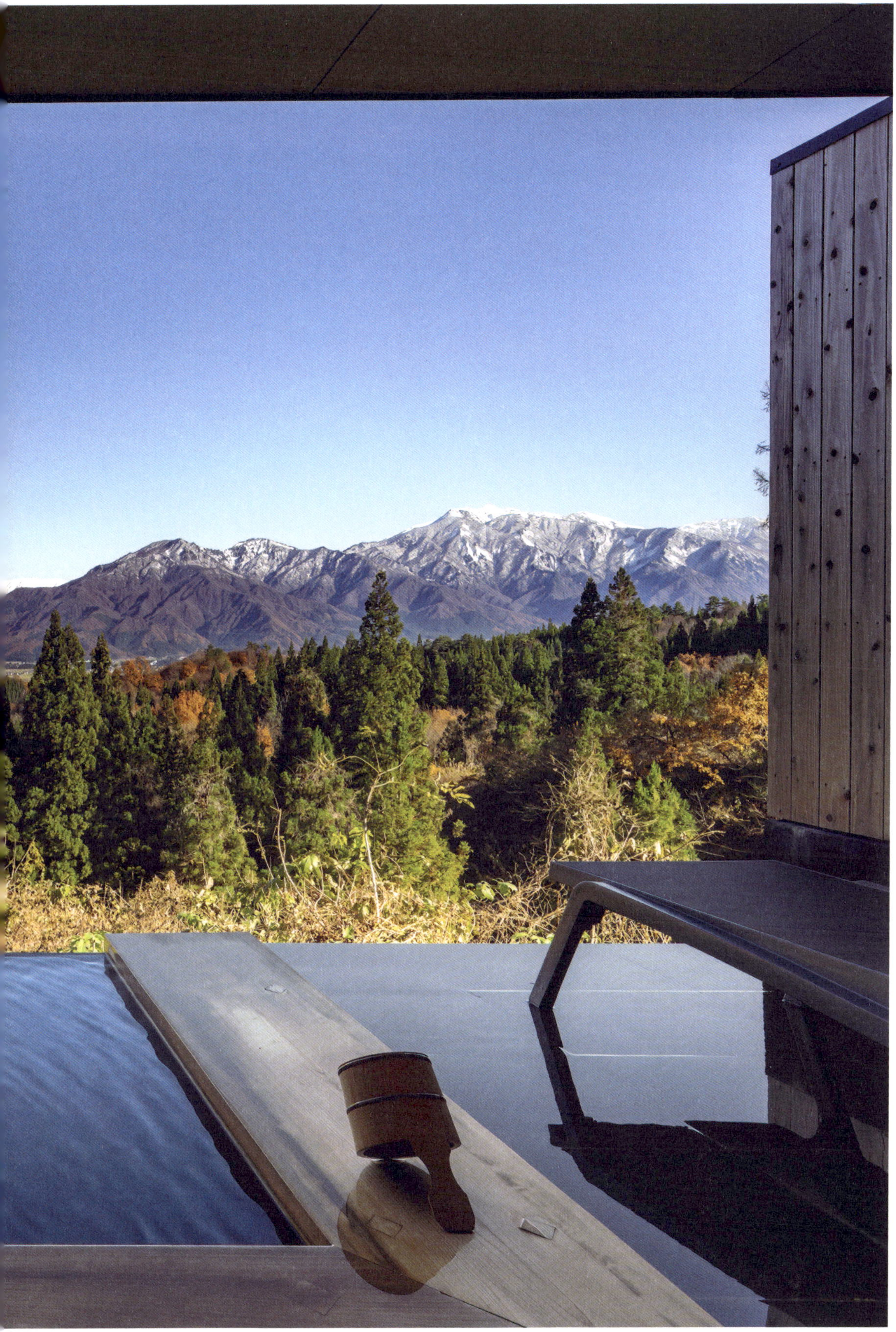

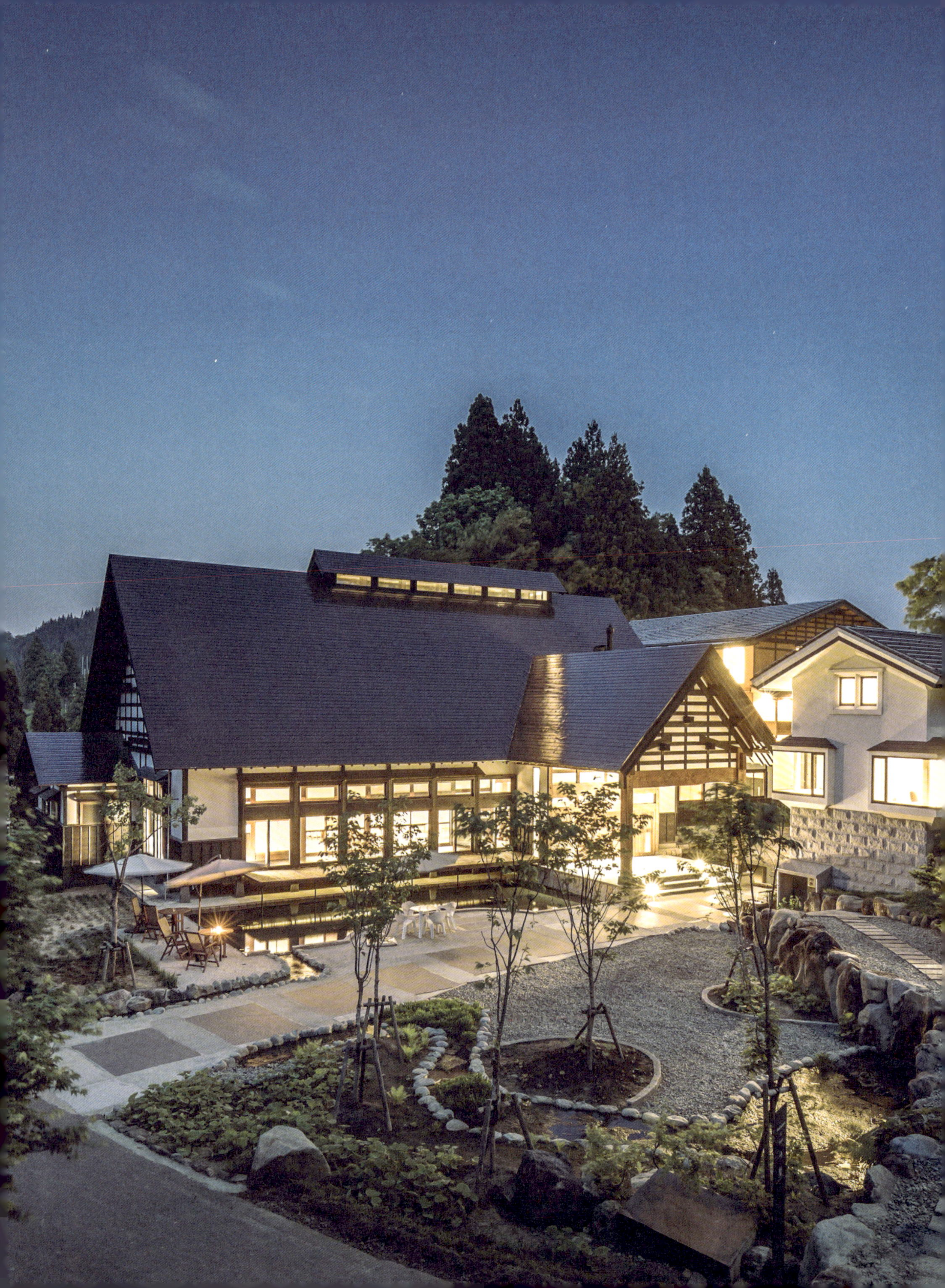

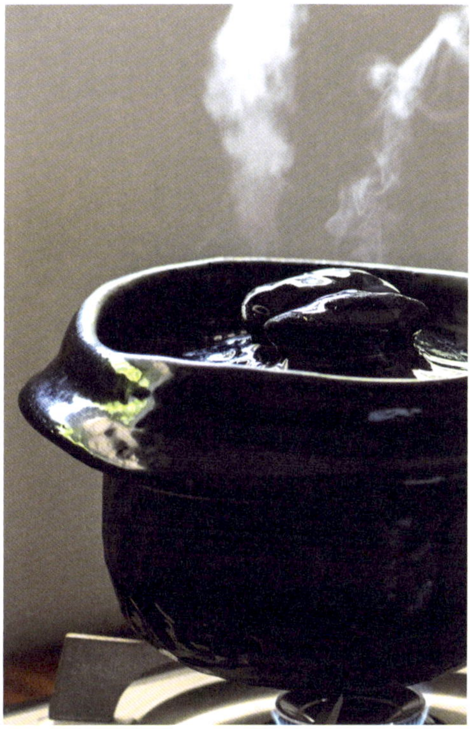

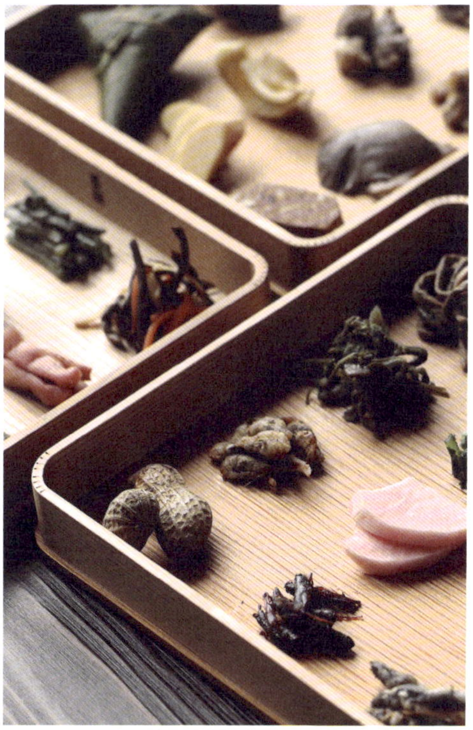

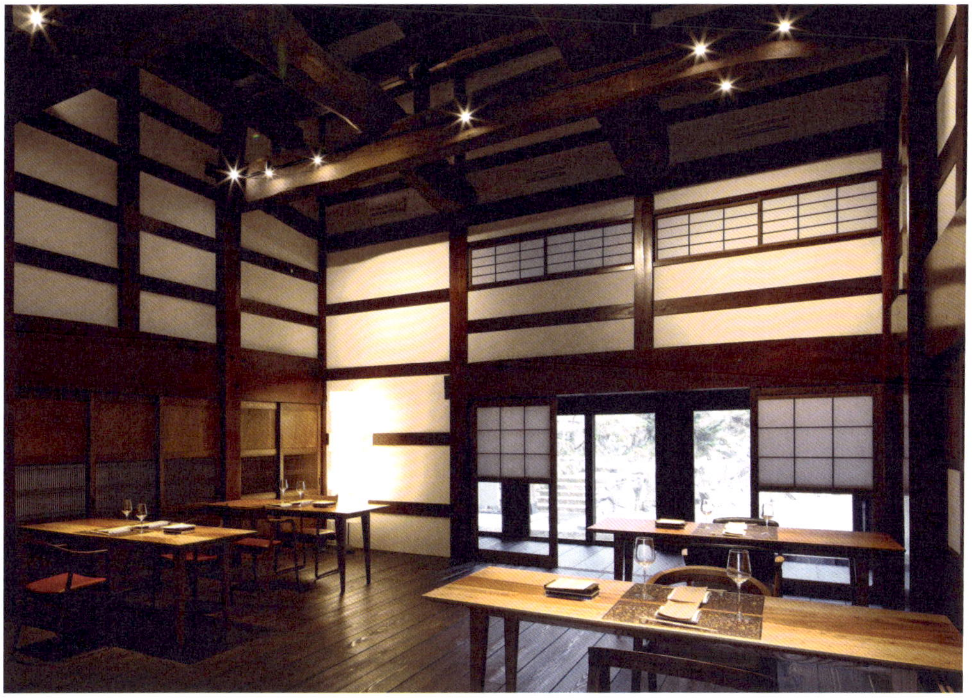

ABOVE The wooden interiors of the *kominka*'s restaurant, where guests taste the flavors of the Minami-uonuma landscape.

Ueyama Ryokan
Himeji ● Hyogo Prefecture

STEP INTO A GHIBLI-ESQUE WORLD JUST OUTSIDE HIMEJI CITY

Spend tranquil days and quiet nights in this onsen refuge located in the popular Kansai region.

Ueyama, Shiota Onsen's first ryokan, was established in 1874, but the source of Shiota Onsen is believed to have been discovered during the Nara period (710–94). Since then, Shiota Onsen has long been a beloved destination, both for its healing baths and its therapeutic, drinkable onsen water. An ancient document states that "many visitors come from the Tamba, Tanshu, Settsu, Bizen, and Shikoku regions, and were cured of all their ailments...amazing is the power of nature."

After the Second World War, Shiota Onsen grew in popularity through word of mouth. Numerous onsen sources were discovered and tapped, and new inns constructed and opened, transforming the site into a thriving onsen town. Sadly, after the collapse of Japan's economy in the 1990s, the devastating Great Hanshin Earthquake in 1995, and various other calamities, five of the newer inns were forced to close, leaving only Ueyama Ryokan.

Ueyama Ryokan's white walls and traditional *kawara* roof tiles stand in vivid contrast to the colors of the mountain backdrop, while its picturesque red bridge over the pond provides a link to a bygone era. The scenery is even more romantic when the light falls just right and the ryokan is reflected in the waters of the pond. The expansive grounds beyond the ryokan that lead to the outdoor onsen baths are also truly impressive, with dappled sunlight falling through the *momiji* (maple trees) onto a carpet of moss and the lovely Inari shrine.

Guests can also enjoy two indoor communal onsen, and a pleasant walk in one's *yukata* leads to a public *rotenburo* framed by more gorgeous red maples. Ueyama also contains two private, outdoor hinoki onsen for families, friends, and couples to bathe together.

One can enjoy several types of stays at Ueyama Ryokan, with the historic east wing overlooking the bridge and pond, and offering simple tatami rooms that retain the elegance and idyllic beauty of both the Taisho and Showa eras. The main building also features slightly larger tatami-style rooms with views of the forest. For those in search of a more intimate, luxurious stay, the separate villa Tsubakikan contains only two rooms, Yamagumo and Keigetsu, each providing their own private onsen baths. At Ueyama, surrounded by the ryokan's traditional, historic interiors decorated with antiques, artifacts, and local crafts, one might feel as though they have entered the fantastical world of a Japanese folktale.

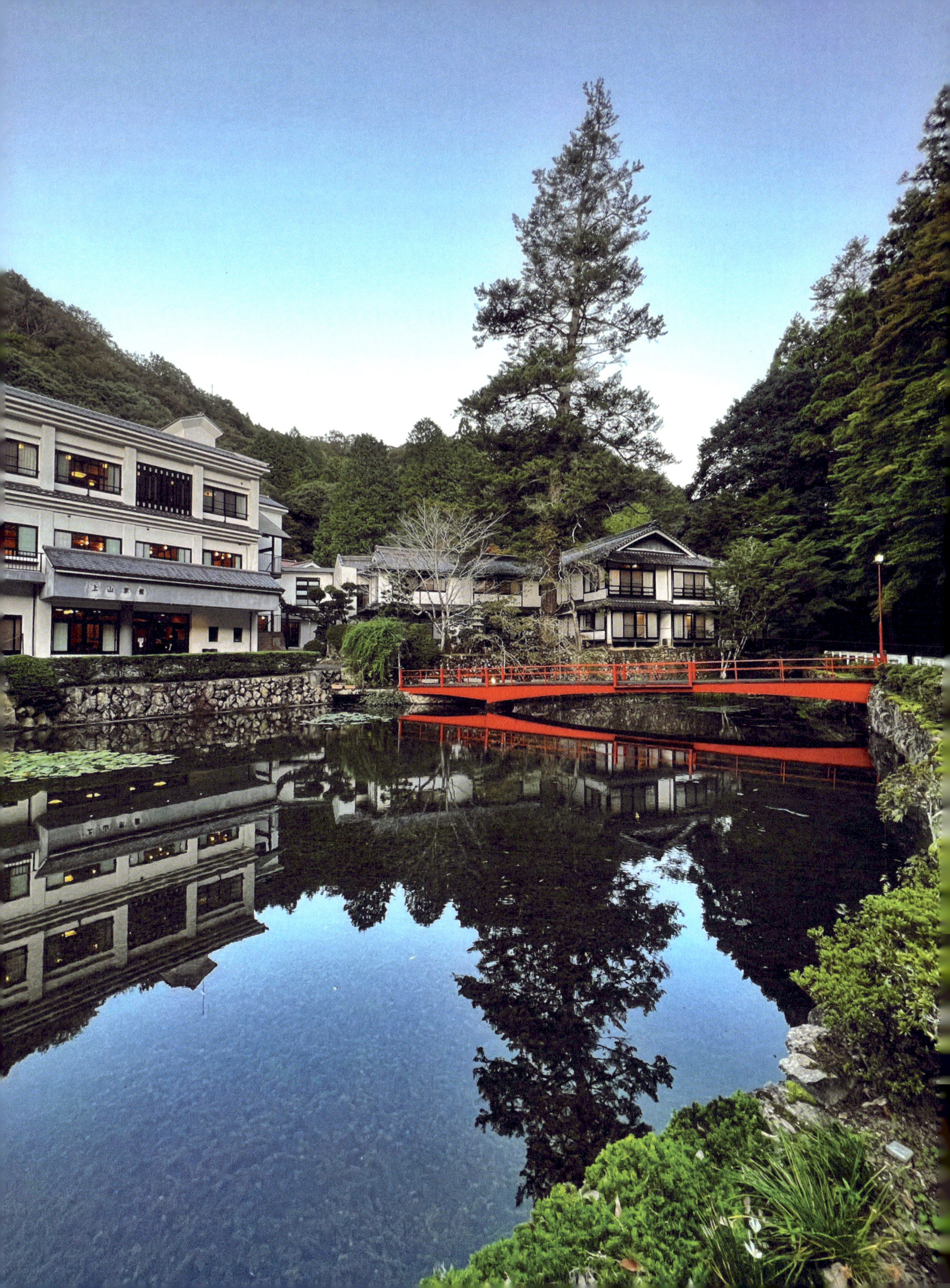

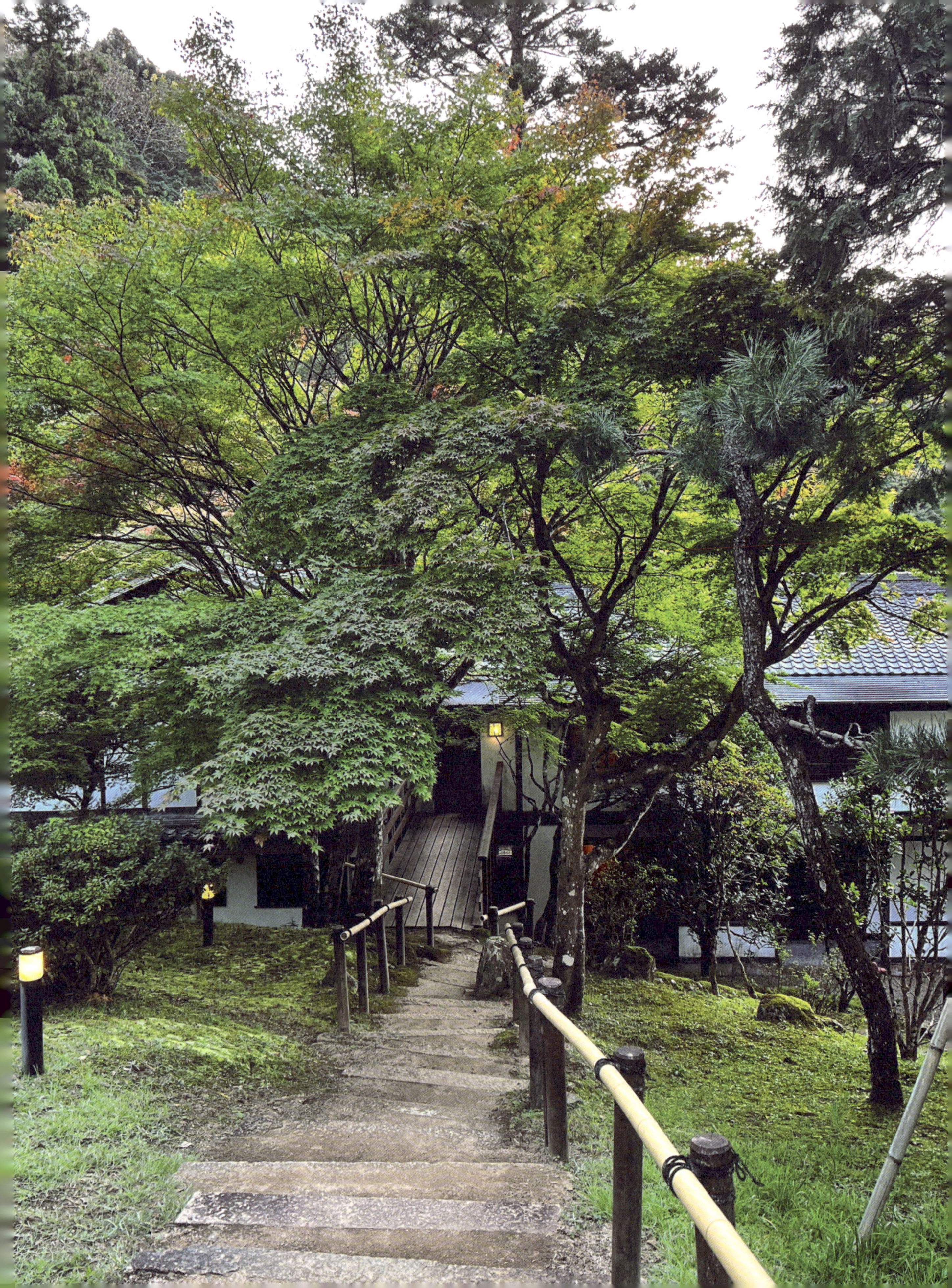

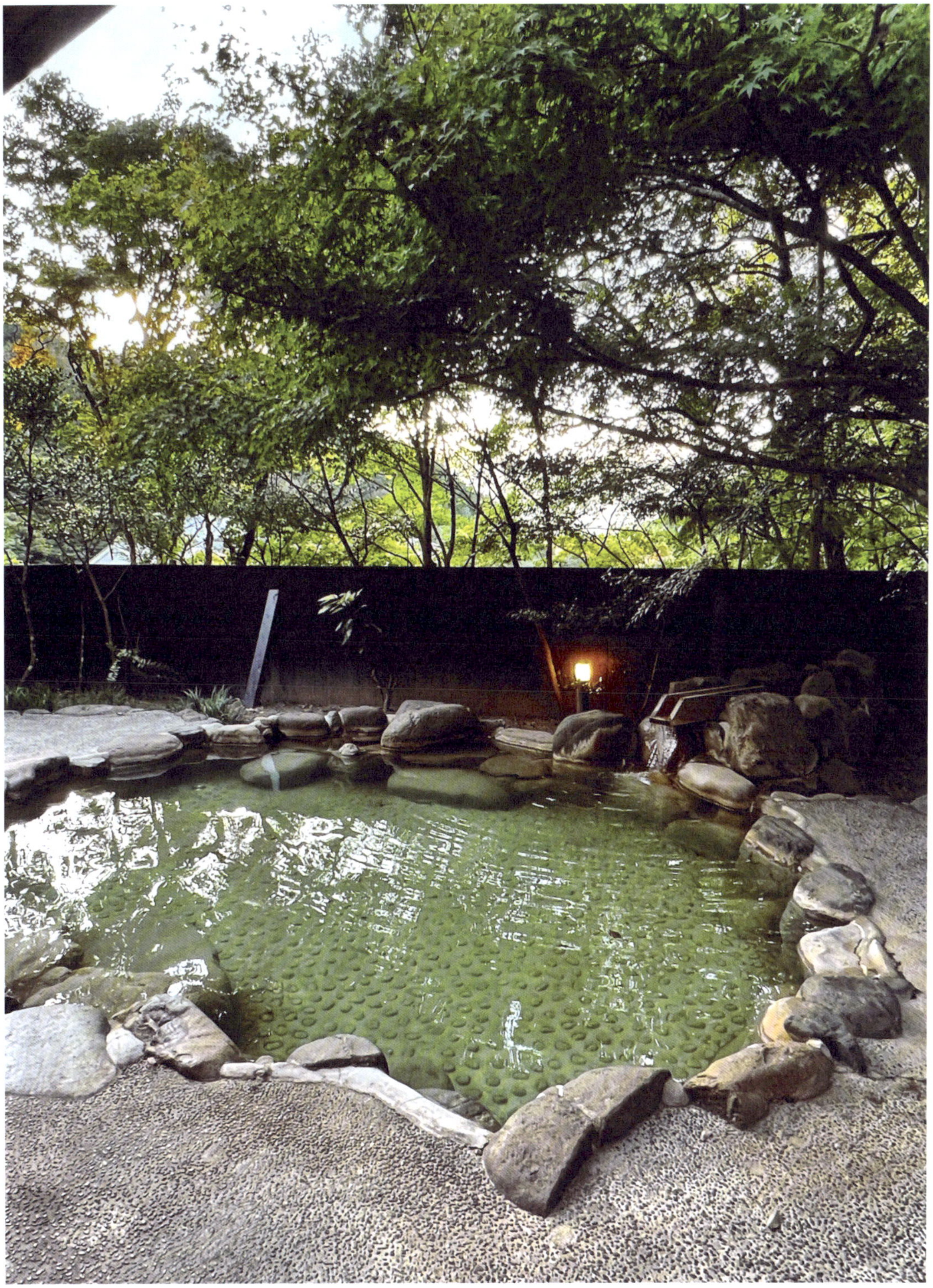

ABOVE One of the public *rotenburo* onsen set within the gardens.

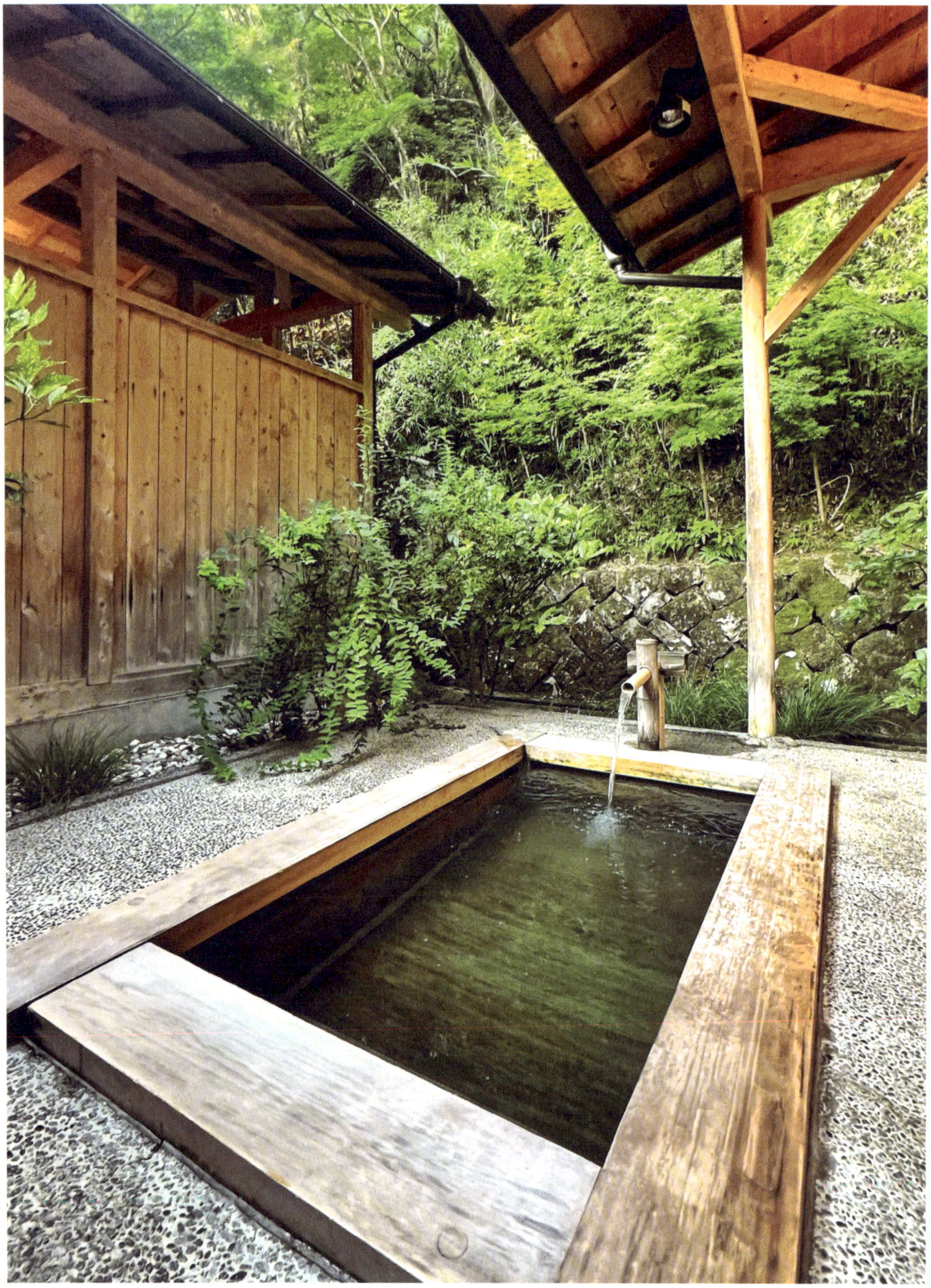

ABOVE A freely reservable, private *kashikiri* onsen for staying guests.

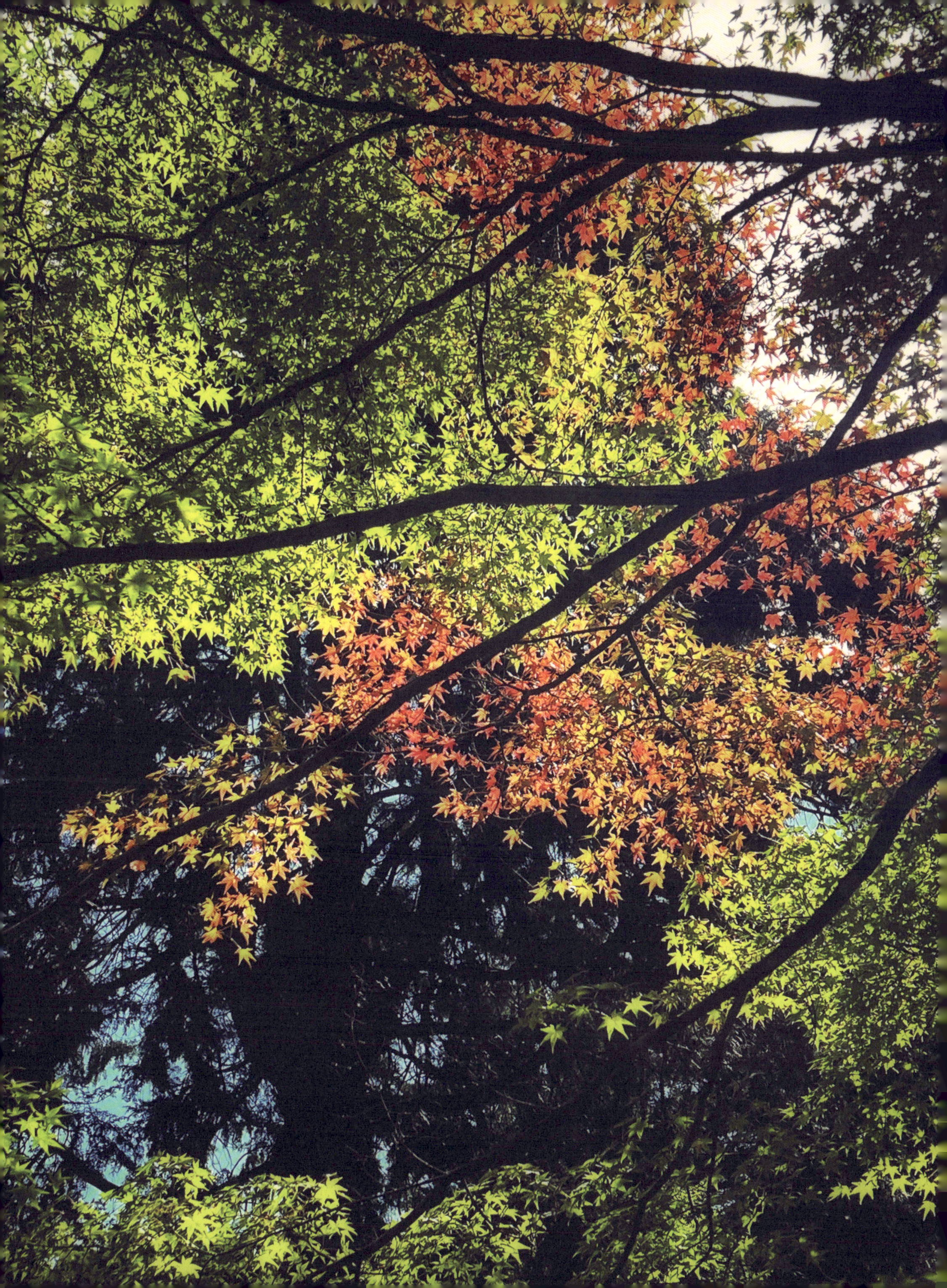

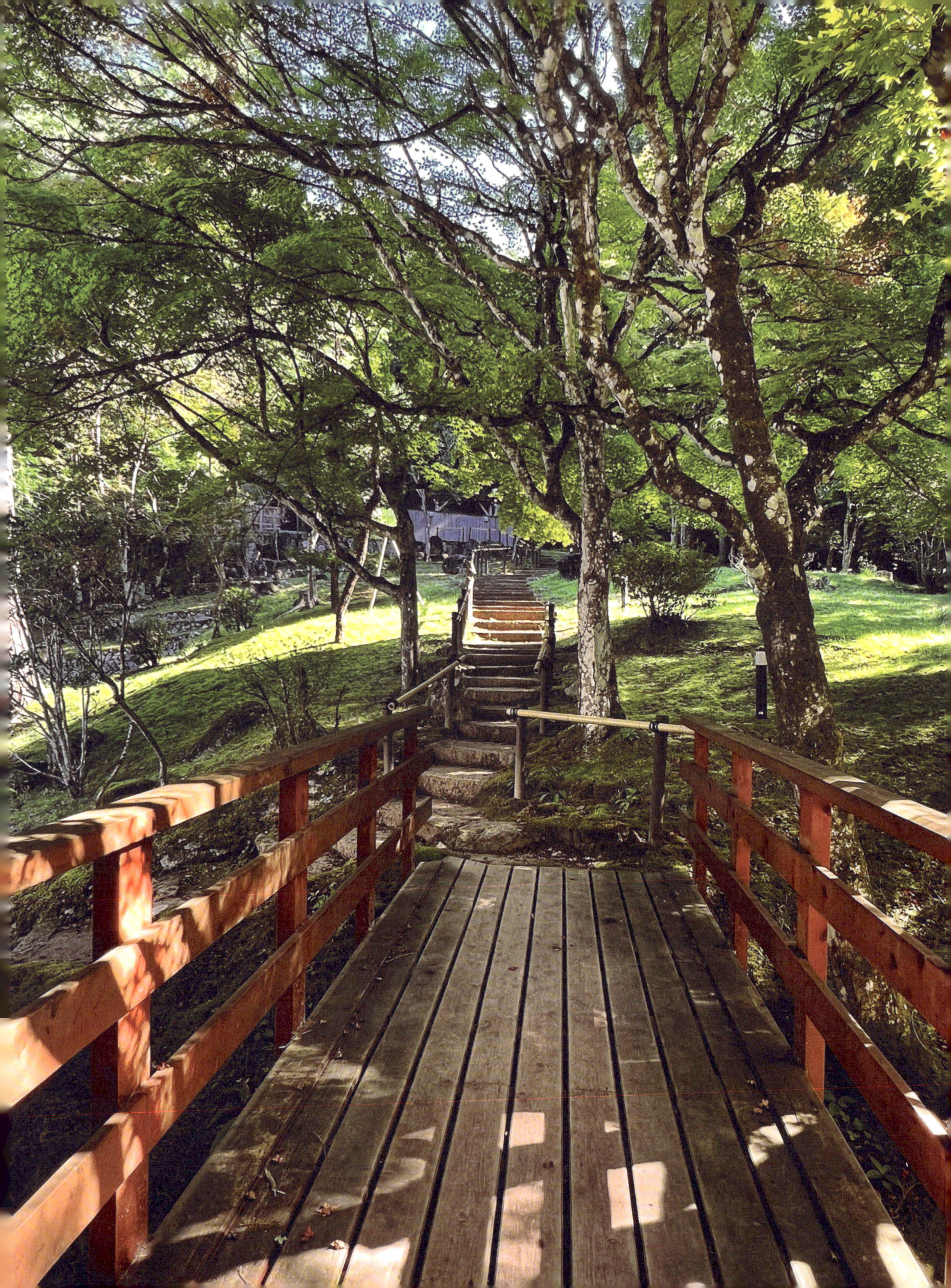

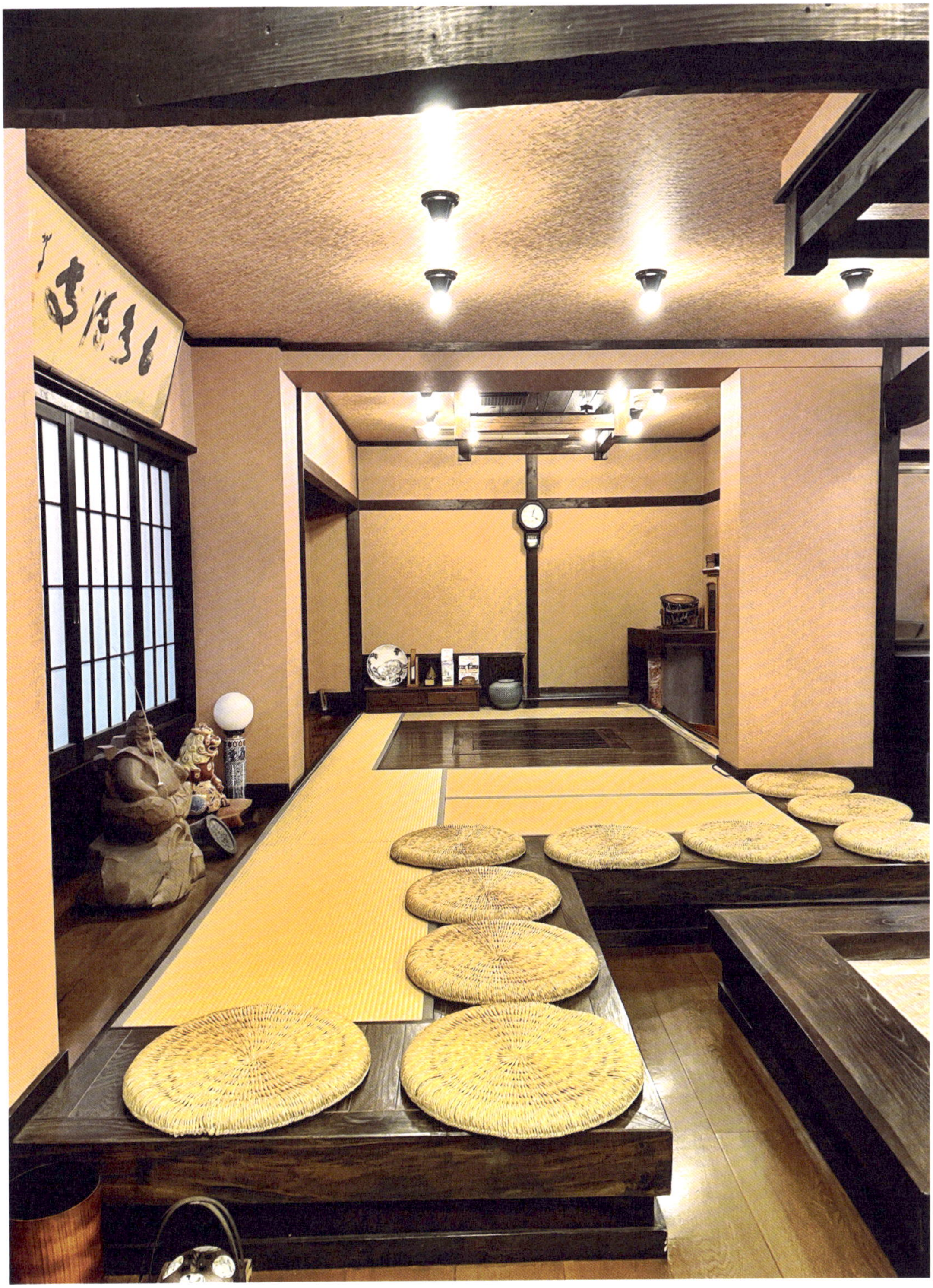

ABOVE Relax in the lobby's communal tea lounge, warmed by a traditional *irori* hearth.

Otani Sanso
Nagato • Yamaguchi Prefecture

UNWIND IN THE COMFORT OF THIS DISTINGUISHED ONSEN RYOKAN

Situated by the banks of the flowing Otozure River, welcoming rest areas and spacious rooms create a peaceful and serene environment.

Entering Otani Sanso's "Mountain Flowers" lobby transports one back to a world of old-school glamour and luxury. The room's towering ceilings, reaching to the second floor, create an open, atrium-like feel, further enhanced by the high, wide windows gazing out onto the calming waterfall garden. As guests check in, they are led to the comfortable, plush armchairs and served Japanese tea and seasonal sweets, setting their minds at ease as their bodies begin to relax. Many guests will stop by the lounge once more in the evening after their *kaiseki* feasts to enjoy a nightcap while listening to the nightly acoustic performances and admiring the evening waterfall illumination.

Established in 1881, the onsen ryokan was originally located opposite Nagato Yumoto's public onsen Onto and was thus called Otani-ya. For five generations, the Otani family has loyally guarded the history and legacy of the town, helping to ensure its preservation for future generations. Today, Otani Kazuhiro, the fifth-generation family head (*godaime*), is at the helm of this proud heritage and was the driving force behind reopening the doors to Onto after it closed in 2017. It was Otani's grandfather, in fact, who moved Otani-ya to its current location on the banks of the Otozure River and gave life to what is today known as Otani Sanso.

Situated by the Otozure's flowing waters, its location is perfect for appreciating the changing seasons, offering a sublime, peaceful environment in which to relax and unwind. Several rest areas are found within the building and its grounds, including a special Kawadoko River terrace right on the water.

Otani Sanso has several room varieties for visitors, but the most sublime are its 21 suites with private, open-air onsen, which feature either river or mountainside views. Spacious and modern, these elegant suites are the epitome of luxury and are even lovelier when viewing the wild, blooming sakura from the balcony or private onsen.

Onsen lovers will absolutely adore the wide variety of baths found within Otani Sanso's Seseragi no Yu and Komorebi no Yu—both public onsen. Each contains saunas, large indoor onsen with overflowing water, lovely nature views, and sleeping onsen baths. Seseragi no Yu also offers an indoor jacuzzi and two outdoor onsen, including a hinoki onsen and a rock *rotenburo;* in contrast, Komorebi no Yu offers an indoor herbal bath and a large, semi-open-air hinoki onsen that faces the mountainside.

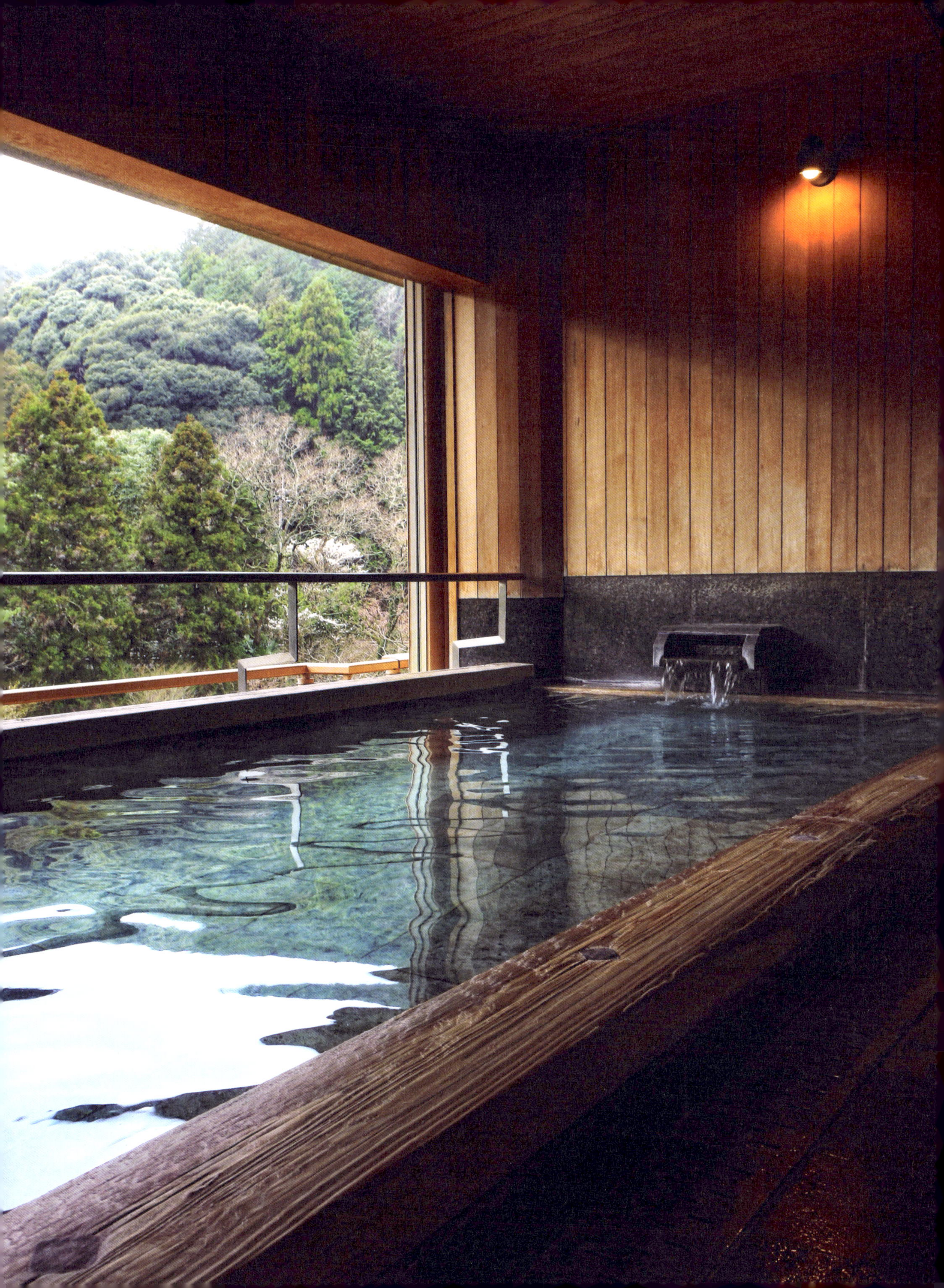

Gaga Onsen
Shibata • Miyagi Prefecture

EMBRACE THE ANCIENT PRACTICE OF ONSEN *TOJI*

In this remote setting, travelers are invited to partake in the wonders of onsen healing.

Gaga Onsen's single ryokan is nestled in a gorge beside a rushing river, deep in the mountains. It was once inhabited by Shugendō Buddhist monks practicing ascetic training upon Mt. Zao, the onsen's waters being close enough to the mountain's peak that the monks could recuperate in the healing onsen after their rigorous morning training.

A destination unto itself, the inn was officially established in 1875, and its first visitors were often physical laborers whose bodies needed rest and rejuvenation. Staying a couple of months or more, they would cook their own meals in the communal kitchen and bring their own bedding, as facilities were rudimentary. Eventually, Gaga Onsen evolved to provide meals, comfortable rooms, and other accommodations to their guests. The site is widely considered one of Japan's top three onsen for the treatment of stomach-related illnesses—one can pour the onsen water continuously over the body (traditionally 100 times) to warm up the stomach and accelerate metabolism, drink the onsen water, or simply absorb its healing properties by soaking.

Helmed by the same family since 1875, it is currently run by sixth-generation owner Takeuchi-san, who has renovated his family's inn to reflect his own personal taste and to create a homey ambiance that maximizes the comfort and relaxation of his guests, eschewing the often stiff formality found in other luxury onsen ryokan.

A cozy, mountain-lodge atmosphere defines the lobby, with its plush chairs and snug nooks surrounding the crackling fireplace, while the guest rooms exude a quiet and elegant tranquility. With both traditional and modern touches, and wide windows offering generous views of the surrounding nature, these tatami rooms are the perfect peaceful getaway.

Proudly carrying on the tradition of the healing practice of *toji*, Gaga Onsen features five different types of onsen, using pure *gensen kakenagashi* (continuously flowing onsen water) direct from the source. The gender-separated onsen have both indoor and outdoor baths, while nearby, an exceptionally picturesque mixed open-air onsen stretches along the river. One can also relax in the rustic open-air onsen Tenku no Yu, created so guests can enjoy the clear night skies and the sounds of the river flowing below.

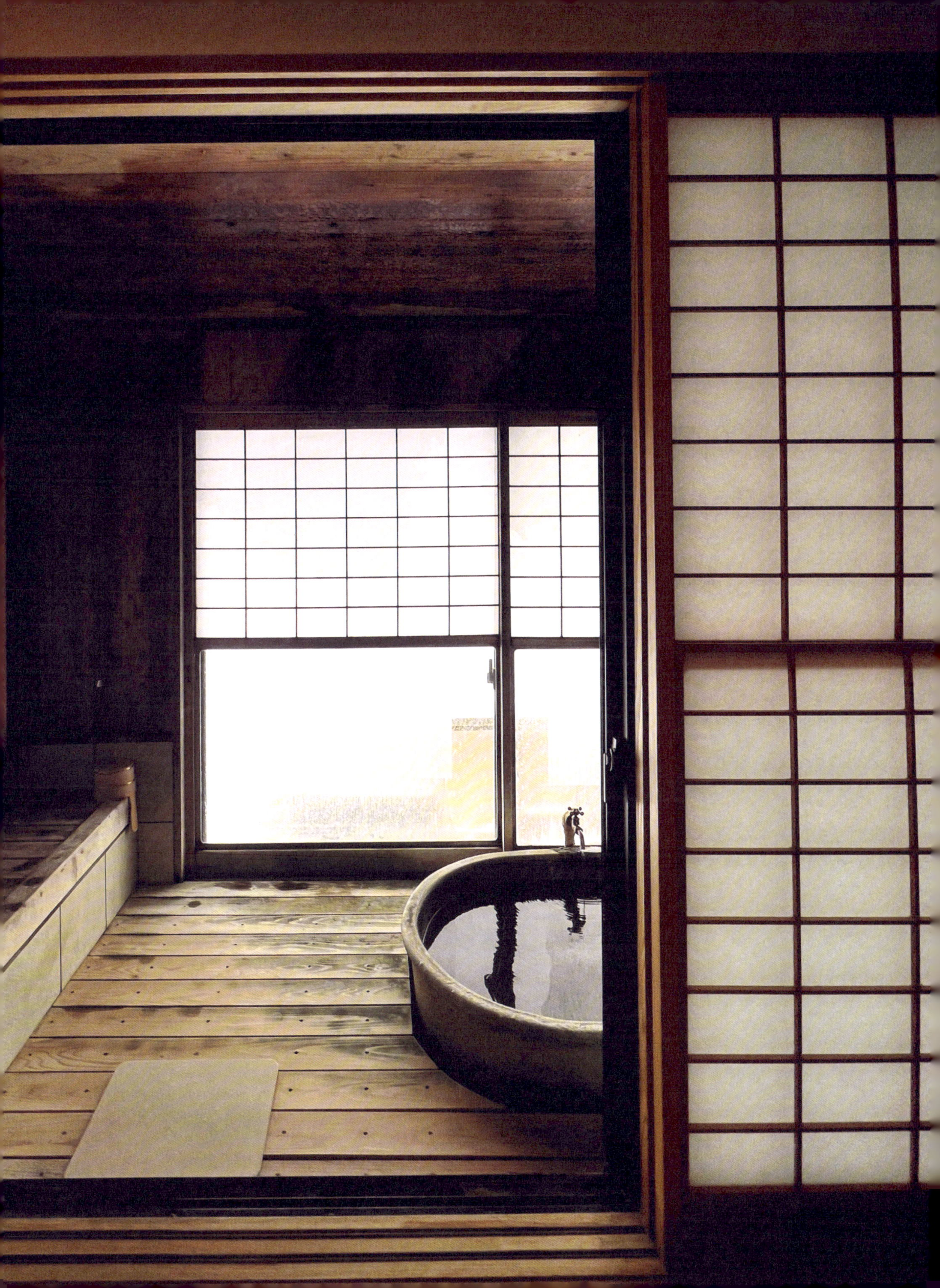

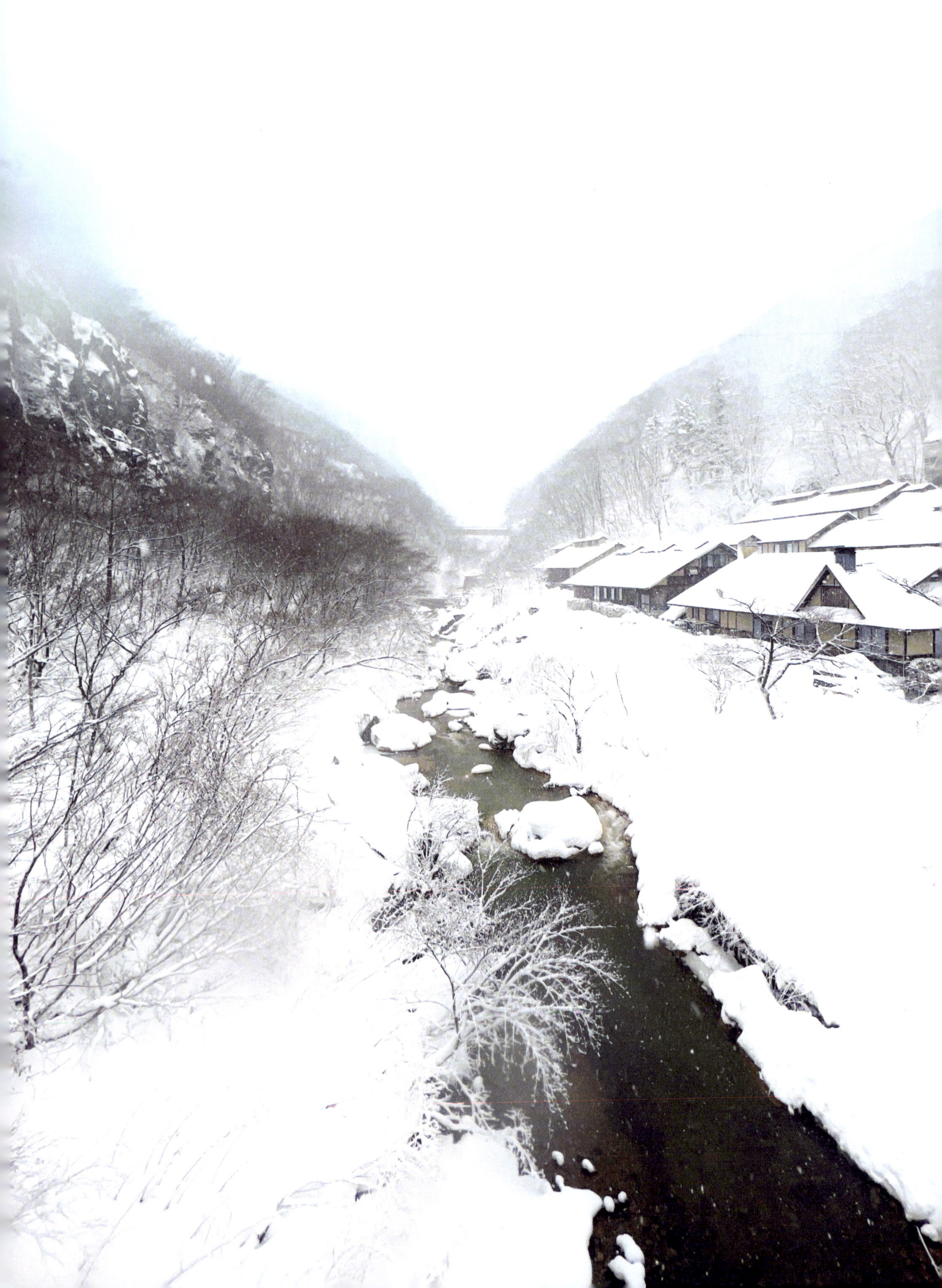

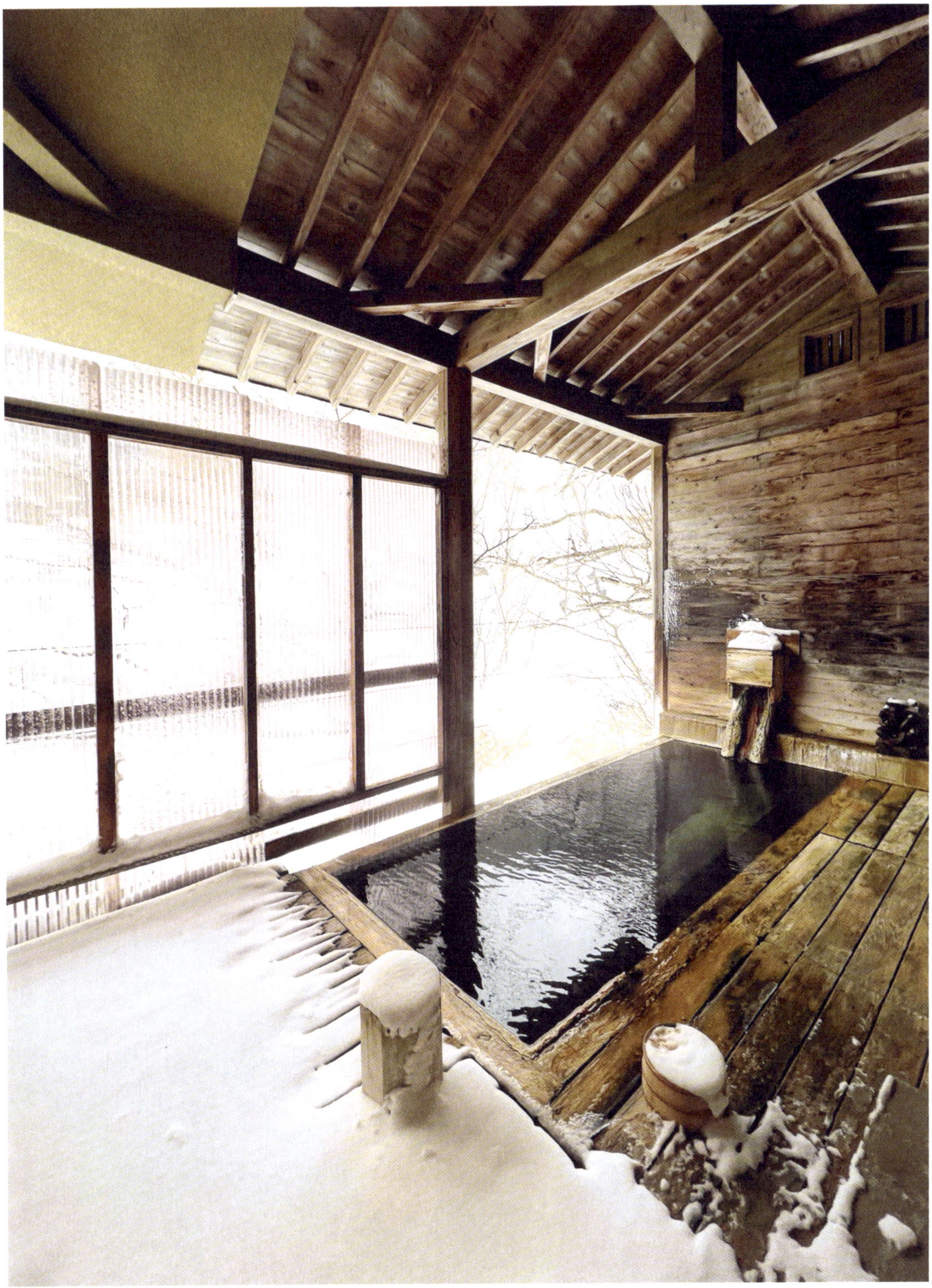

ABOVE Gaga Onsen's Tenku no Yu is a private onsen situated in a standalone building.

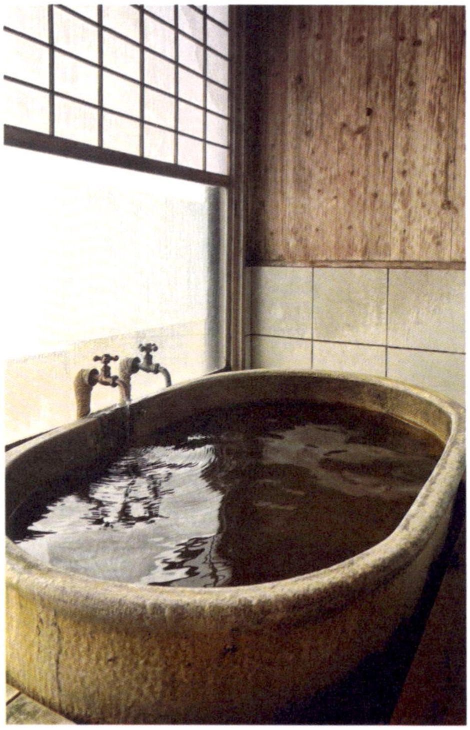

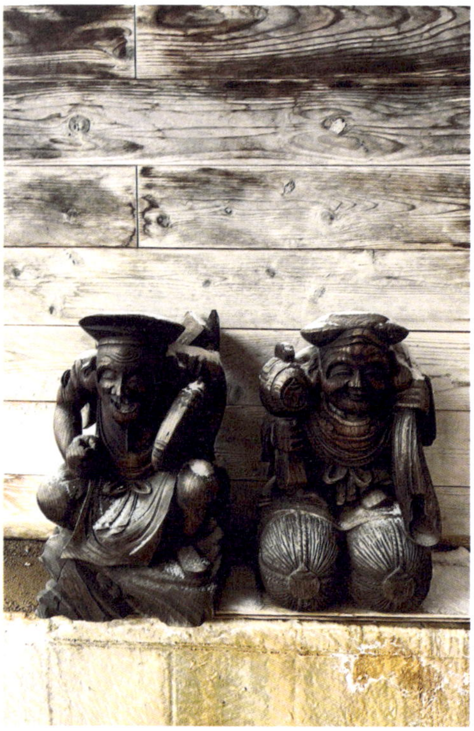

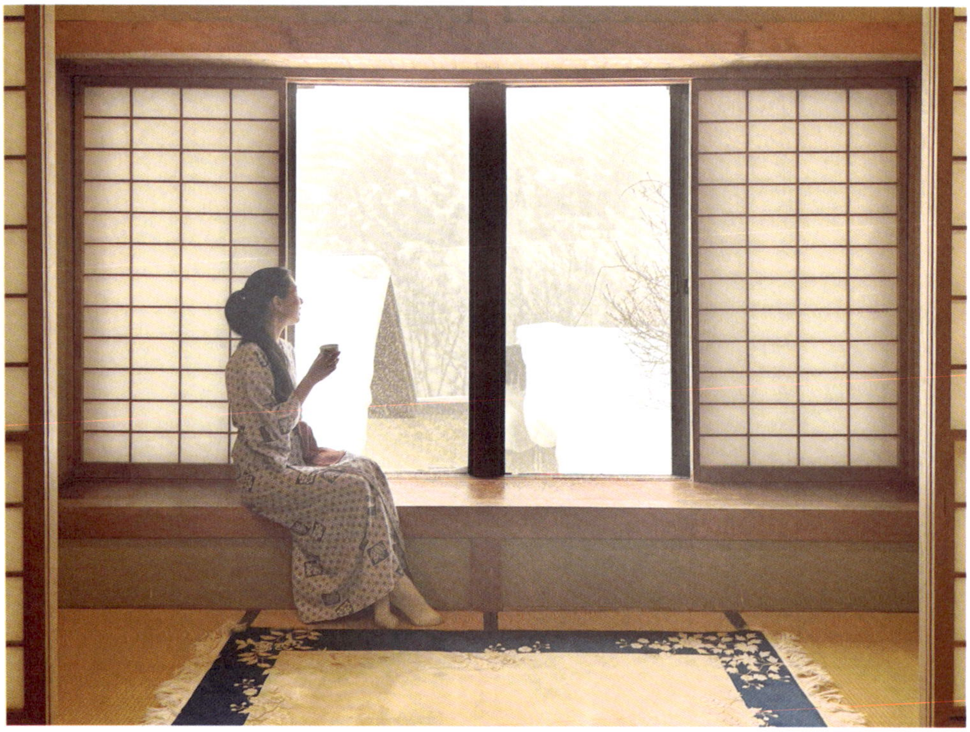

ABOVE Appreciate the quiet solitude of the spacious, wide-windowed rooms.

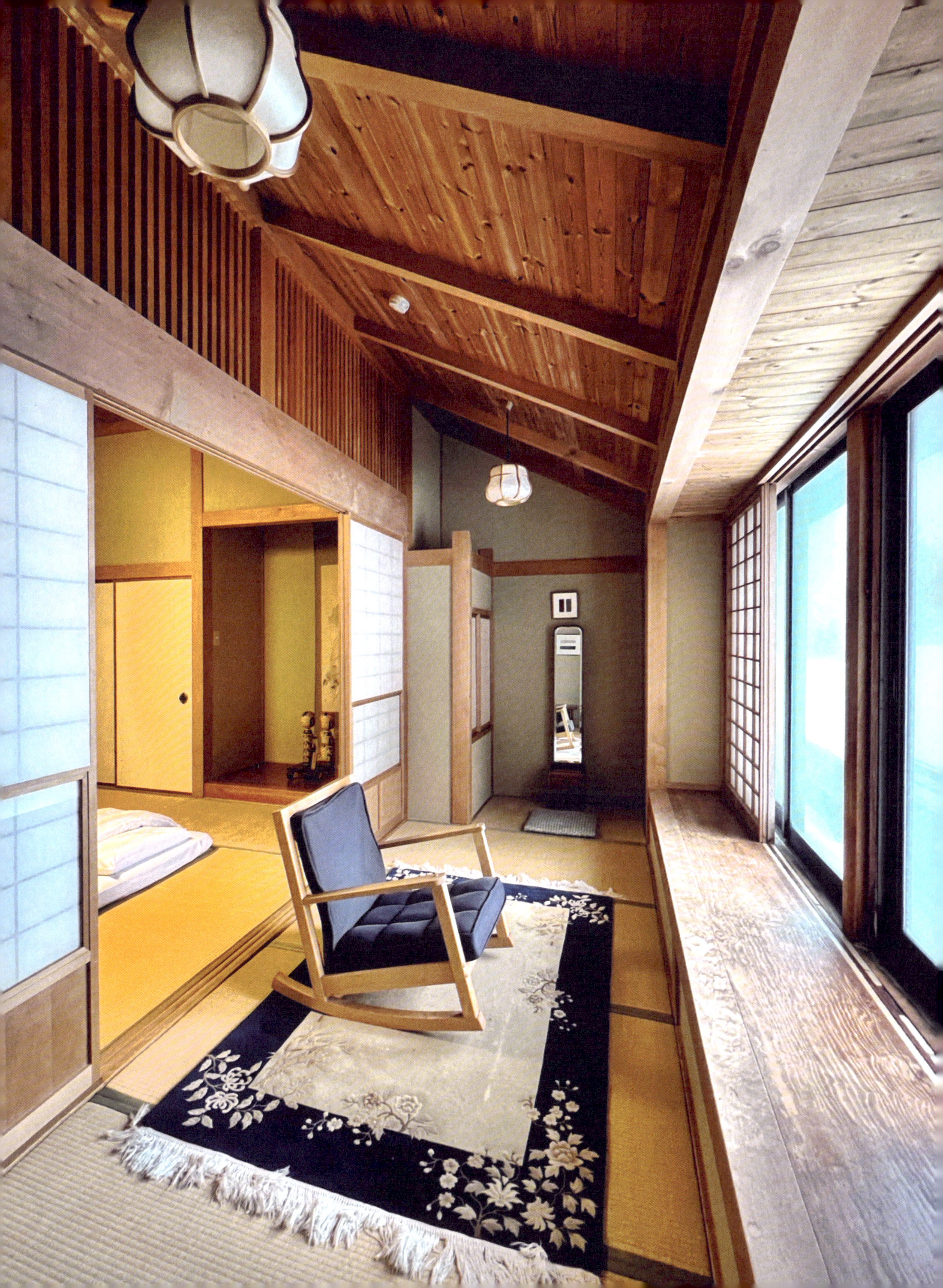

Maguse Onsen
Kijimadaira Village • Nagano Prefecture

RELAX IN AN ONSEN OVERLOOKING THE MOUNTAINS

A mini road trip through the peaceful countryside and up along winding mountain roads leads to this much-loved outdoor onsen.

One of the largest prefectures in the country, Nagano is home to vast areas of breathtaking nature, including a stretch of the stunning Japanese Alps. An outdoor enthusiast's dream, Nagano is beloved for its many mountain hiking trails, winter snow sports, pure water, and numerous remote onsen.

Set inside the scenic Maguse Hot Spring Park in Ogo, Kijimadaira Village, Maguse Onsen is a day-use-only destination, accessible most easily via car or taxi. The drive up the winding roads to Maguse gives visitors an inspired display of rural countryside life you'll pass numerous terraced rice fields, apple orchards, and groups of children making their way to and from school.

Maguse Onsen first opened its baths in 1987, and in the 2024 Hot Spring General Election, it was voted the best onsen in the central Chūbu region. For lovers of pure onsen, Maguse's waters are categorized as *gensen kakenagashi,* as they flow directly from the onsen source and are not regulated for temperature or recycled. Maguse derives its name from the kanji characters for "horse" and "turns," as the original road to Maguse was full of sharp ascents and treacherous switchbacks. It is also aptly named, as the spirit of the local Kannon deity is said to be a horse that looks after weary travelers.

Recently renovated, the premises are a perfect place to while away a morning or afternoon, either in the indoor rest area, where one can enjoy local ice cream, or on the outdoor observation terrace, where multiple seating areas offer a place to enjoy the incredible beauty of the northern Nagano seasons.

Most guests, however, will want to seek immediate immersion in Maguse's soothing onsen waters, both in the indoor hinoki onsen or outdoor stone *rotenburo,* which is a favorite of most visitors. A large, spacious outdoor onsen, the *rotenburo* offers breathtaking views of Nagano City with the Northern Alps (part of the Hida Mountain range) in the distance, framed by lush trees and foliage. The hardest decision one faces at Maguse is simply in which season to visit—during the verdant spring and summer, the crisp and reflective fall, or the white, snow-graced winter.

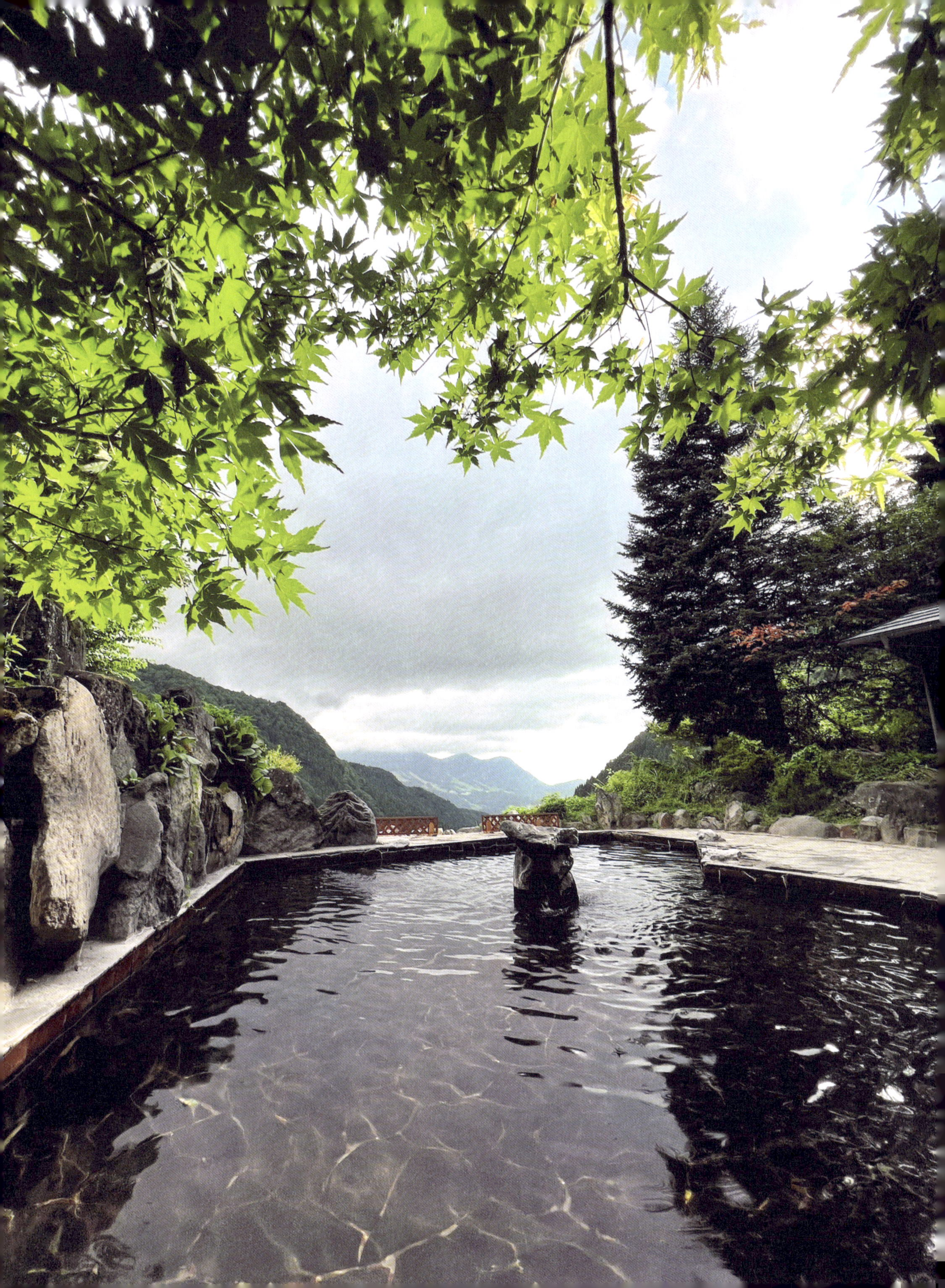

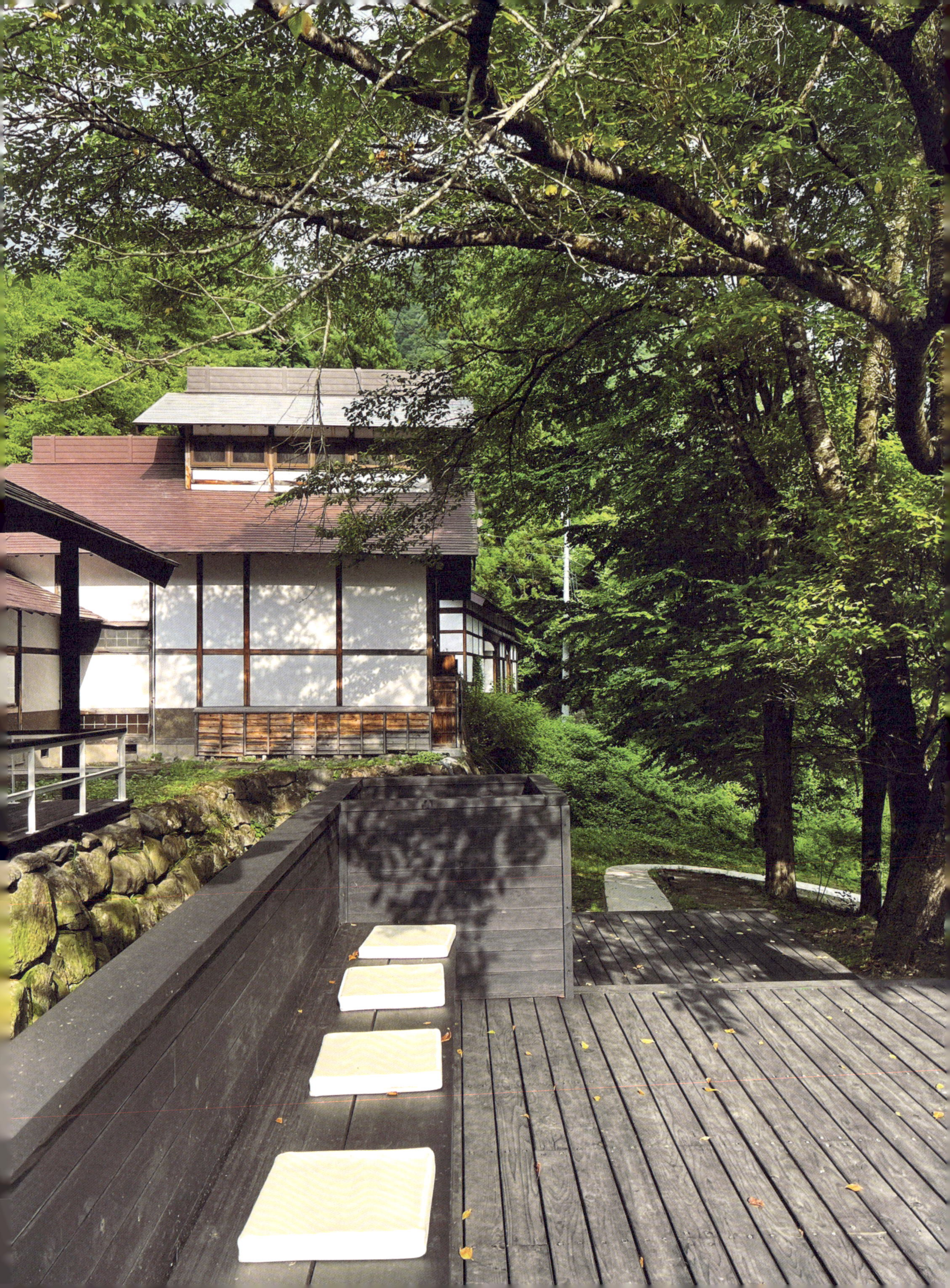

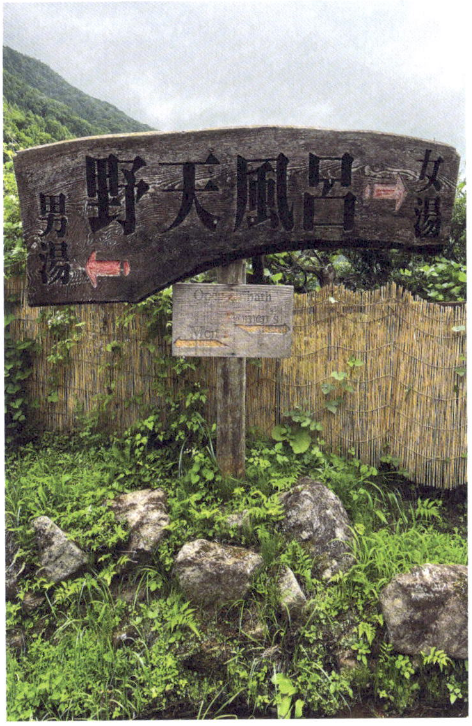

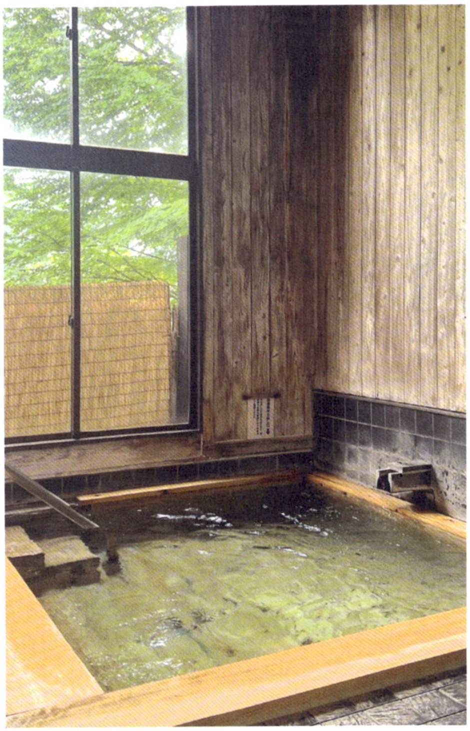
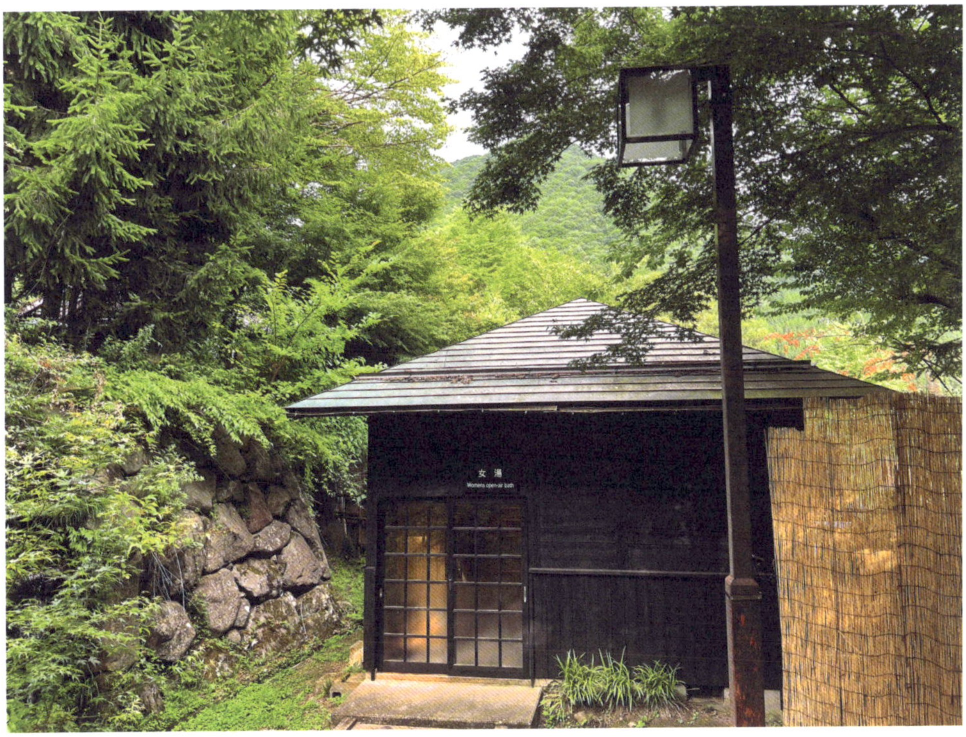

LEFT After bathing, enjoy the wooden outdoor terrace of Maguse Onsen.

Misasa Onsen
Misasa • Tottori Prefecture

SOME OF THE WORLD'S RAREST ONSEN WATERS

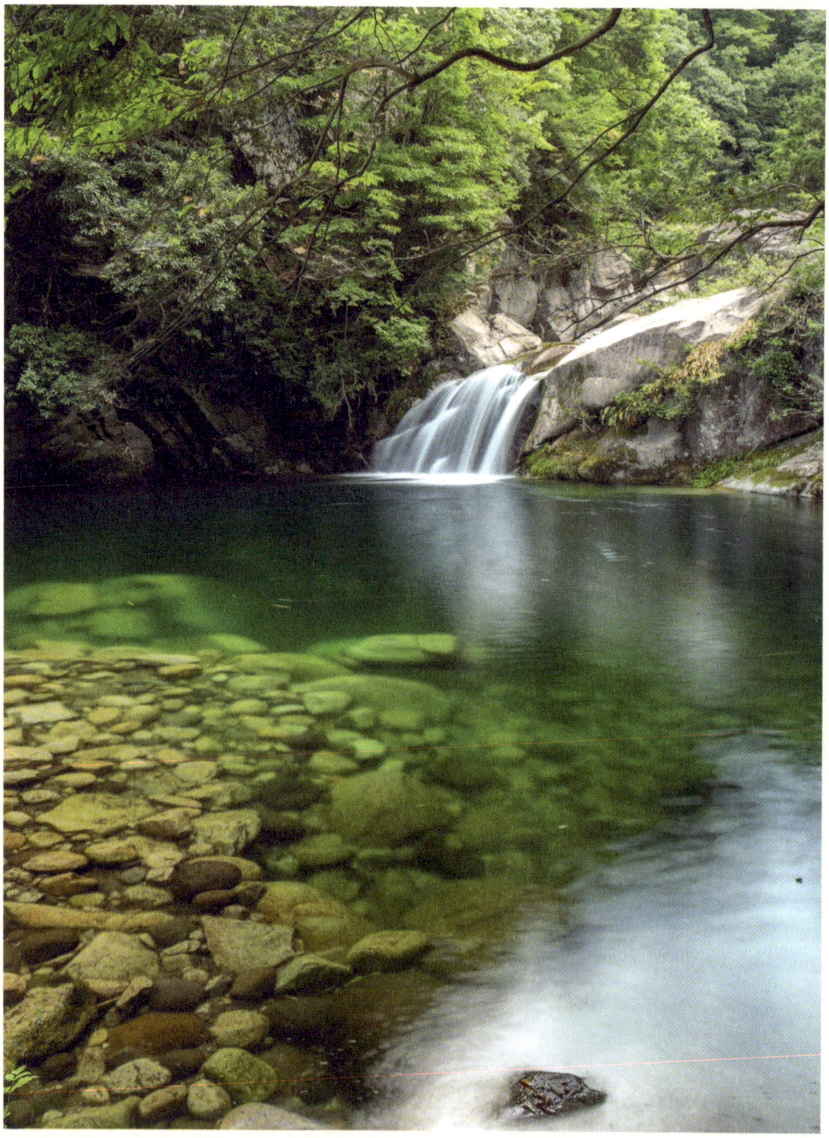

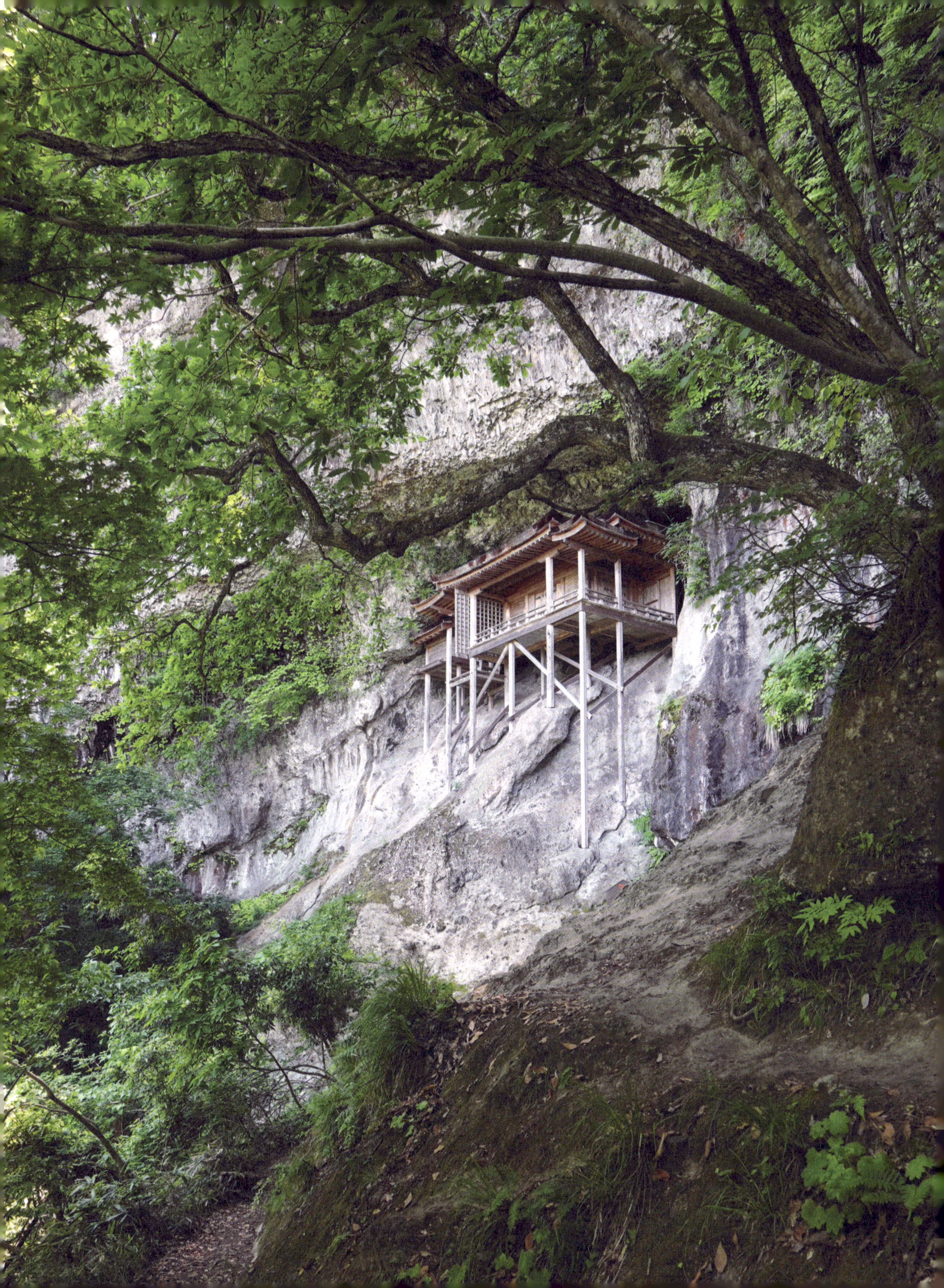

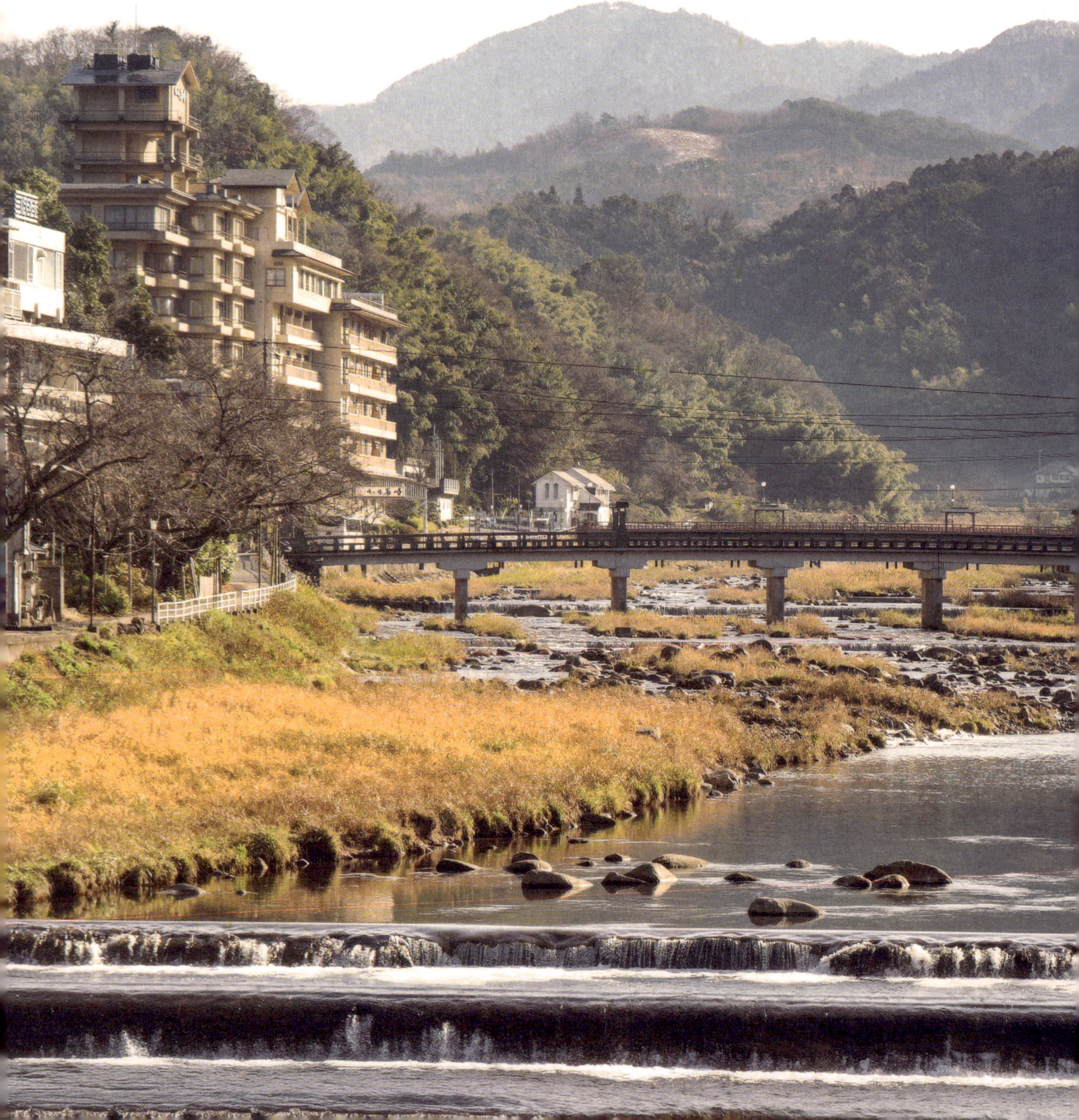

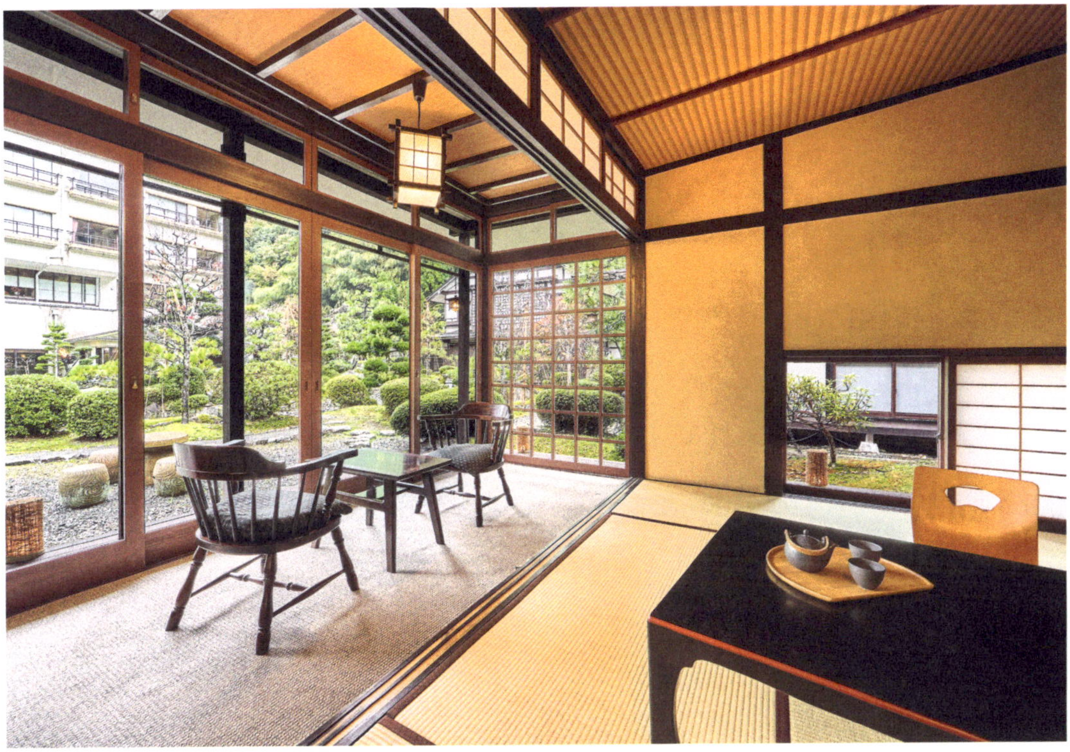

LEFT Meander across one of Misasa's three bridges to take in the full beauty of the landscape.

Soak in the therapeutic, radon-rich waters, and delve deep into a history rich with lore, national treasures, and breathtaking nature.

A captivating tale from the Heian period tells of samurai Okubo Samanosuke, who came across an elderly white wolf under a camphor tree. Okubo-san believed it would be an act of disrespect to take a wolf's life, as it could possibly be an incarnation of a god, so he let it live as he continued on his pilgrimage. As he slept, the great Buddha Myokan Daibosatu visited him in his dream and informed the samurai, in gratitude for his act of kindness and mercy, that the camphor tree held an onsen source beneath it. Once he awoke, Okubo-san conveyed the whereabouts of the onsen spring to the villagers who, after soaking in the water, were cured of many illnesses.

The ancient camphor tree from the tale still exists today. From beneath its roots flows the town's original onsen source. The public onsen Kabuyu, with its onsen drinking spring, has been constructed around this same tree. It is believed that drinking the mineral-rich onsen water has a cleansing effect and promotes better health, especially in the digestive tract.

Misasa Onsen is one of the most radioactive onsen in the world, which is curiously part of its allure. The waters hold a high concentration of radon (although not levels harmful to the human body), which, according to the theory of hormesis, activates the body's metabolism, enhances immunity, and prevents aging and other lifestyle-related diseases. This radon is created by the decomposition of uranium, producing a very weak radiation that stimulates cells throughout the body and promotes its natural functions.

Equally important and closely intertwined with Misasa is the sacred mountain Mt. Mitoku, which is deeply tied to the esoteric Shugendō faith (a blending

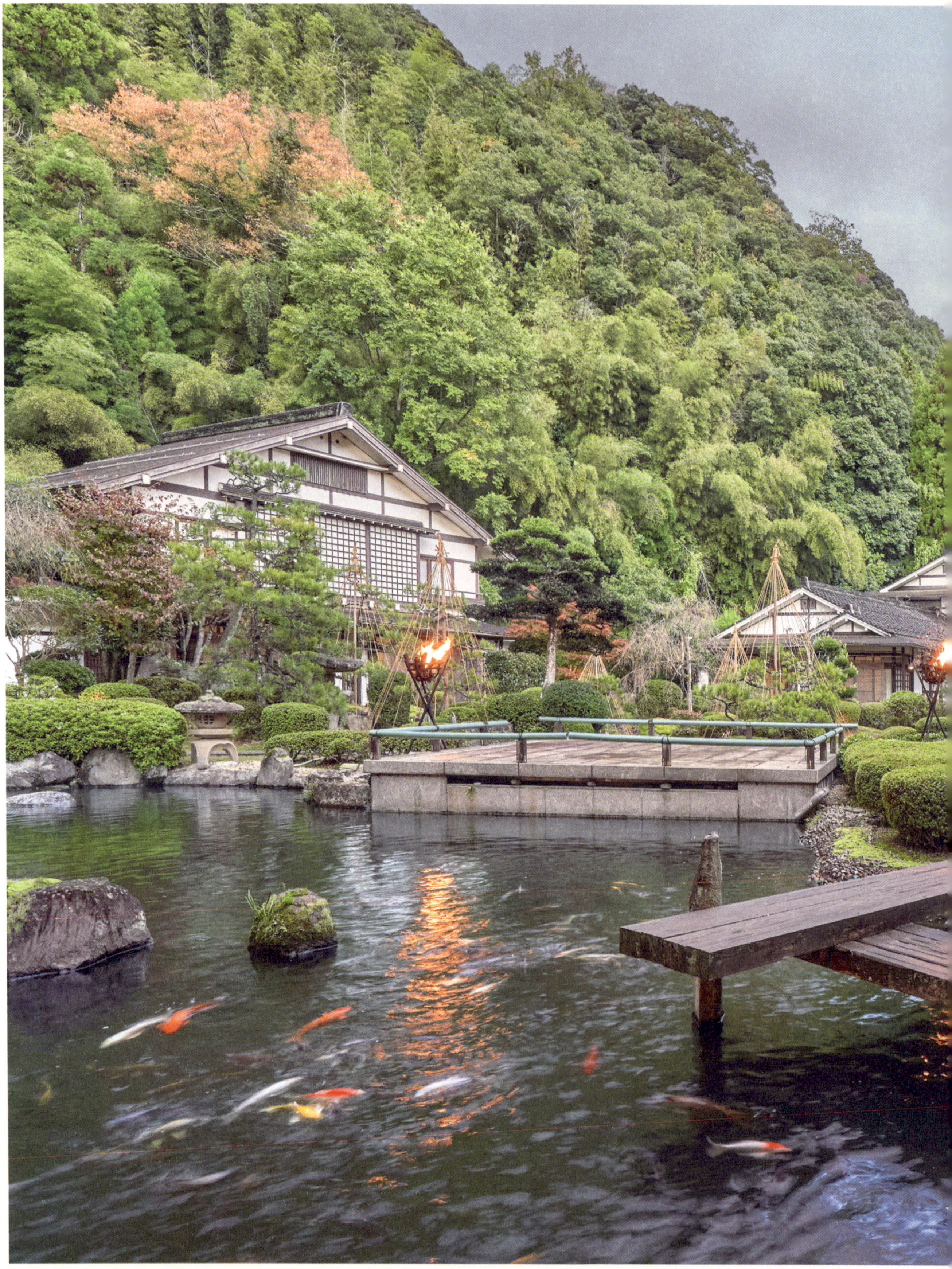

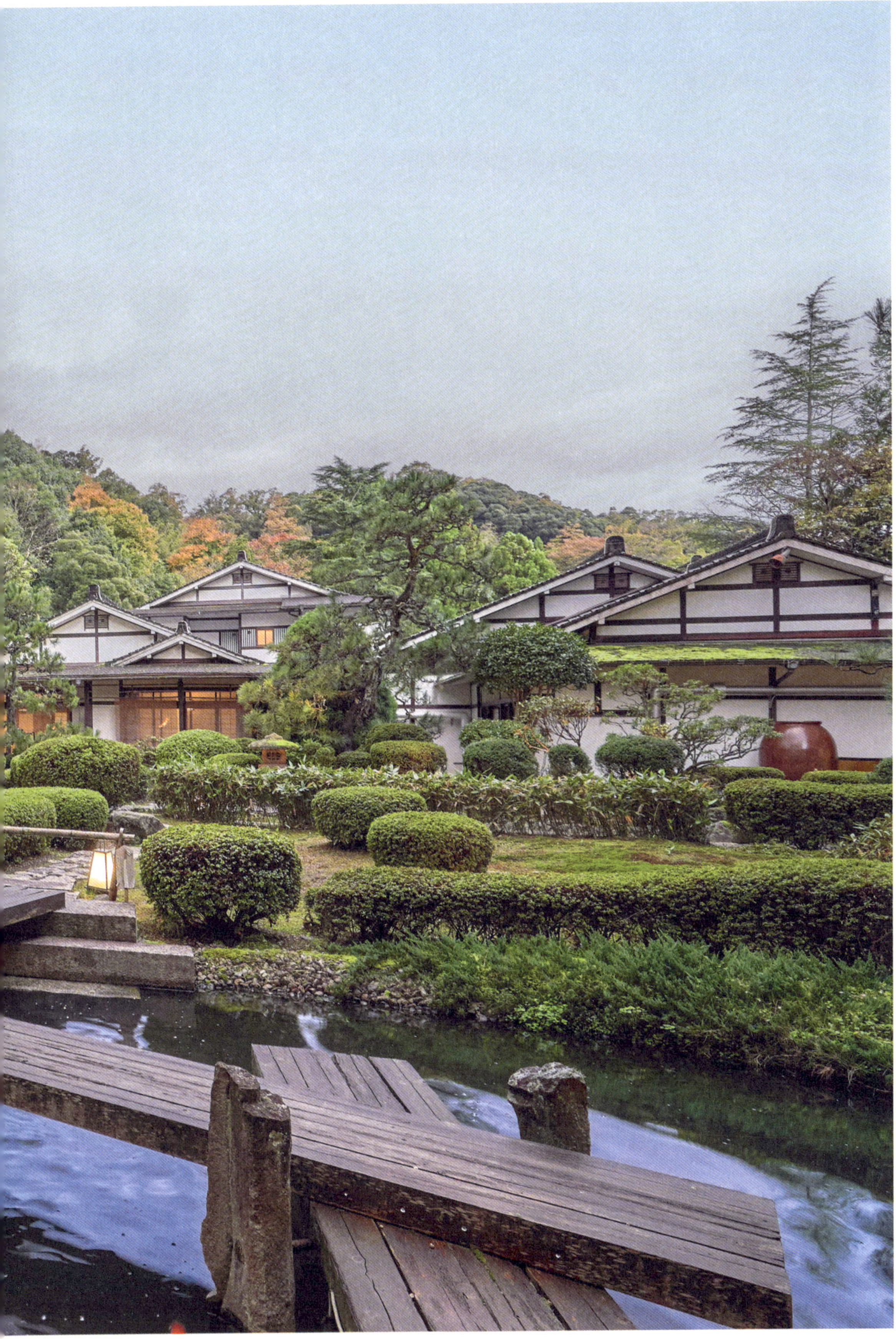

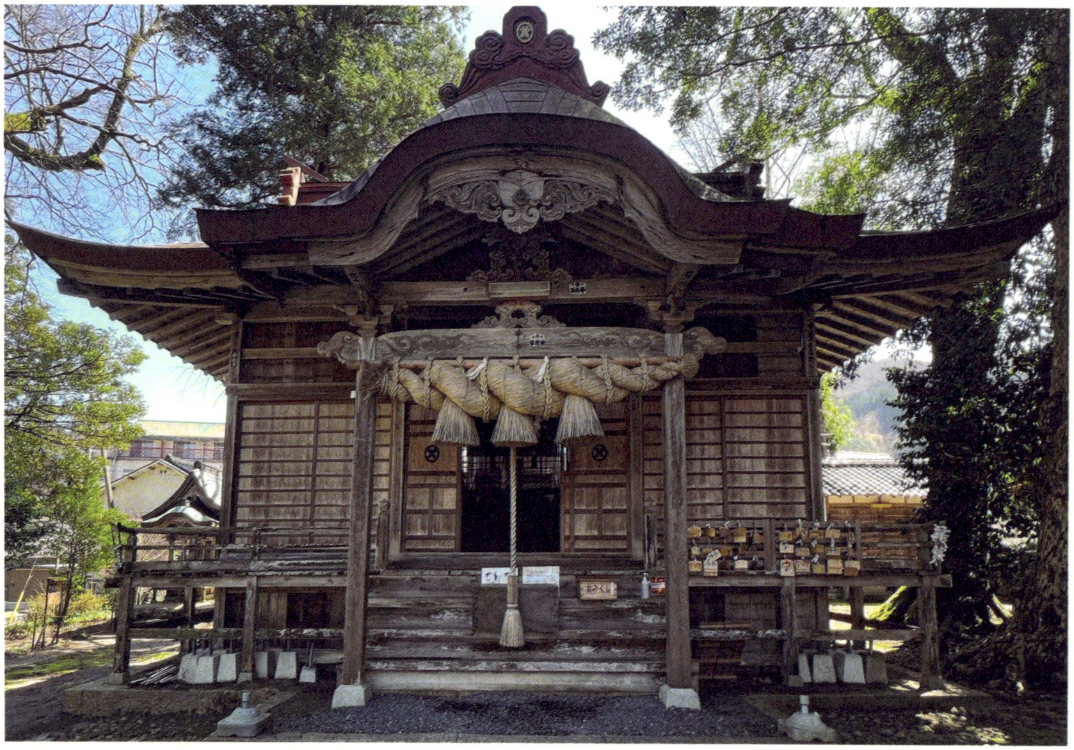

ABOVE Take the time to visit Misasa Shrine, whose deity guards Misasa Onsen.

of Buddhism, Taoism, Shinto, and mountain worship). Roughly 1,300 years ago, the founder of Shugendō, En no Gyōja, threw three lotus petals into the air so that they "should fly down to places related to gods and Buddhas." It is said that one landed at Yoshino in Nara Prefecture, another in Ishizuchiyama in Ehime Prefecture, and the last at Mt. Mitoku.

No visit to Misasa Onsen is complete without hiking up Mt. Mitoku on a sacred pilgrimage to its temple complex that culminates in the beloved Nageiredō Hall. The complex is built inside a cave on the mountain cliff and it is believed that using the power of Buddhism and Shugendō, En no Gyōja threw the temple into the mountain cave, hence its name Nageiredō (thrown-in temple).

The pilgrimage is slightly perilous, as one must clamber over giant tree roots, boulders, and sharp rock ridges to reach Nageiredō. The journey requires calm strength, heightened awareness, and intense focus, and this struggle is known as the "way of the ascetics." To begin the pilgrimage in one's purest form, Shugendō beliefs dictate that one should first bathe in Misasa's onsen waters, cleansing one's spirit before attempting the sacred ascension up Mt. Mitoku. Once the temple complex has been reached and the descent is completed, one should bathe once more in the healing onsen. In Misasa, it is recommended to bathe for at least three mornings, in keeping with the town's namesake. This practice embraces the ideas of *rokkan chiyu* (healing of the six senses) and *rokkon shojo* (purification of the six roots of perception), both of which are fundamental to Mt. Mitoku and Misasa Onsen.

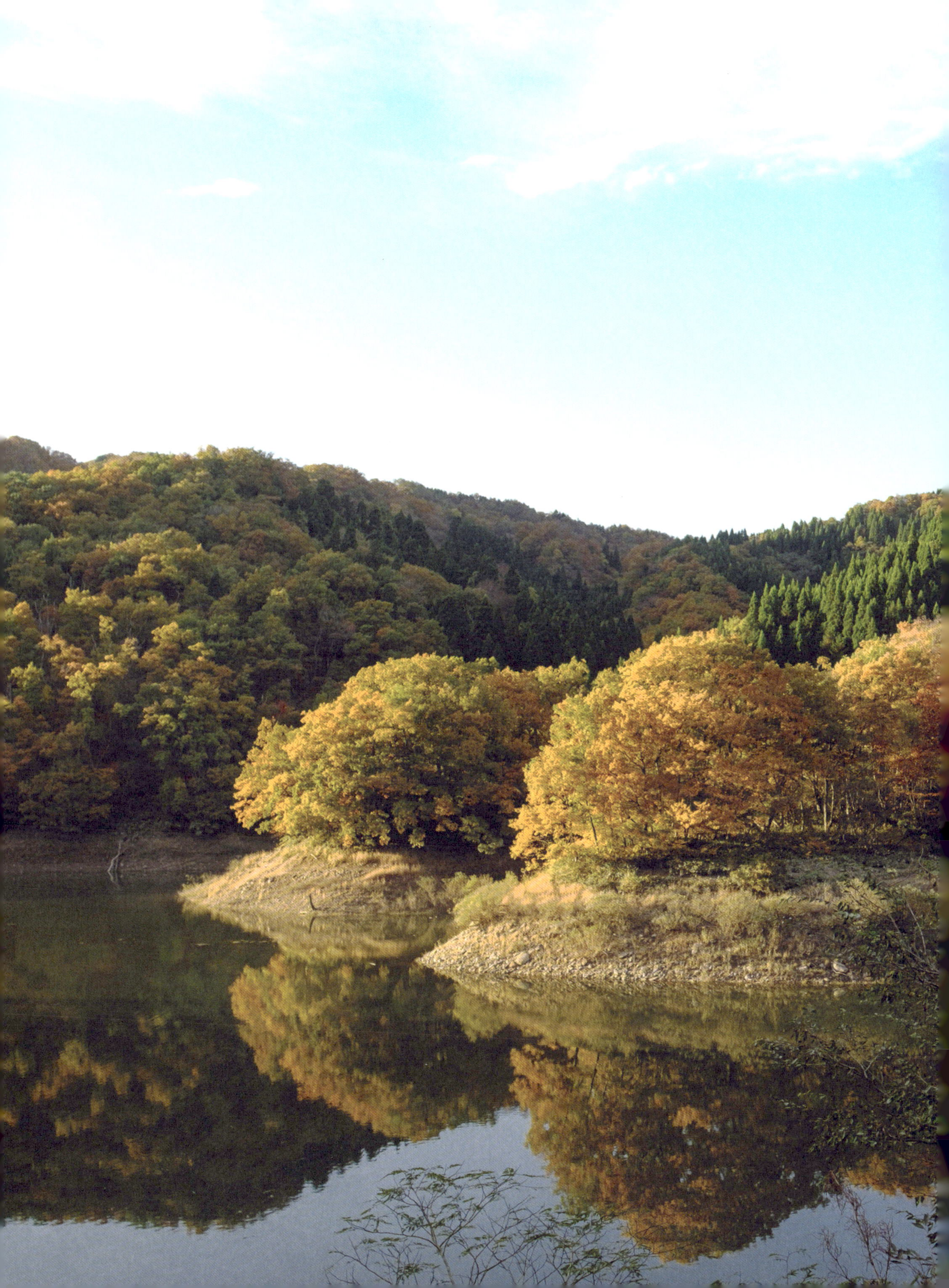

Ryokan Sanga
Miaminoguni • Kumamoto Prefecture

REVITALIZE THE SPIRIT IN THIS FOREST ABODE

Sequestered amid lush mountain scenery, this peaceful retreat provides an ideal opportunity to practice *shinrin-yoku.*

At Kurokawa, a beloved onsen town situated in the mountains of Kumamoto Prefecture, a multitude of onsen ryokan provide accommodations for visitors. One of the loveliest of these is Ryokan Sanga, which is a little further up the mountain from the town's center, found by following along the forested mountain stream until the first glimpses of this traditional abode appears.

Hidden amid the trees, the ryokan has a historic, folk-like style—wooden buildings with *kawara* tile roofs and earthy, sandy-hued walls—that blends effortlessly with the natural environment. The main building is lit from within with warm, soft light; inside, guests will find a cozy lobby and lounge area, where dark, wooden interiors are enhanced by antiques, handmade decor, and an *irori* hearth. Comfortable tatami rooms featuring spacious *engawa* are located in the main building, while several more luxurious, private villas dot the grounds. These villas are spacious, with multiple tatami rooms decorated with beautiful antique treasures, and feature their own private open-air onsen, indoor onsen, or both—perfect for those traveling in larger groups or in search of private bathing. All provide a serene, tranquil space to relax and unwind while experiencing the very best of *omotenashi.* And with only 15 rooms available, one is bound to have an intimate, singular experience.

The onsen water of Ryokan Sanga is drawn from two sources: a medicinal onsen that has been used for generations and a newer onsen, whose source is more alkaline and said to beautify the skin. Wander down in the provided *yukata* to the grounds, crossing straw-covered paths (in winter) en route to a dip in the glorious outdoor *rotenburo,* which is found by the river amid the trees. Moyai no Yu is for male guests, whereas Shiki no Yu is for women—both have their own indoor onsen, Yakushi no Yu.

Another wonderful feature of Ryokan Sanga is the three *kashikiri*—private onsen baths freely available for staying guests. Two are private indoor onsen, one of hinoki cypress and the other of cut stone. To reach the third, one crosses a small bridge over a babbling stream, then heads up a tiny hill where a marvelous (and huge) Shigaraki pottery bath sits, offering views of the river and seasonal foliage.

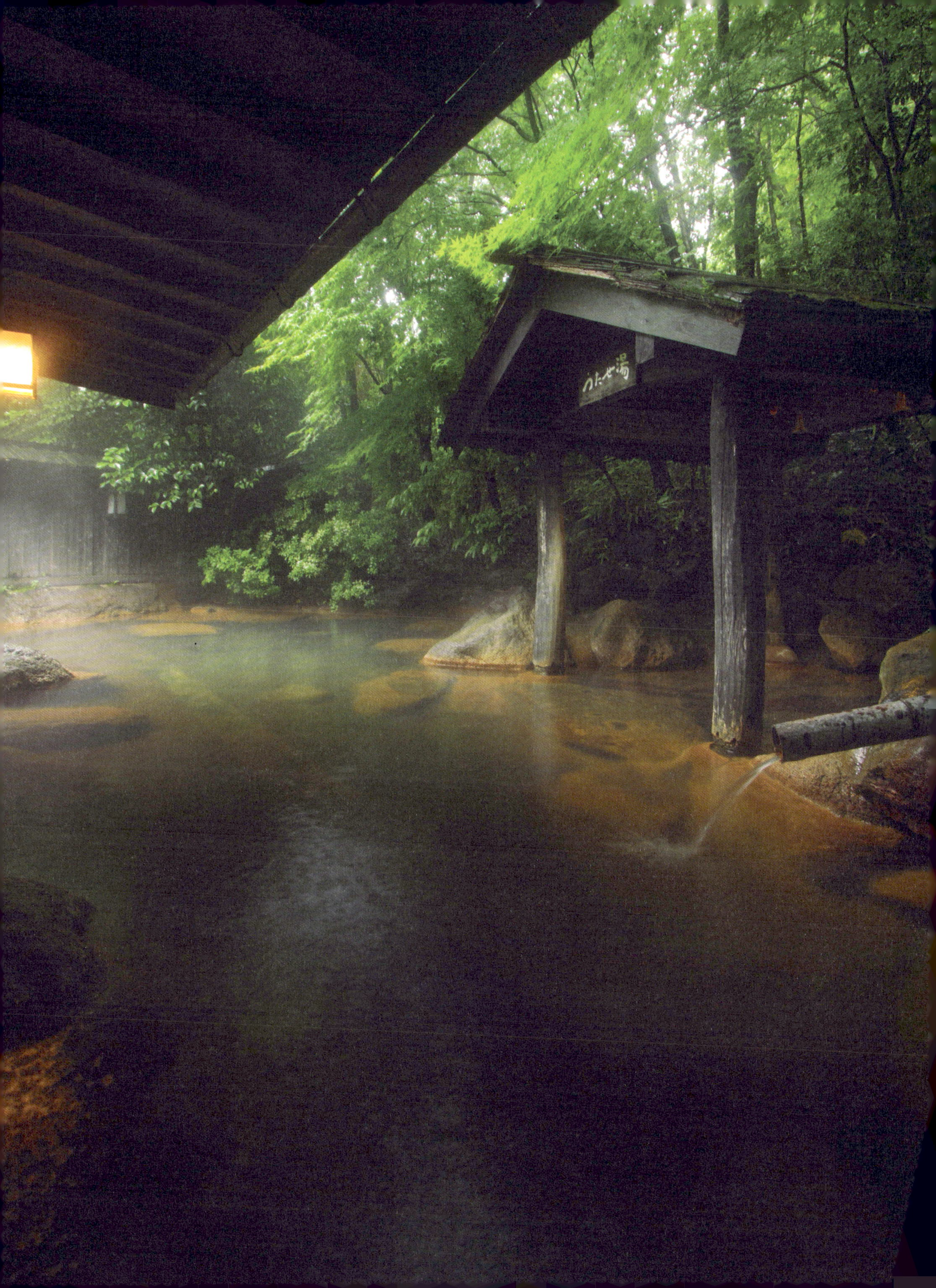
うたせ湯

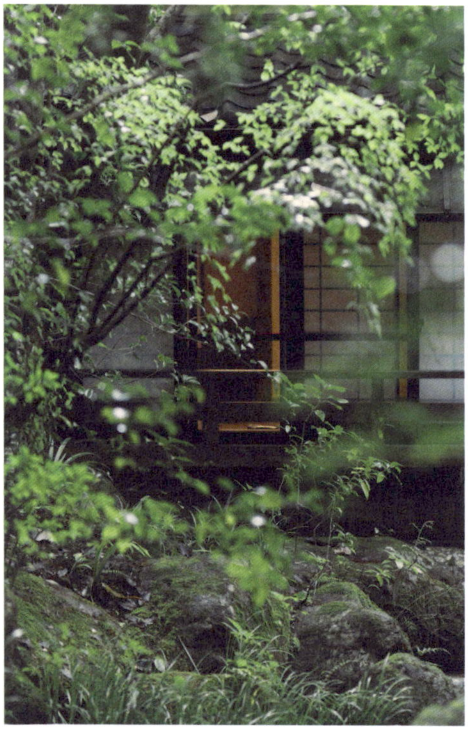

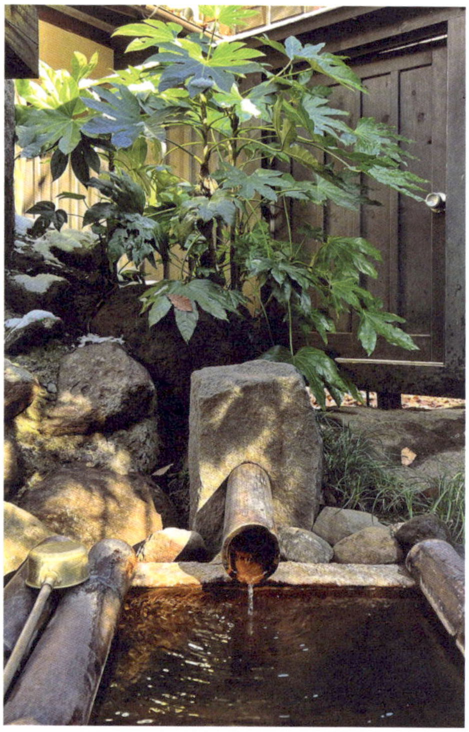

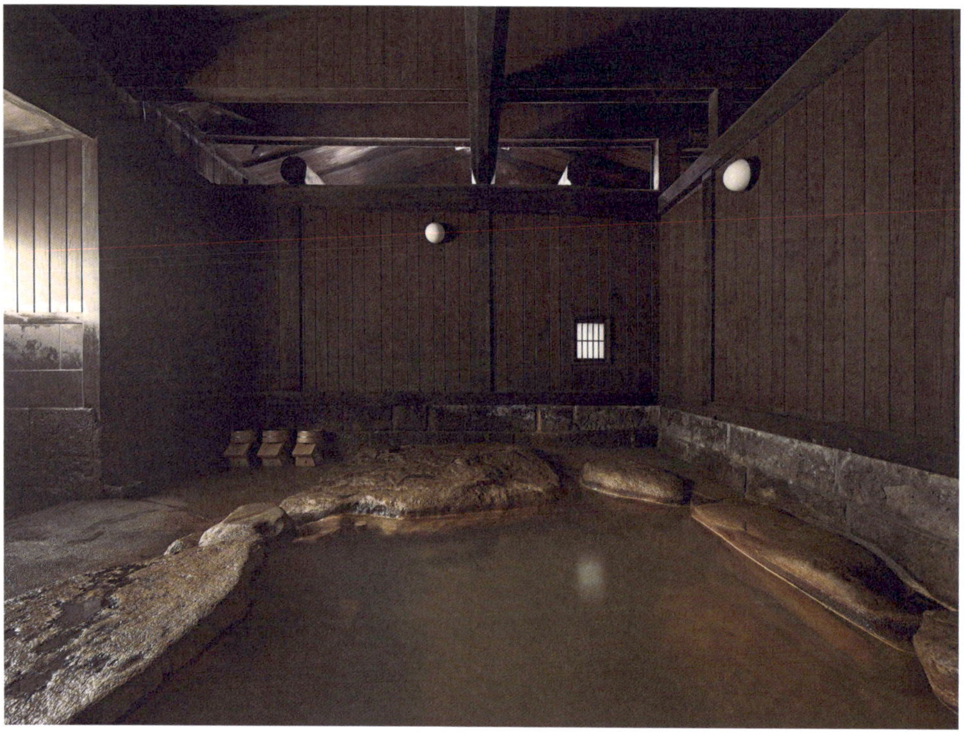

RIGHT Light and shadow delightfully combine in the tatami rooms of Ryokan Sanga.

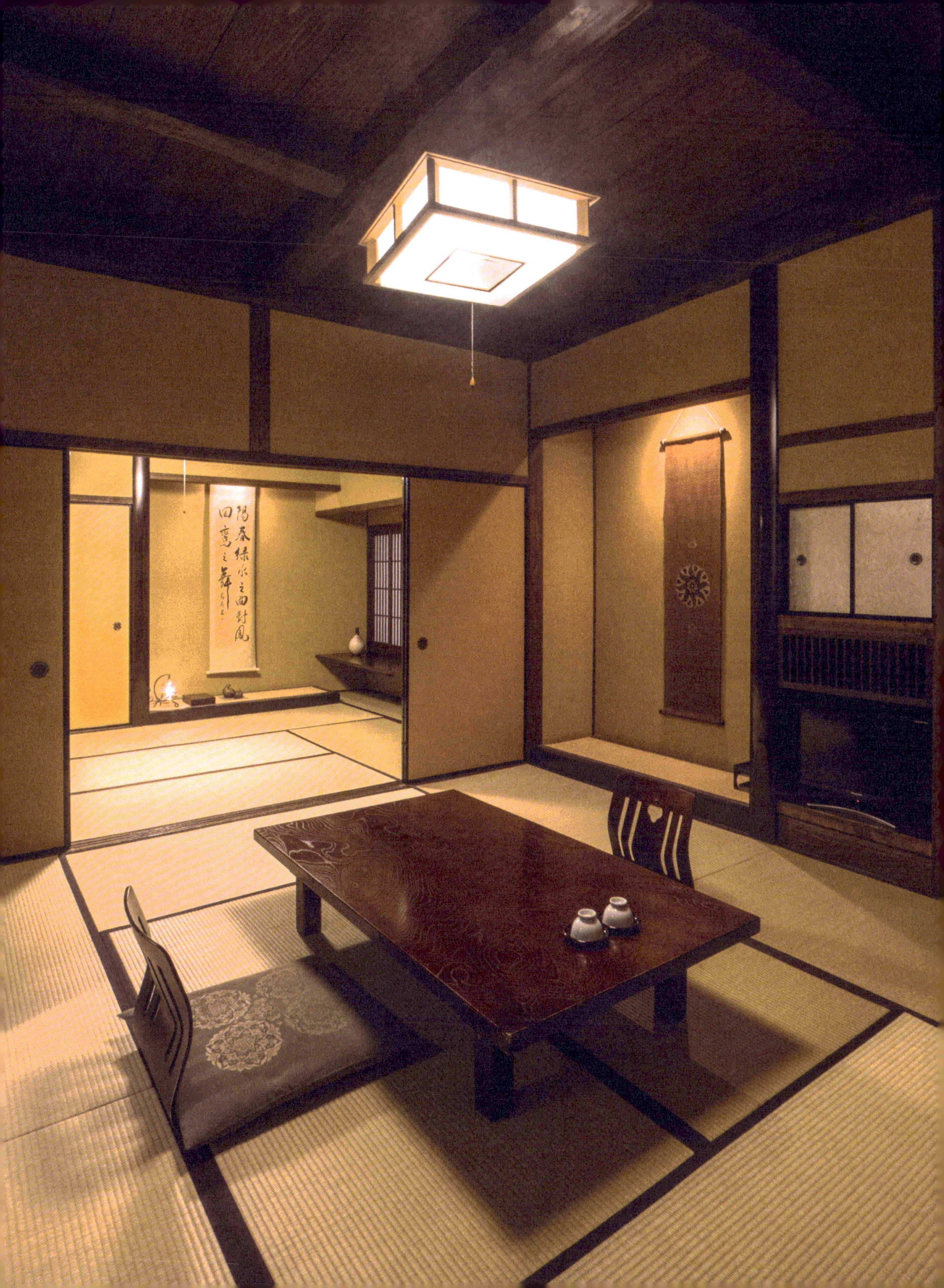

Isaribi

Okawa • Shizuoka Prefecture

ENJOY A BLISSFUL INTERLUDE BY THE WATER

The sea's relaxing sounds and refreshing salty scent drift gently up to this small onsen ryokan in a charming oceanside village.

The notion that one should, on occasion, spend time doing absolutely nothing finds its perfect, peaceful expression at Isaribi ryokan. A tiny, quiet seaside village on the Izu Peninsula, Okawa is found at the peninsula's midpoint, in an area blessed with delightful views of the sea and an overflow of pastoral beauty. The journey to Okawa, either via express or local train, is a slow adventure unto itself, as you pass from an urban landscape to a rural countryside of rice paddies, countless trees, glimpses of Mt. Fuji, and ocean views.

Established in 1970, Isaribi Ryokan is a peaceful adults-only inn with 12 rooms, all featuring pleasing views of the region's beloved Sagami Bay from their own private, open-air onsen baths. Named after the golden fires that local fishermen traditionally lit at night to attract fish to their boats, Isaribi draws its inspiration from the soothing beauty of the sea and the fresh bounty it provides. The ryokan asks only that its guests completely immerse themselves in the practice of doing nothing, giving their bodies and minds a chance to reset and recharge.

The inn's 12 rooms have been designed in a myriad of styles, combining touches of traditional ryokan aesthetics, furnishings in warm, rich colors, patterns and textures popular in the romantic Taisho Roman era, and modern Western comforts. Each private, open-air onsen is different in shape and material, with some built from local stone and others from hinoki wood. Early birds can slowly awaken by soaking in their onsen as they watch the sunrise over the sea in summer; other seasons reveal the early blooming Kawazusakura flowers or the fruiting of the mandarin orange trees.

Isaribi additionally has two large, communal onsen, which can be reserved for guests' private use. Dim, muted lighting graces the indoor onsen, whose designs echo those favored during the Showa era, with both baths connecting to a generously sized outdoor *rotenburo.* Encircled by trees and pretty shrubbery, these outdoor baths encourage one to feel at home among the natural world and to focus, by doing nothing at all, on enjoying the present moment.

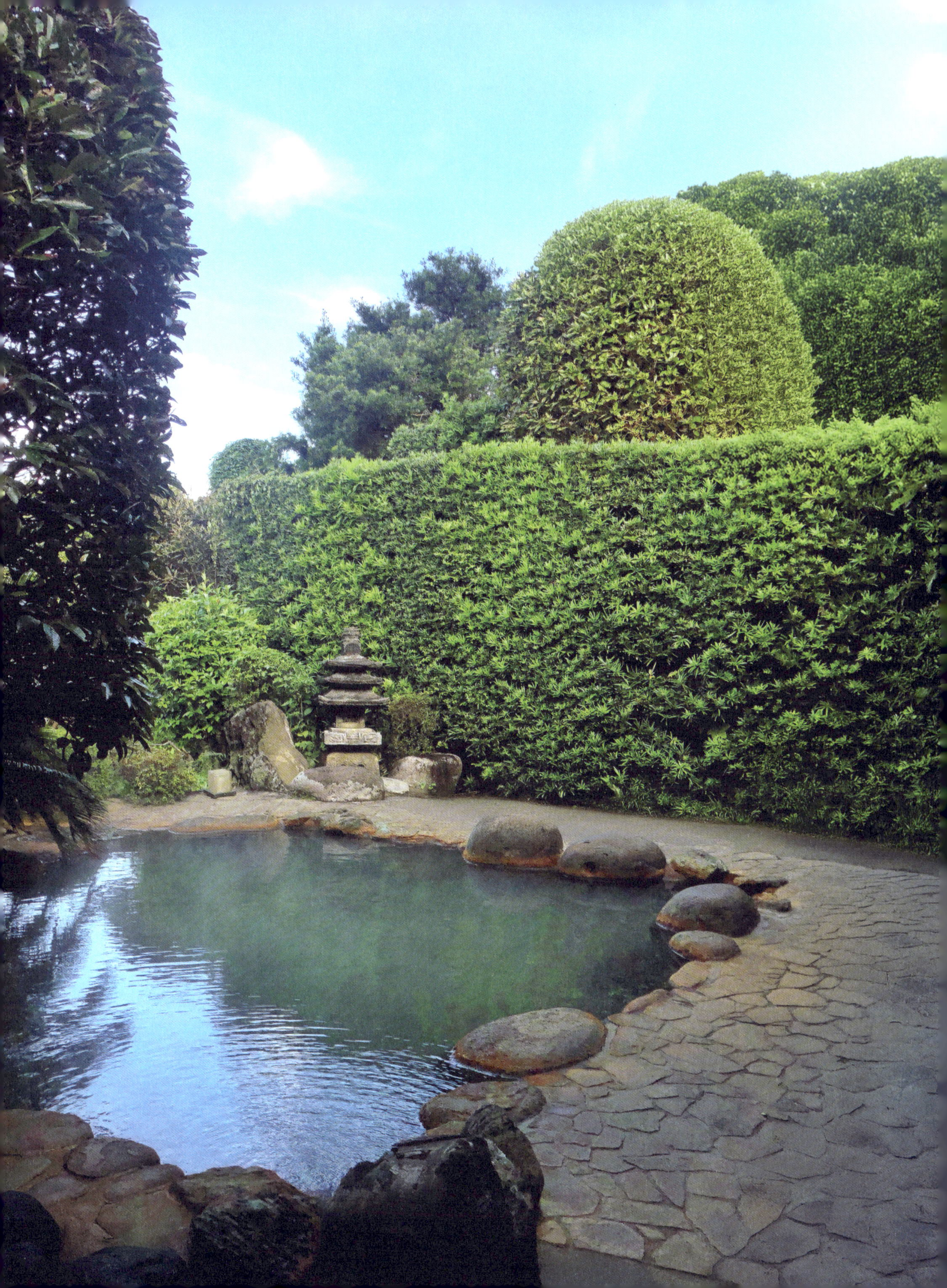

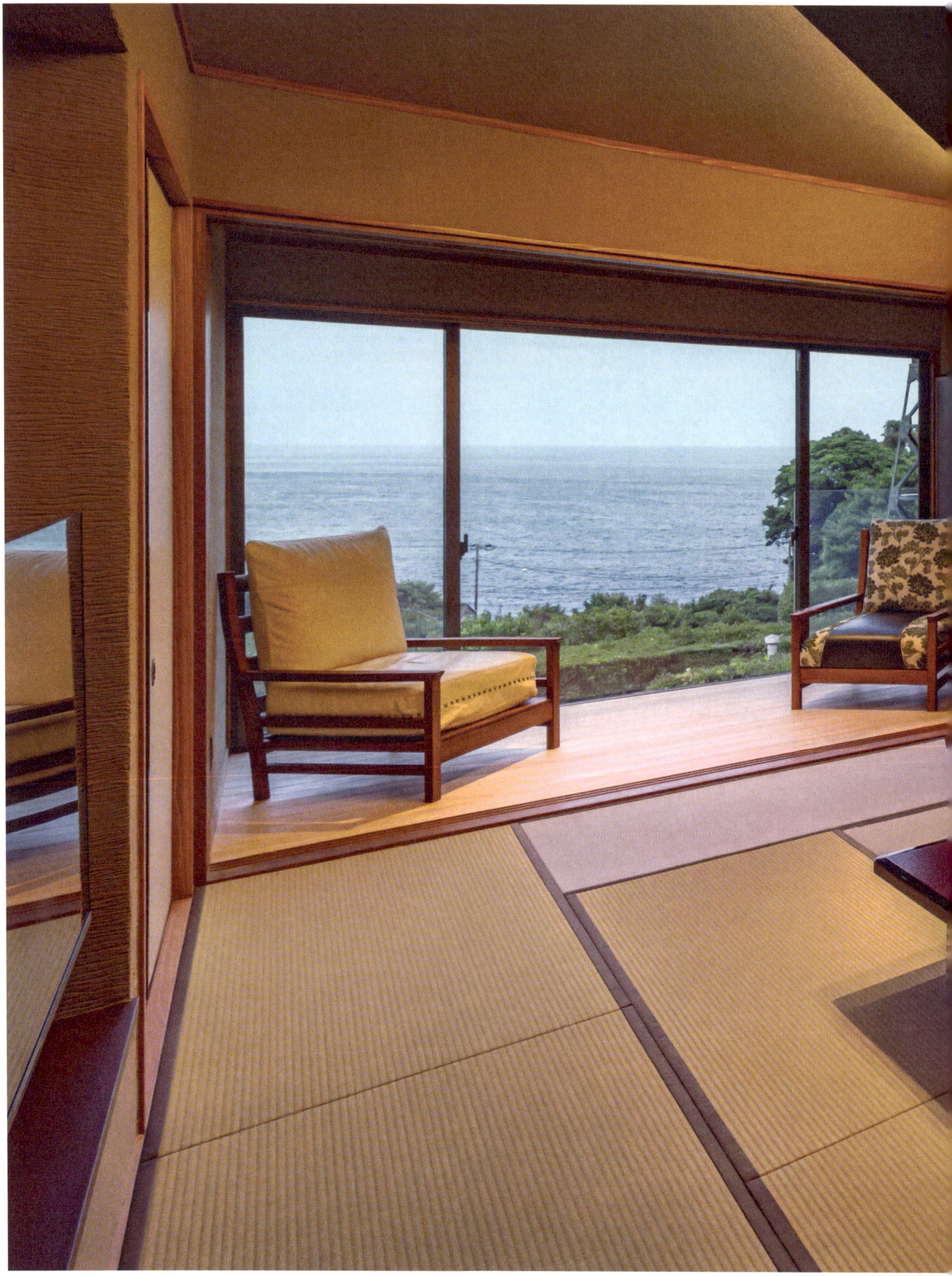

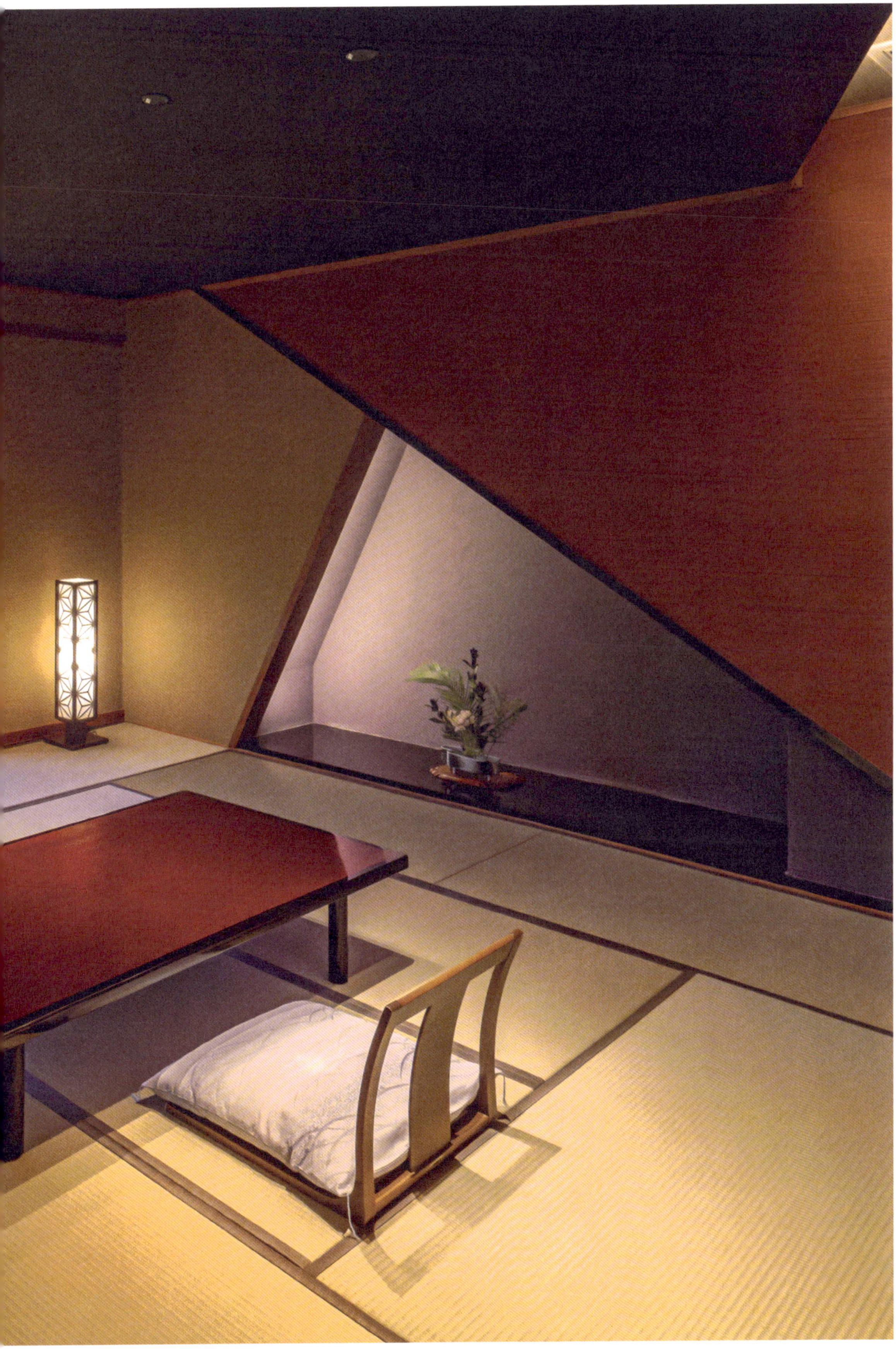

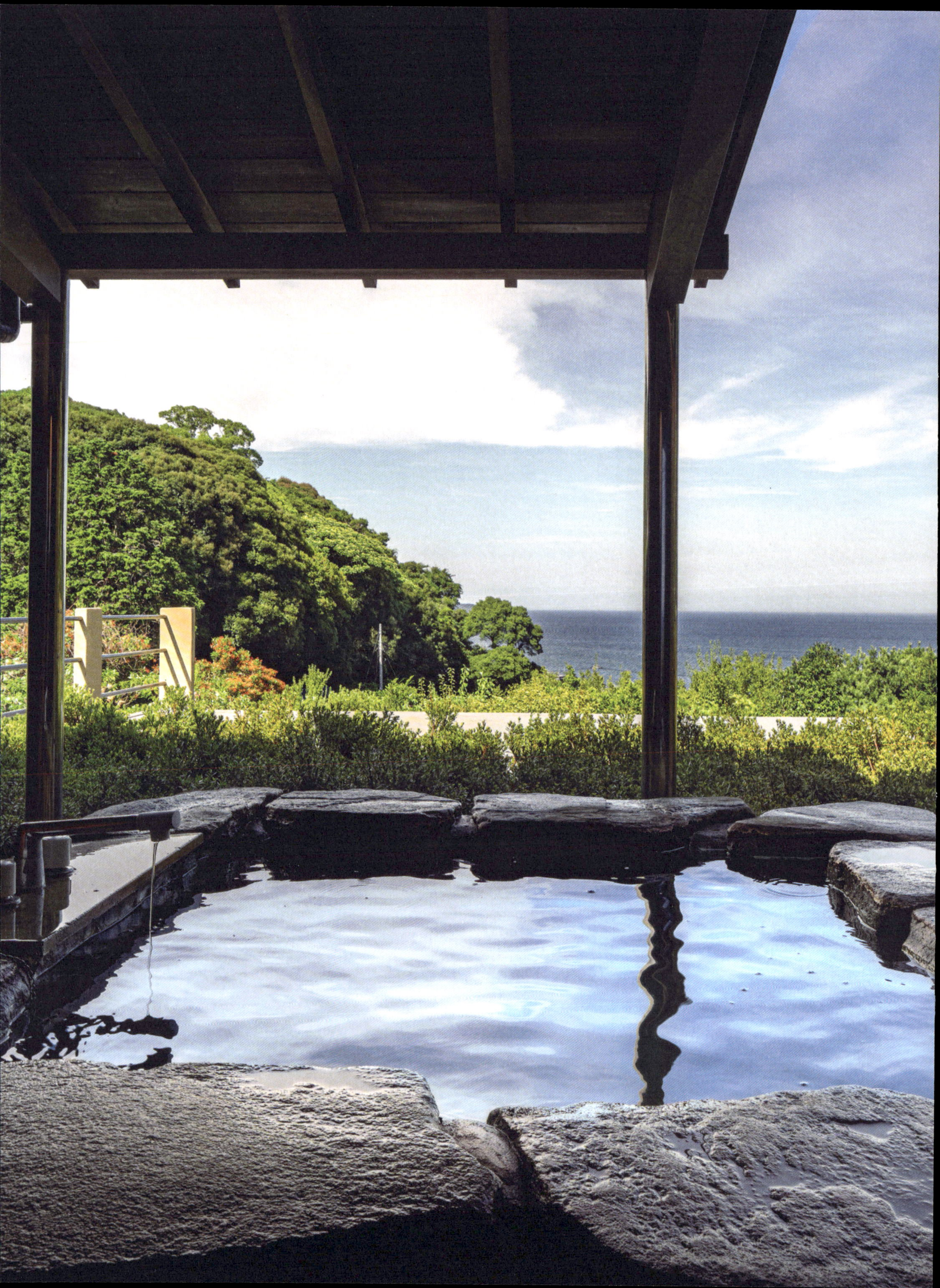

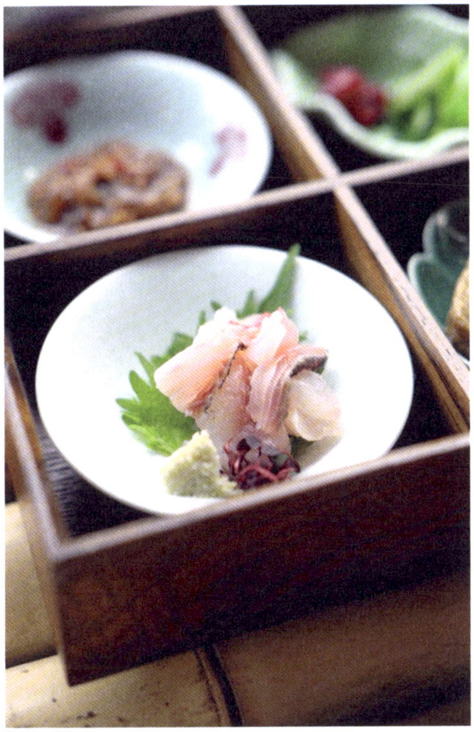

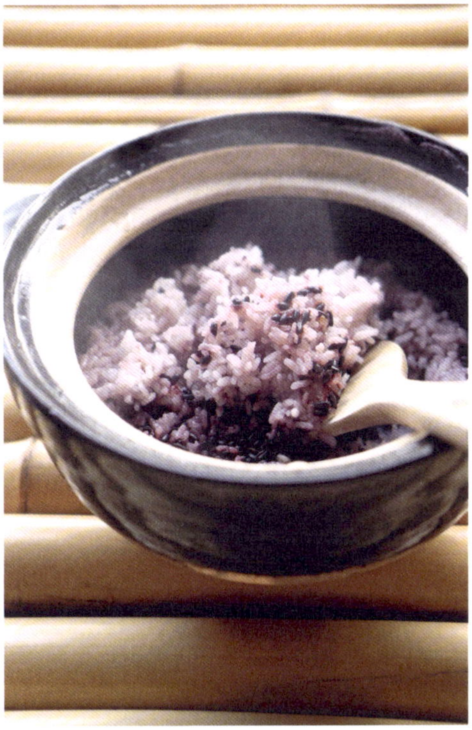

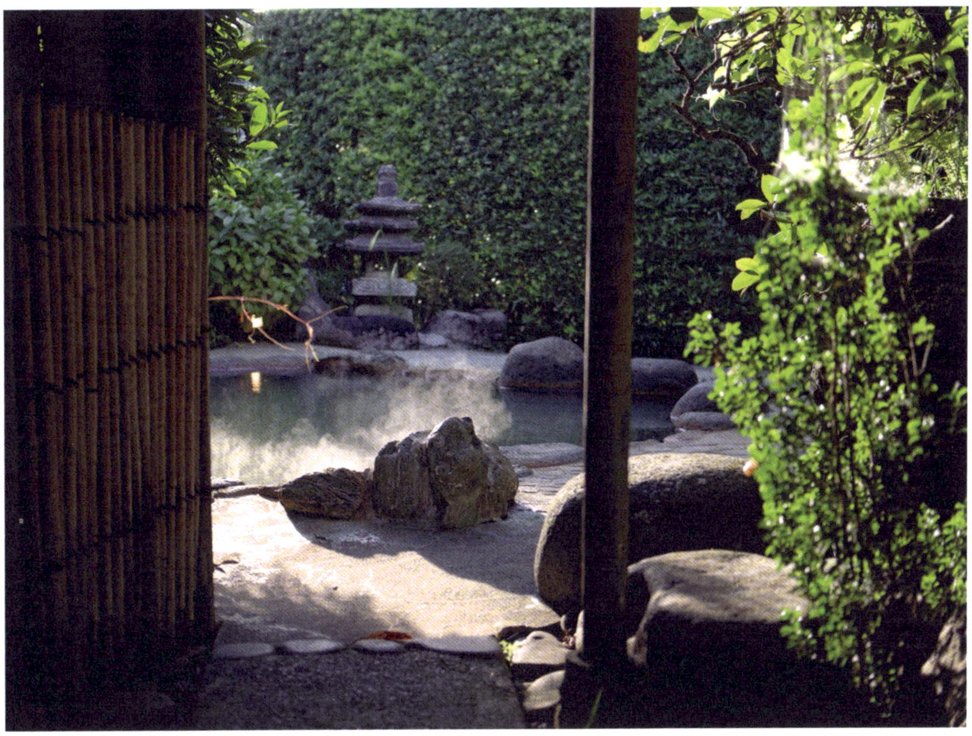

LEFT Ocean views at one of Isaribi's private, open-air onsen.

Tsuboyu
Yunomine Onsen, Tanabe • Wakayama Prefecture

THE WORLD'S FIRST ONSEN REGISTERED AS A UNESCO WORLD HERITAGE SITE

Said to be one of Japan's oldest and most revered onsen, this bath is a popular stop for travelers on the Kumano Kodō pilgrimage route.

In the Kumano Mountains, a secluded valley along the Yunotani River shelters the tiny village of Yunomine Onsen, a place where time stands still. This quaint town, which seems to have avoided modernity entirely, houses a collection of small wooden *minshuku* and onsen ryokan along the river.

Yunomine is adored for its authentic, rustic ambiance, and many pilgrims on the Kumano Kodō come to soak at Tsuboyu. The onsen sits at the head of the river, enclosed in a cozy wooden cabin near the village center. Tsuboyu is considered one of the oldest onsen in Japan, and the only one in the world listed as a UNESCO World Heritage Site.

Discovered some 1,800 years ago, the healing properties of Tsuboyu became known throughout the land when the 15th lord of Oguri Castle, Oguri Hangan, suffered poisoning from bandits and subsequently was saved by the maiden Princess Terute who, along with the Priest Yugyo, led Oguri to Tsuboyu's waters where he was subsequently healed. In addition to providing Tsuboyu with its founding legend, the fascinating story of Oguri Hangan also forms the basis for a popular work of Kabuki theater. Today, Tsuboyu is the site of another story: locals swear that any couples bathing in its waters hugely improve their chances of having children.

Descending the rough-hewn stone steps to Tsuboyu leads one to its wooden entrance door. Leave your shoes outside, hang your numbered bathing card on the hook, and enter the small cabin. Dimly lit, with small rays of sunlight sifting through the thin gaps of the wooden planks, the enclosure features a small series of steps leading down to the onsen.

Carved from the natural rock, Tsuboyu was once open to the river and its elements, but today its sturdy enclosure allows for a more structured, private onsen experience. Visitors pay at the main bathhouse entrance, whereupon one receives a numbered bathing card. Turns are taken every 30 minutes for groups of two or three; many return multiple times in the hopes of glimpsing the changing color of the water, said to turn seven different hues over the course of the day. Depending on the color, the rock wall is sometimes beautifully reflected on the surface of the onsen water, creating an illusion of endless depth. At these times, until one steps in, one cannot be completely certain of how far down the onsen goes.

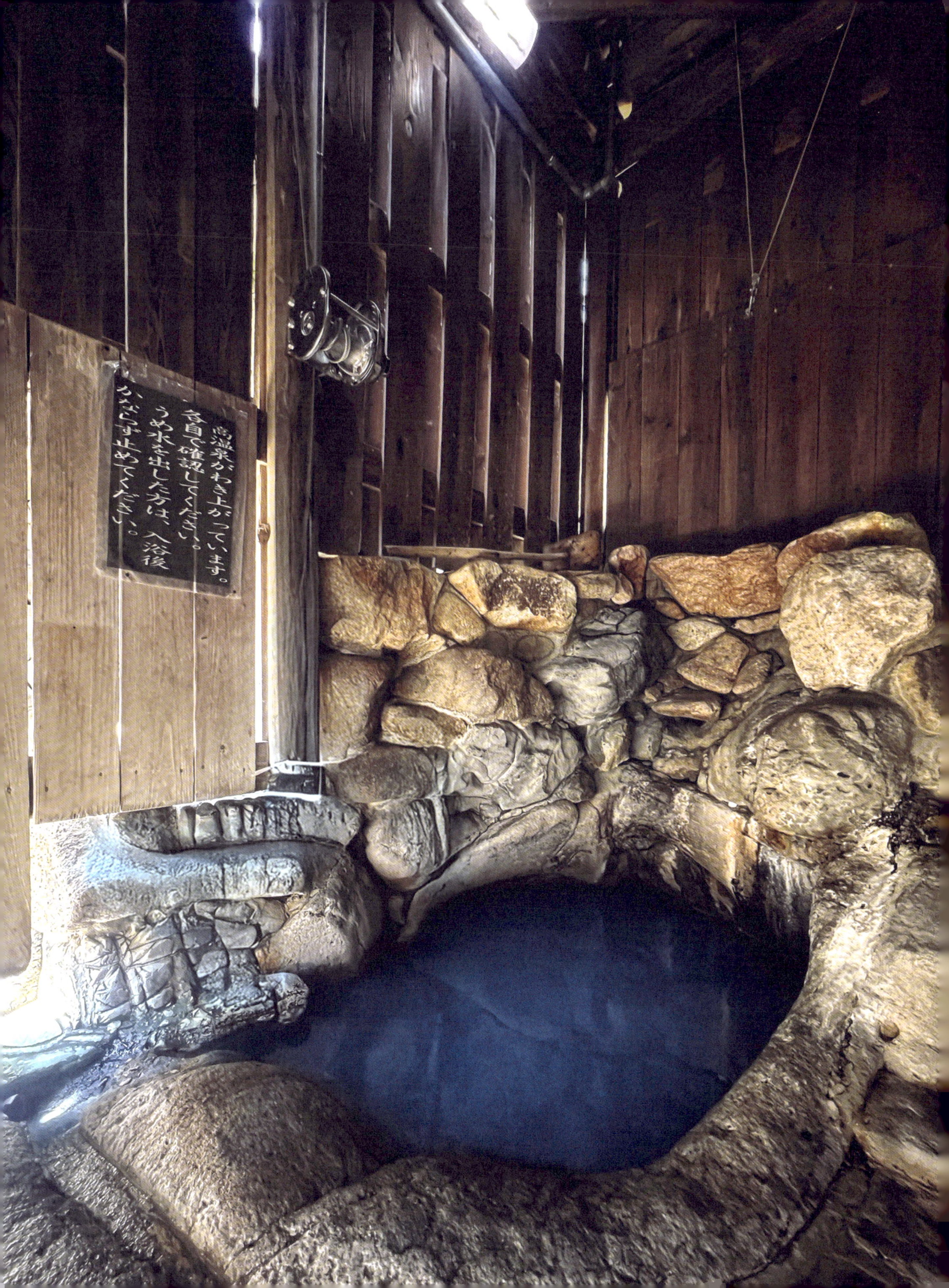
高温泉がわき上がっています。
各自で確認してください。
うめ水を出した方は、入浴後
かならず止めてください。

Yunosuke no Yado Chorakuen
Tamatsukuri • Shimane Prefecture

SOAK IN THE HEALING WATERS OF THE GODS

Steeped in history and lore, this onsen ryokan is found at the very birthplace of Japan's deities—making a stay here unforgettable.

Shimane, the westernmost prefecture on the main island of Honshu, is justly known as "the Land of the Gods." While Miyazaki Prefecture is thought to be the birthplace of the first Emperor Jimmu—a descendant of the gods—Shimane Prefecture is known as the birthplace of the primordial gods Izanami and Izanagi, who created the land of Japan itself. Legend tells that once a year during the 10th lunar month—locally known as Kamiari-zuki—all of Shinto's eight million deities descend upon Shimane's venerated Izumo Taisha shrine for an annual gathering, joyfully immersing themselves in the rich, rejuvenating onsen waters of Tamatsukuri, also known as "the Bath of the Gods."

With a history tracing back to the 8th century, Tamatsukuri is one of the oldest onsen towns in the country and lore has it that the gods Sukunahikona (the onsen deity) and Okuninushi (head of the earth gods) were the first to discover the onsen. The Nara period saw the region become popular with the people, whilst during the Edo period under the Matsue Domain, "Yunosuke" (the name given to the individual) was officially appointed to run the town and the baths. The first manager was a distinguished man from the Hasegawa family, whose ancestor Hasegawa Toshikata settled in Tamatsukuri and founded Daizenji Temple. In 1868, after the feudal system was officially abolished, Hasegawa's descendants began to landscape a Japanese garden and operate an onsen inn which would later become today's Yunosuke no Yado Chorakuen.

The year 1910 saw the ryokan's massive garden completed, along with the large open-air onsen bath called Ryugu no Yu. Literally translated as "the bath of the dragon god's palace," this immense, open-air onsen bath is not only Japan's largest outdoor onsen, but also the largest outdoor *konyoku* mixed onsen. This entirely natural onsen soothes and heals, as overnight guests soak away in the tranquil setting and the rising onsen steam provides a shield of privacy. Women enter Ryugu no Yu via a private onsen corridor and wear a cotton cover provided by Chorakuen. An open-air hinoki onsen and an open-air rock *rotenburo* offer differing hours for men and women, and for those who prefer utter privacy, a family *kashikiri* onsen can be reserved. Several rooms also contain their own private, open-air onsen.

However one chooses to enjoy "the Bath of the Gods," local lore states that "if you wash once, your appearance will be perfect, and if you bathe again, all illnesses will be cured instantly."

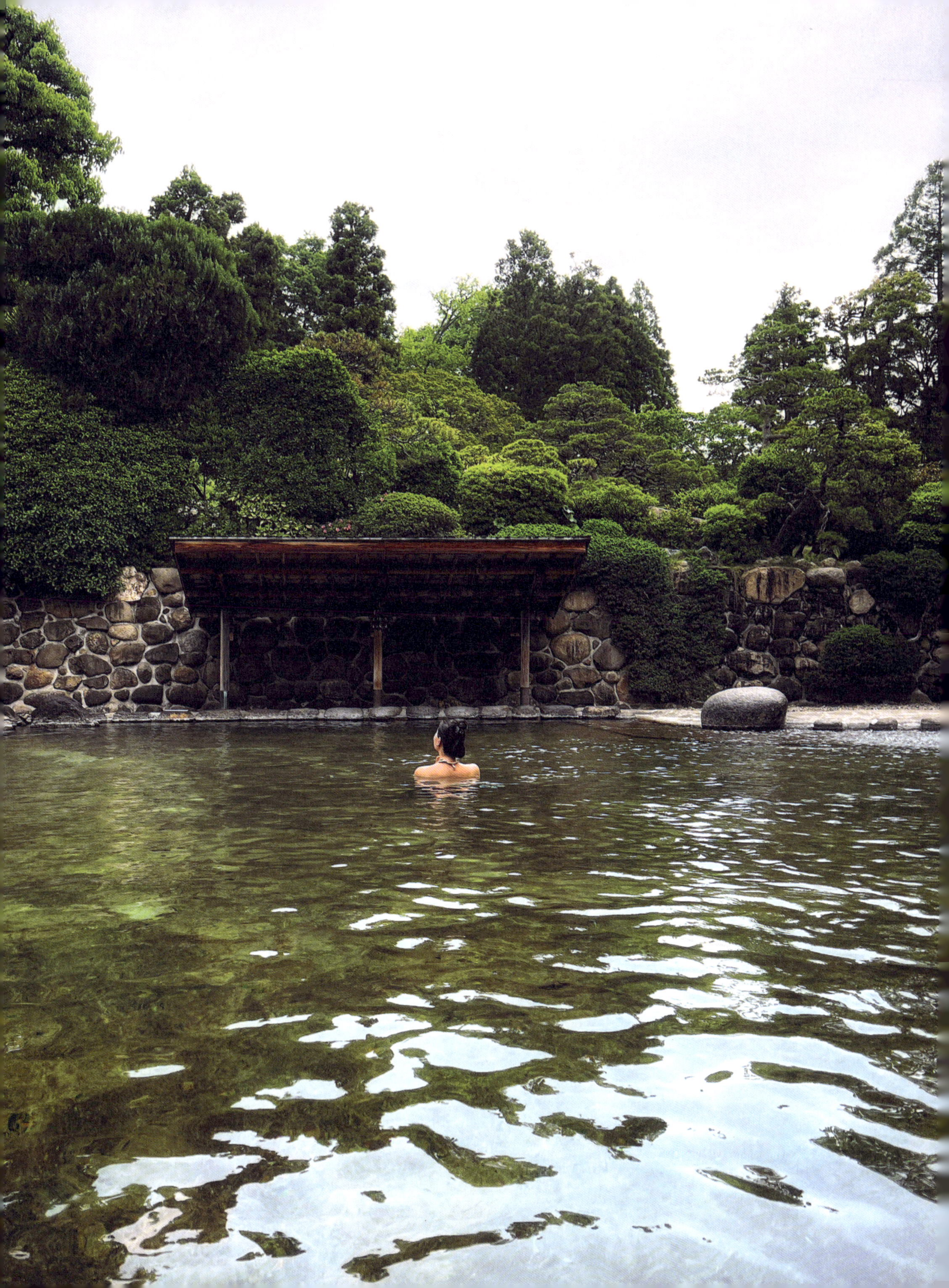

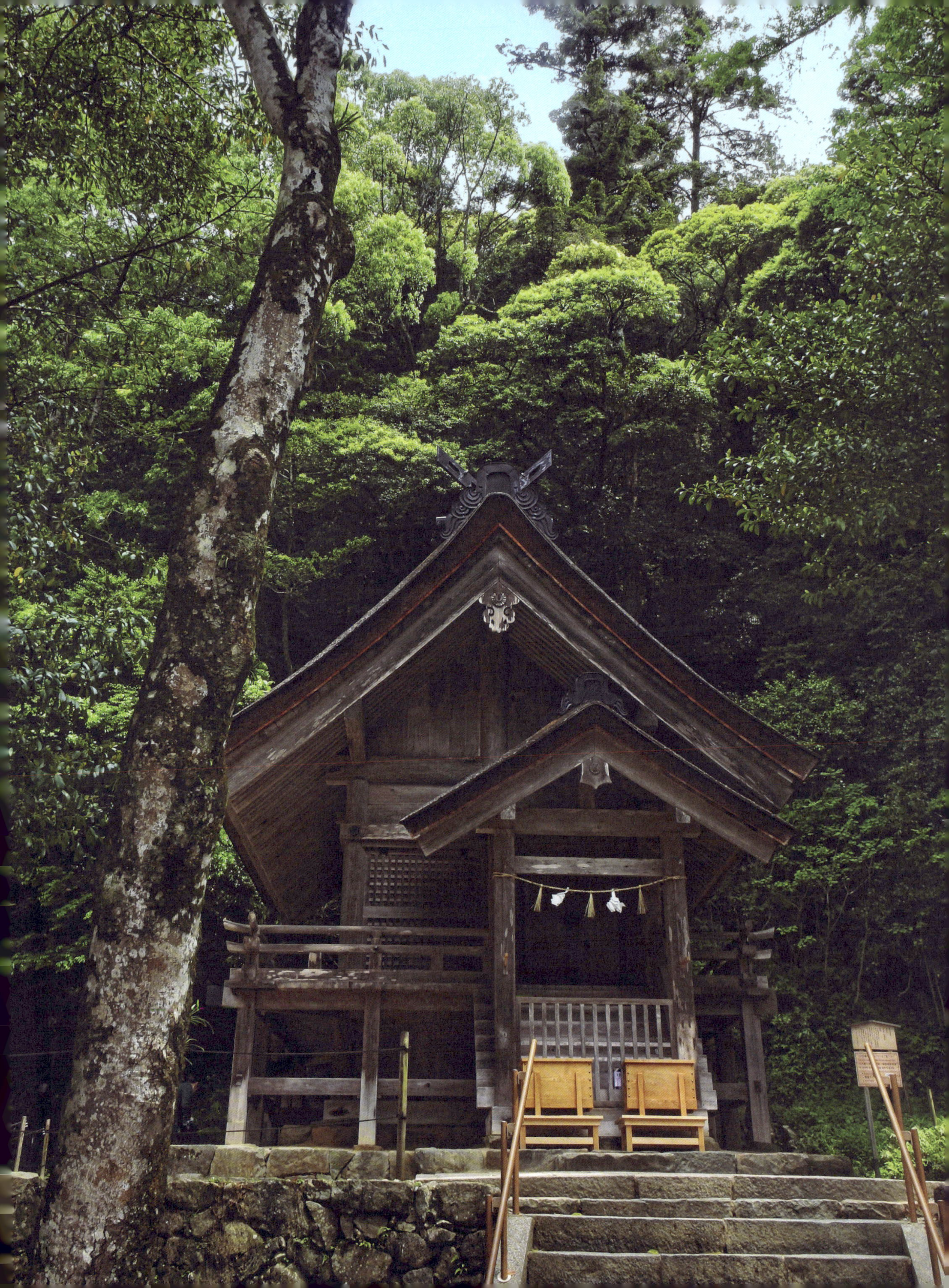

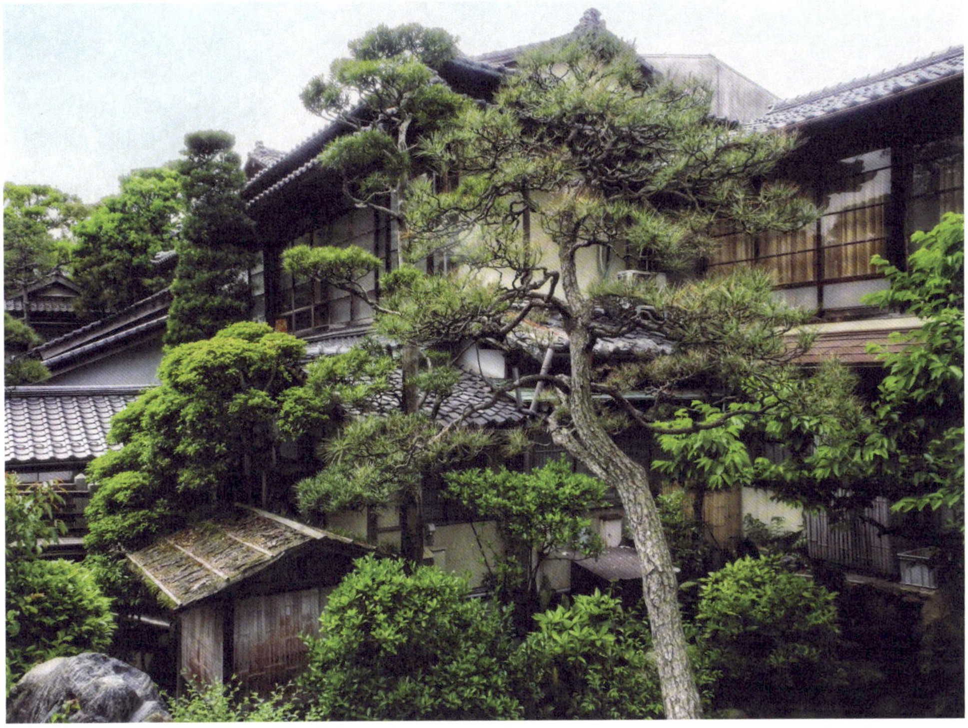

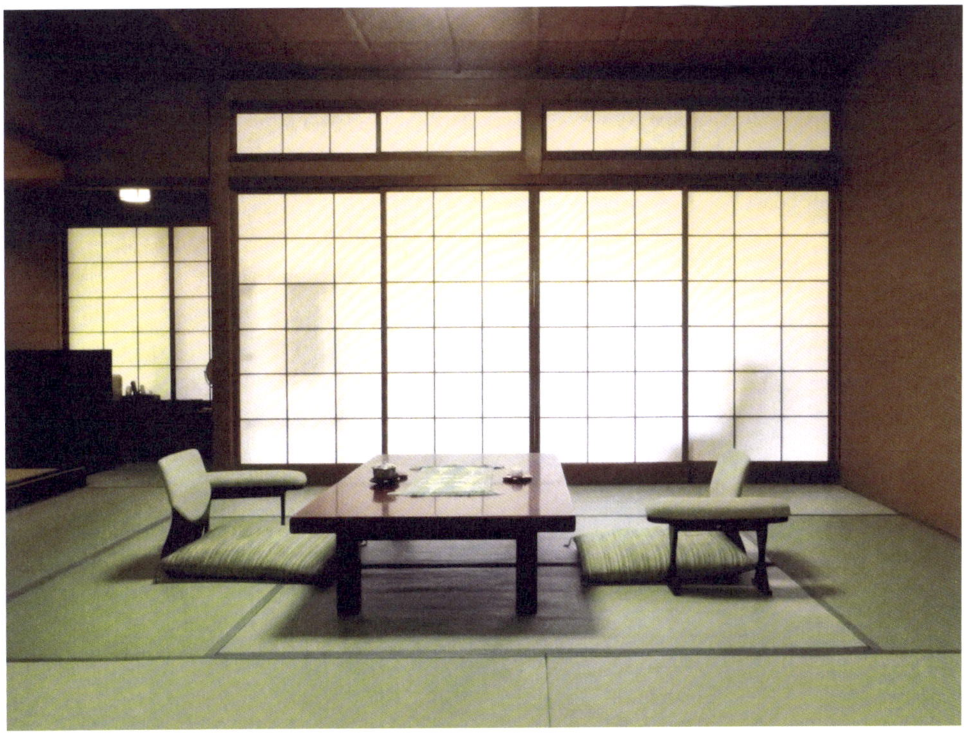

LEFT Soganoyashiro Shrine is an important pilgrimage site within Izumo-taisha's grounds.

KAI Yufuin
Yufu • Oita Prefecture

A RETREAT SET WITHIN A SCULPTED LANDSCAPE OF PASTORAL BEAUTY

Paying homage to the rich, agricultural history of Oita Prefecture, this ryokan invites guests to relax amid the changing colors of terraced rice fields.

Oita Prefecture, whose kanji characters translate to "grand rice field," is a region notable for its abundance of picturesque, natural environments. It has also been dubbed the "onsen prefecture," due to its plentiful onsen sources. Located at the foot of Mt. Yufu surrounded by countryside scenery and countless terraced rice fields, Yufuin Onsen is one of the region's most popular onsen destination. Within Yufuin, the luxury onsen ryokan KAI Yufuin honors the prefecture's strong ties to traditional Japanese agriculture.

Designed by the architect Kengo Kuma, the premises of KAI Yufuin were greatly inspired by the area's rural countryside vistas; as such, the property sits nestled amid a weaving, tiered platform of rice fields, an artfully landscaped site that offers stunning views in any season.

Independent cottage suites containing open-air onsen baths are placed intermittently throughout the fields, offering guests communion with both the lush landscape and the vast sky above. Other traditional rooms are found in the main building, while the Kunugi annex villas lie within the forest grounds. One distinguishing interior feature of the main building's rooms is the tatami floor, made from the rare *shichitoi* grass grown in the Kunisaki Peninsula of Oita. Its delicate scent immediately imparts a feeling of peaceful refuge. Several rooms also have their own private, open-air onsen, whereas the ryokan's public onsen gives guests an opportunity to soak away their days in indoor and outdoor settings, with the latter featuring views of Mt. Yufu.

Particularly charming at the KAI properties are the cultural workshops provided to guests; at KAI Yufuin, one can try their hand at making a rice-straw amulet, which farmers would traditionally make during the off-season. Afterward, one might find tranquil moments relaxing on the Rice Terrace Deck in the center of the property. The panoramic views from here are remarkable in all the seasons, but especially in spring when the sky and landscape are reflected on the water that fills the rice fields.

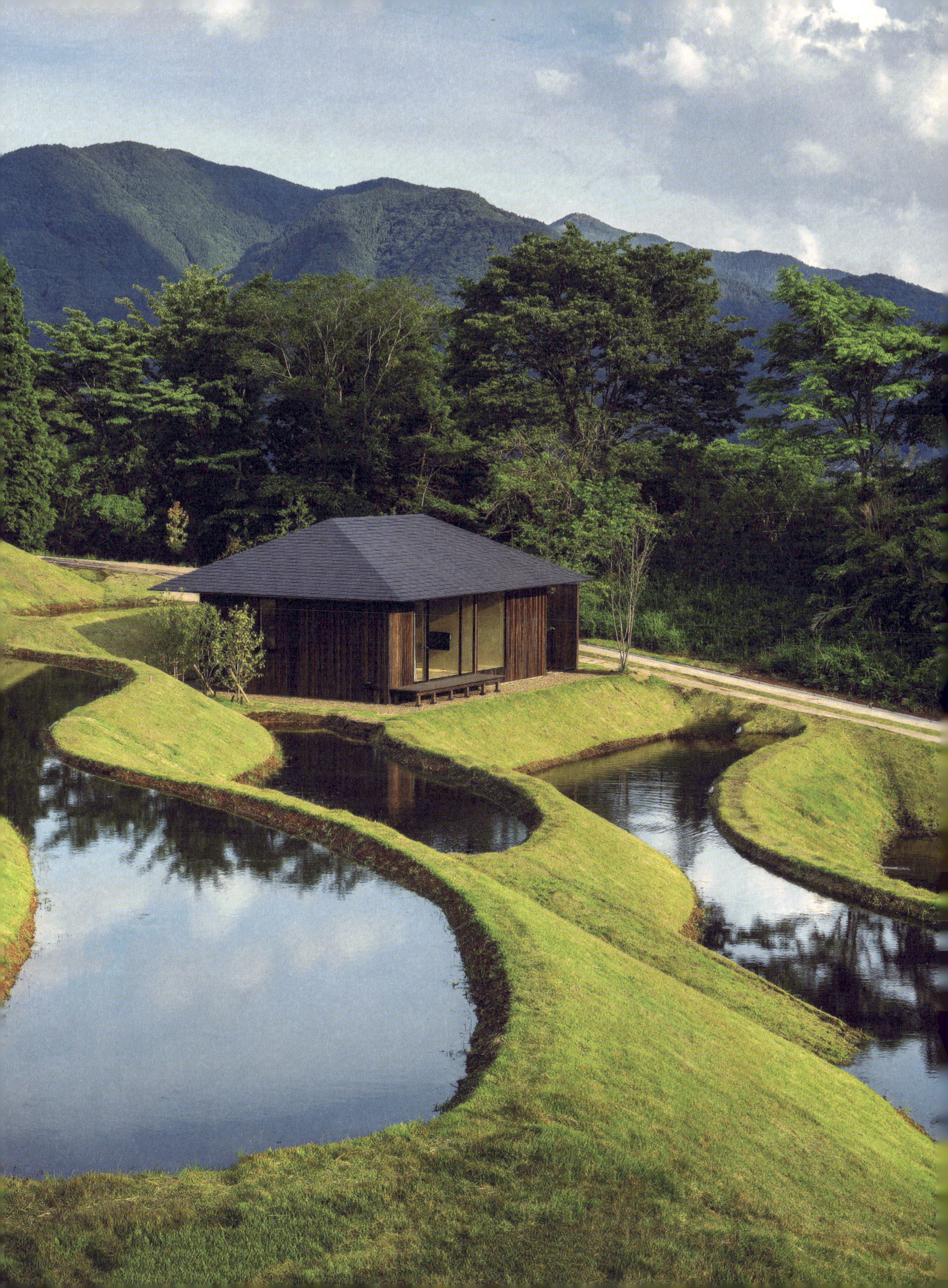

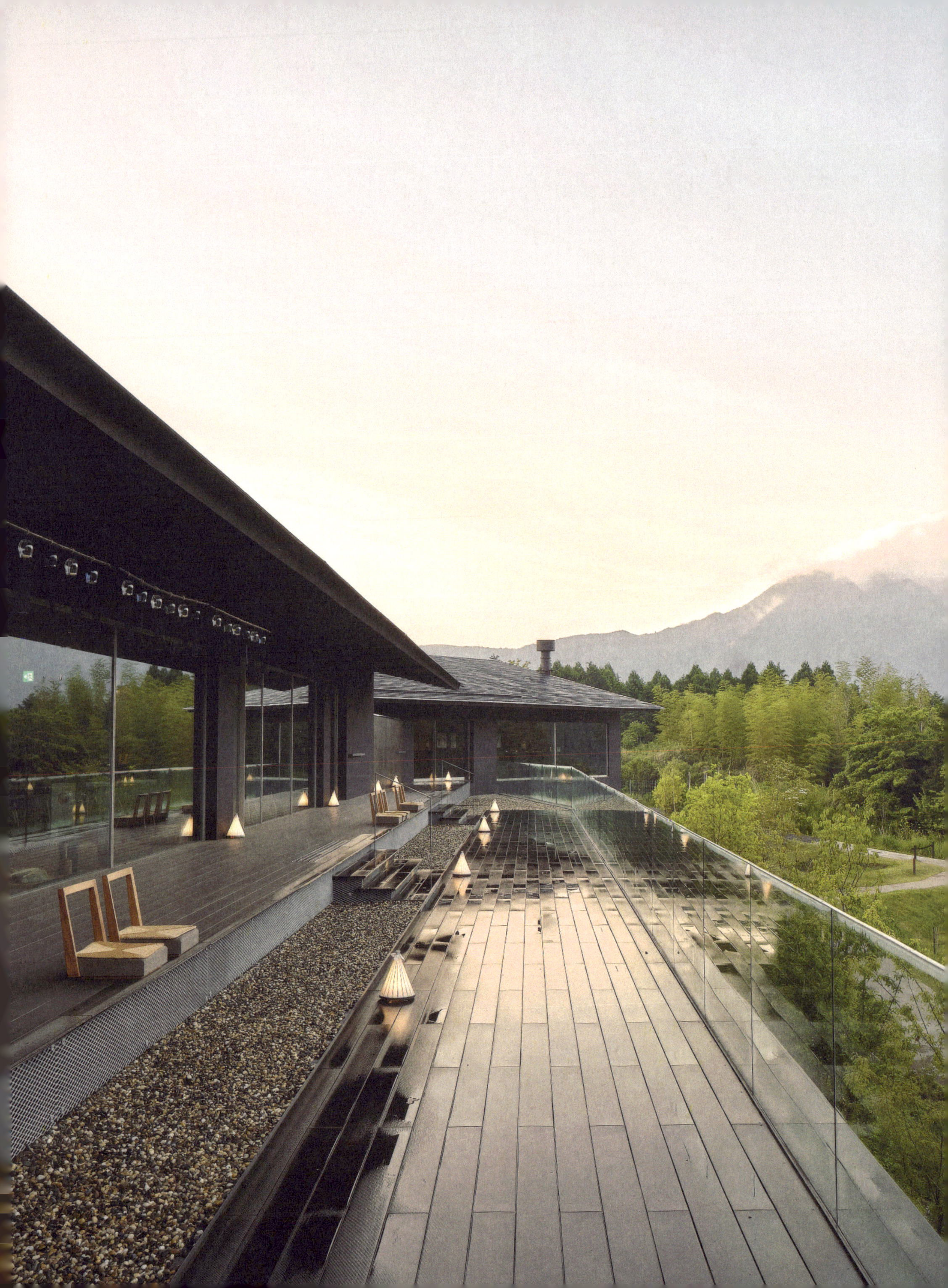

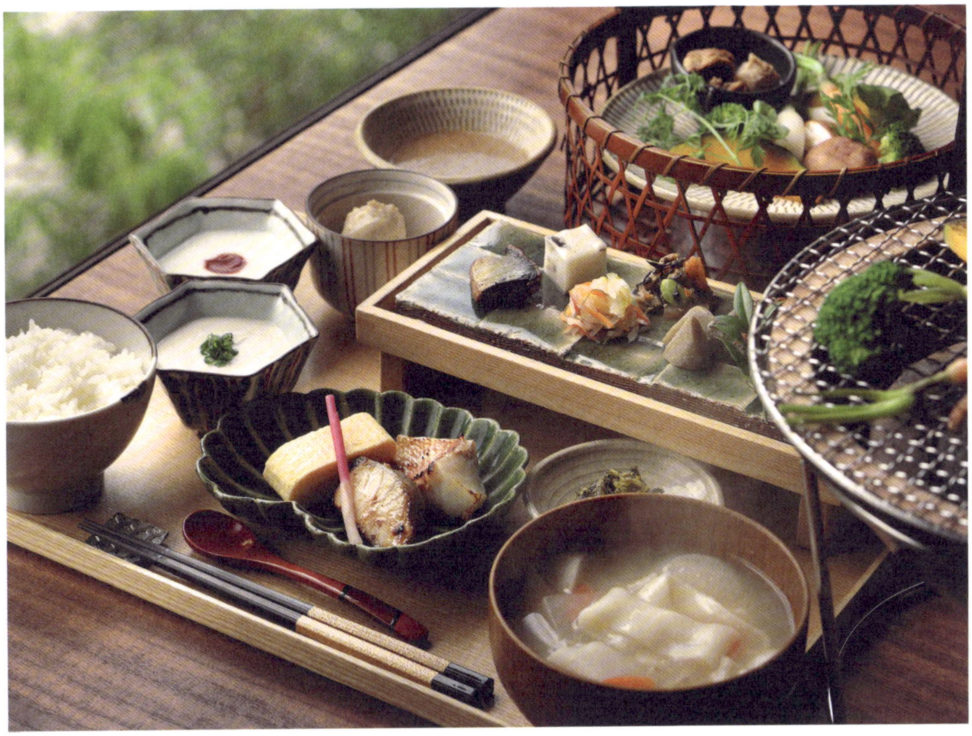

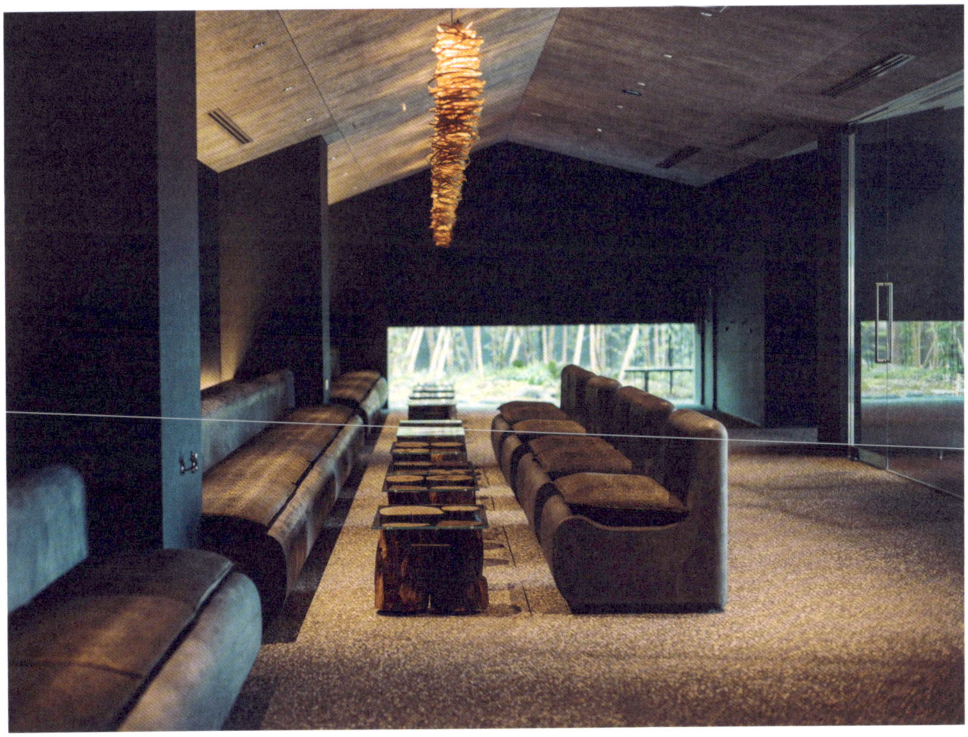

LEFT Panoramic views of the rice terraces can be appreciated from the aptly named "Rice Terrace Deck."

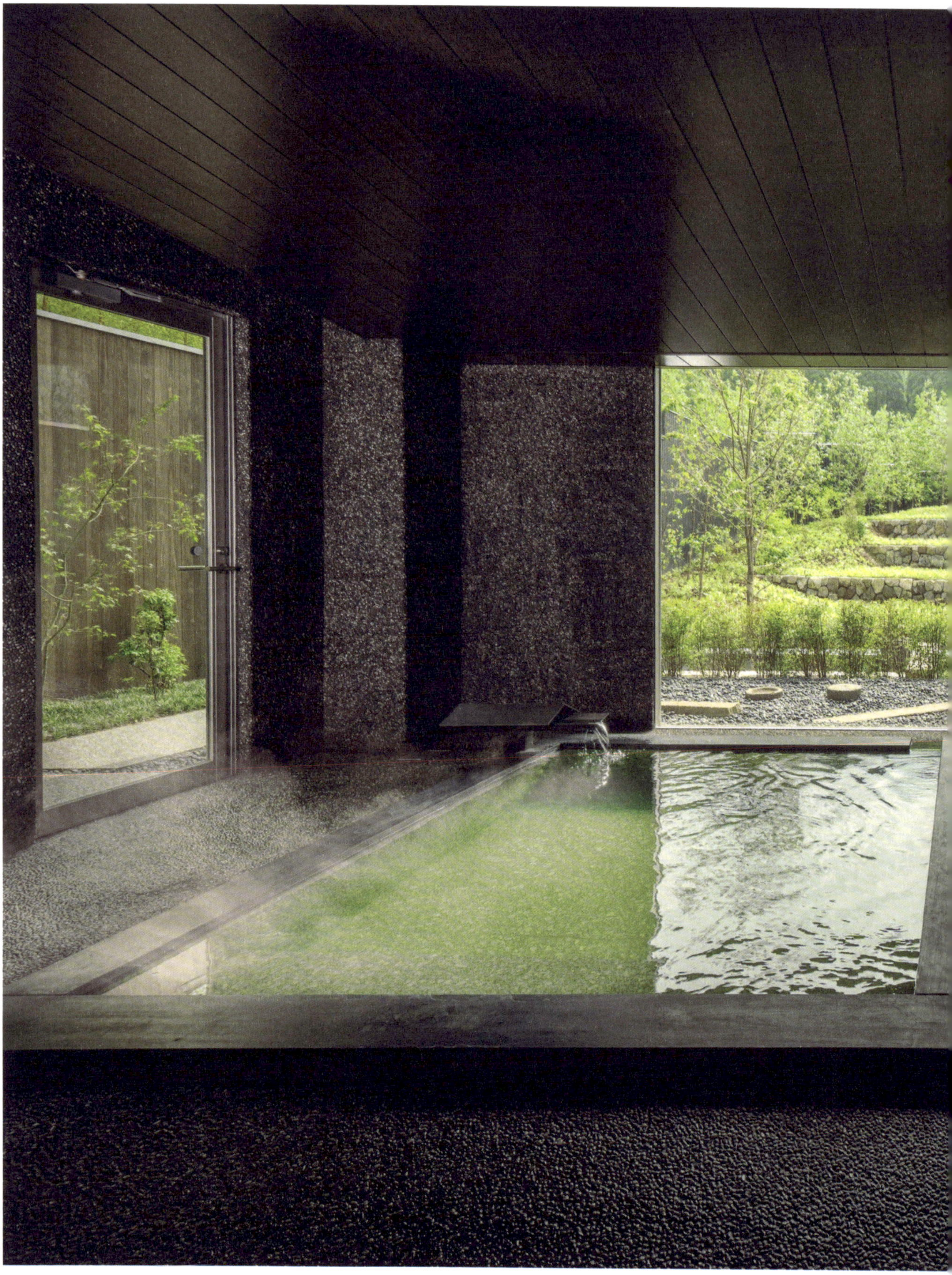

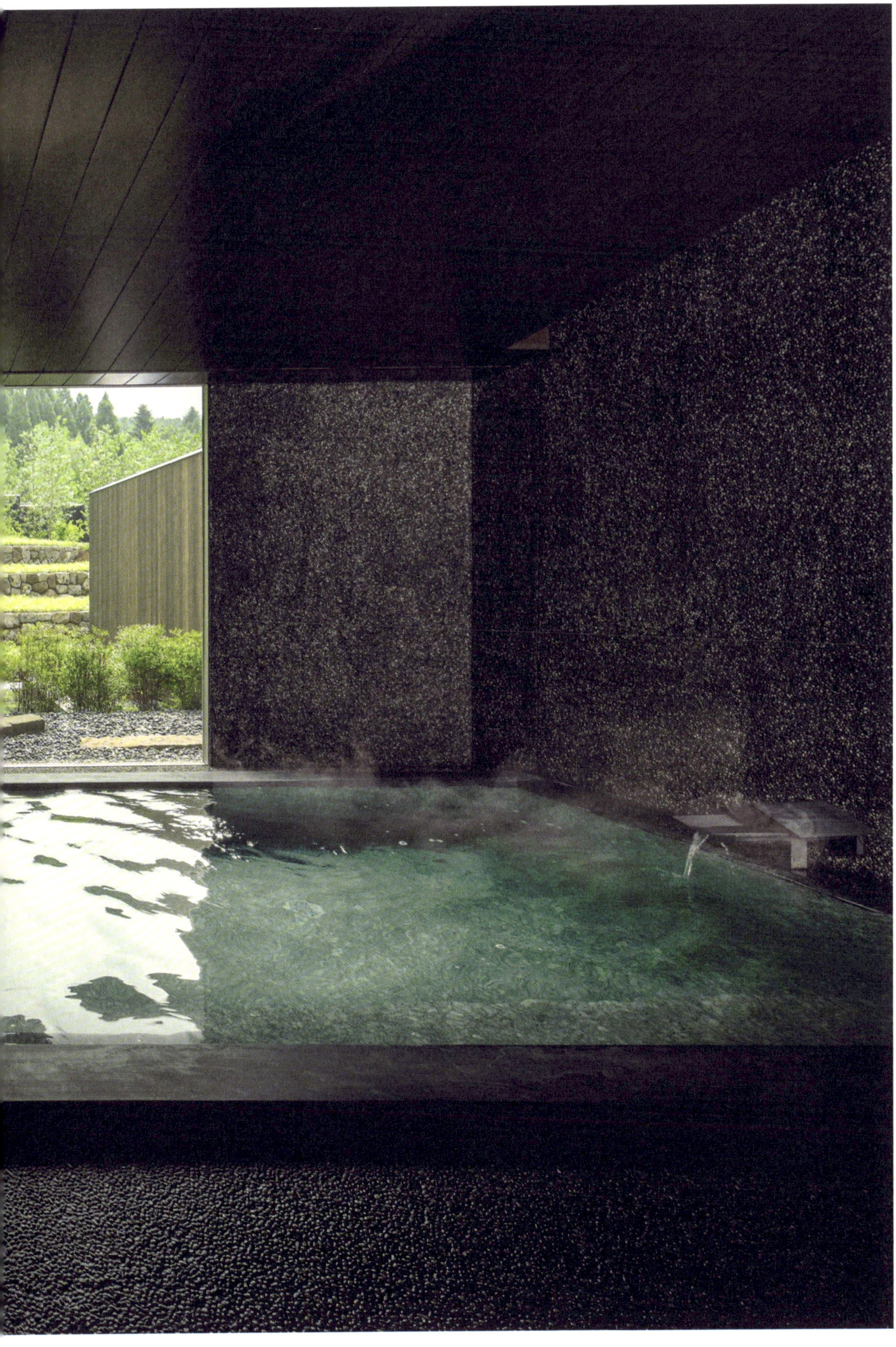

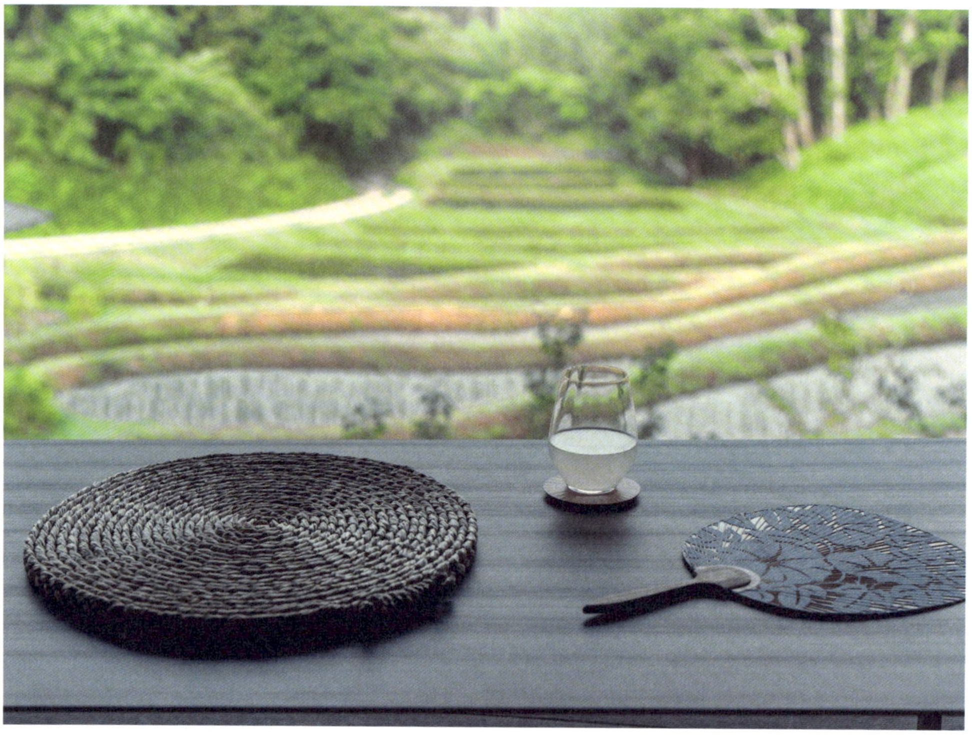

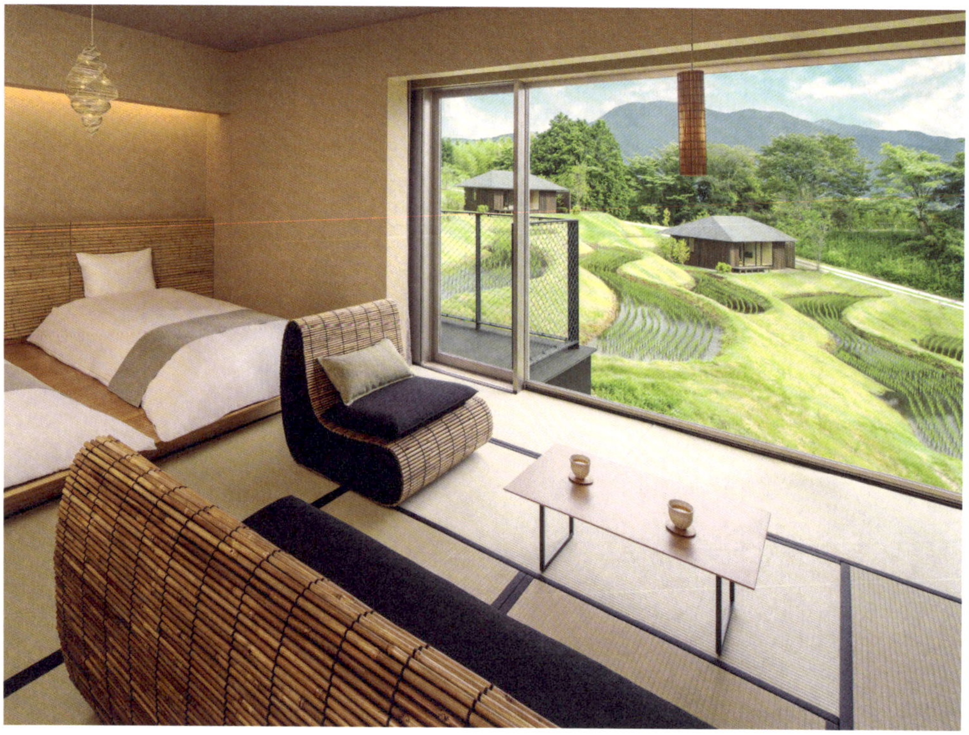

RIGHT Views of Mt. Yufu from the public onsen bath.

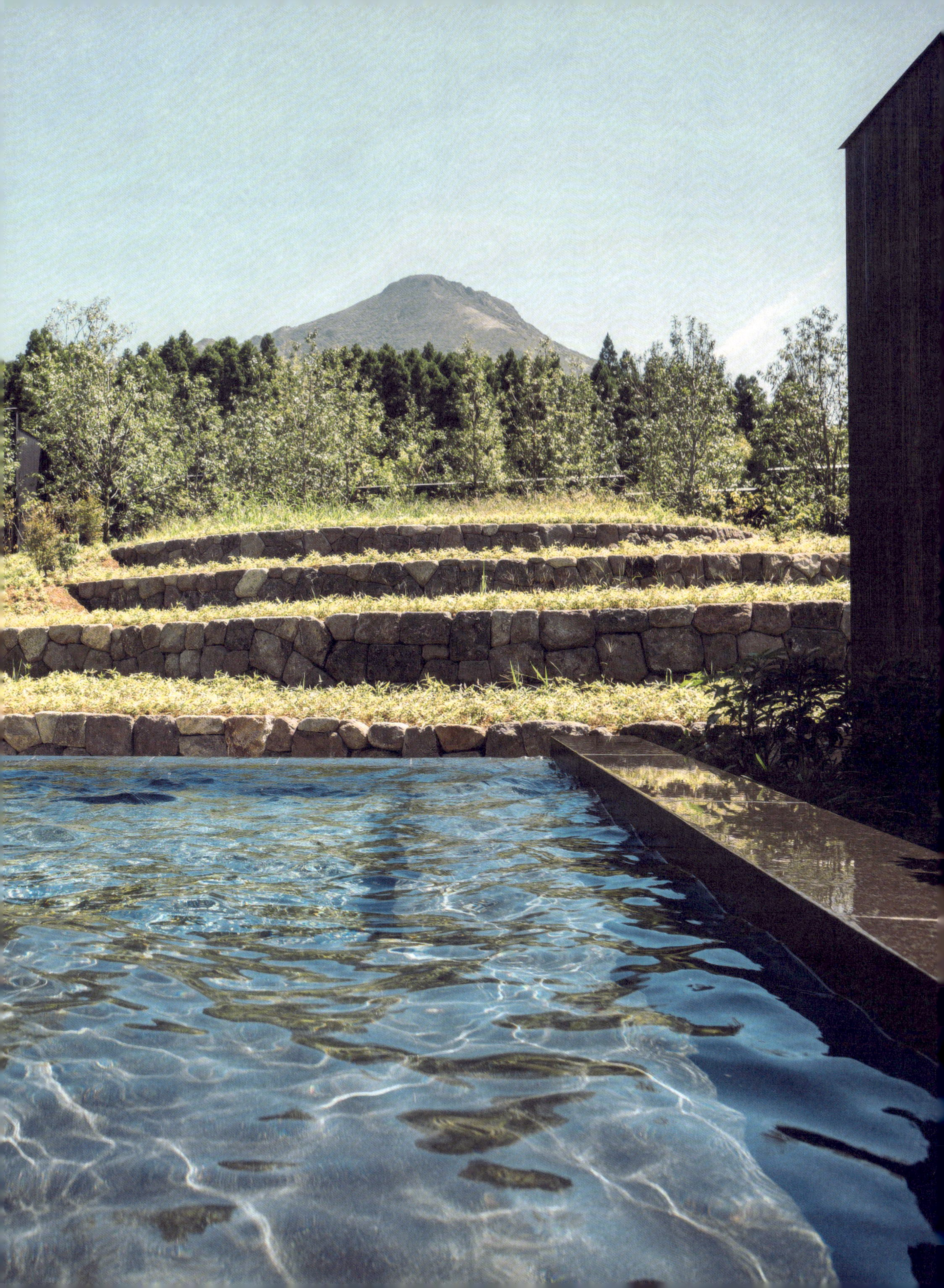

Hokkawa Onsen: Kuroneiwaburo
Higashiizu • Shizuoka Prefecture

A SEASIDE PUBLIC ONSEN CHERISHED BY LOCALS

This beloved open-air onsen allows visitors a chance to soak in harmony with the nearby ocean.

With Hokkawa Onsen, Shizuoka Prefecture offers an underrated gem of an onsen destination, especially as it's an easy getaway from Tokyo. The Izu Peninsula is dotted with an abundance of tiny, quaint onsen villages and hamlets filled with boutique lodgings, family-run properties, and various Airbnbs featuring private onsen. Though the peninsula contains several famous onsen towns such as Atami, Ito, and Shuzenji, many of the sleepy local train stations are home to their own mini onsen suburbs where one finds delicious seaside restaurants, farmer's markets, small onsen ryokan, and oceanside public baths.

One of these hamlets can be accessed via Izu-Hokkawa station (many of the stations with an Izu prefix tend to have some wonderful onsen ryokan and public onsen to explore), from which a short 15-minute walk brings one to the similarly named Hokkawa Onsen. Here one finds a small street beside the ocean offering, once night falls, a view of the "Moon Road," a path of moonlight stretching across the sea to the horizon. Only five onsen ryokan are situated around this small street, ranging from simple and affordable to very luxurious. Many guests will also pay a visit to Hokkawa Onsen's public, open-air onsen bath set right beside the sea.

Popular with visitors and locals alike, Hokkawa Onsen's Kuroneiwaburo bath sits on the shore at a level not much higher than the sea so that bathers feel a profound connection with both the onsen and the ocean. Ranked in the top 10 for hot springs in natural surroundings, Hokkawa Onsen has two outdoor onsen baths—a large *rotenburo* made of black rocks that blends into the shoreline, and a smaller, circular onsen made with lovely stone tiling inspired by Turkish baths. In the past, the rock *rotenburo* was a mixed *konyoku* onsen, while the circular stone onsen would switch between male and female guests depending on the day or time. Today, the rock *rotenburo* has become the male bath, while the circular stone onsen is the domain of female bathers. Harkening back to the old days, Hokkawa offers no shower or spa amenities, only a simple changing room for each bath. Visitors should take care to use the *yu-oke* to pour onsen water over their bodies a few times before entering.

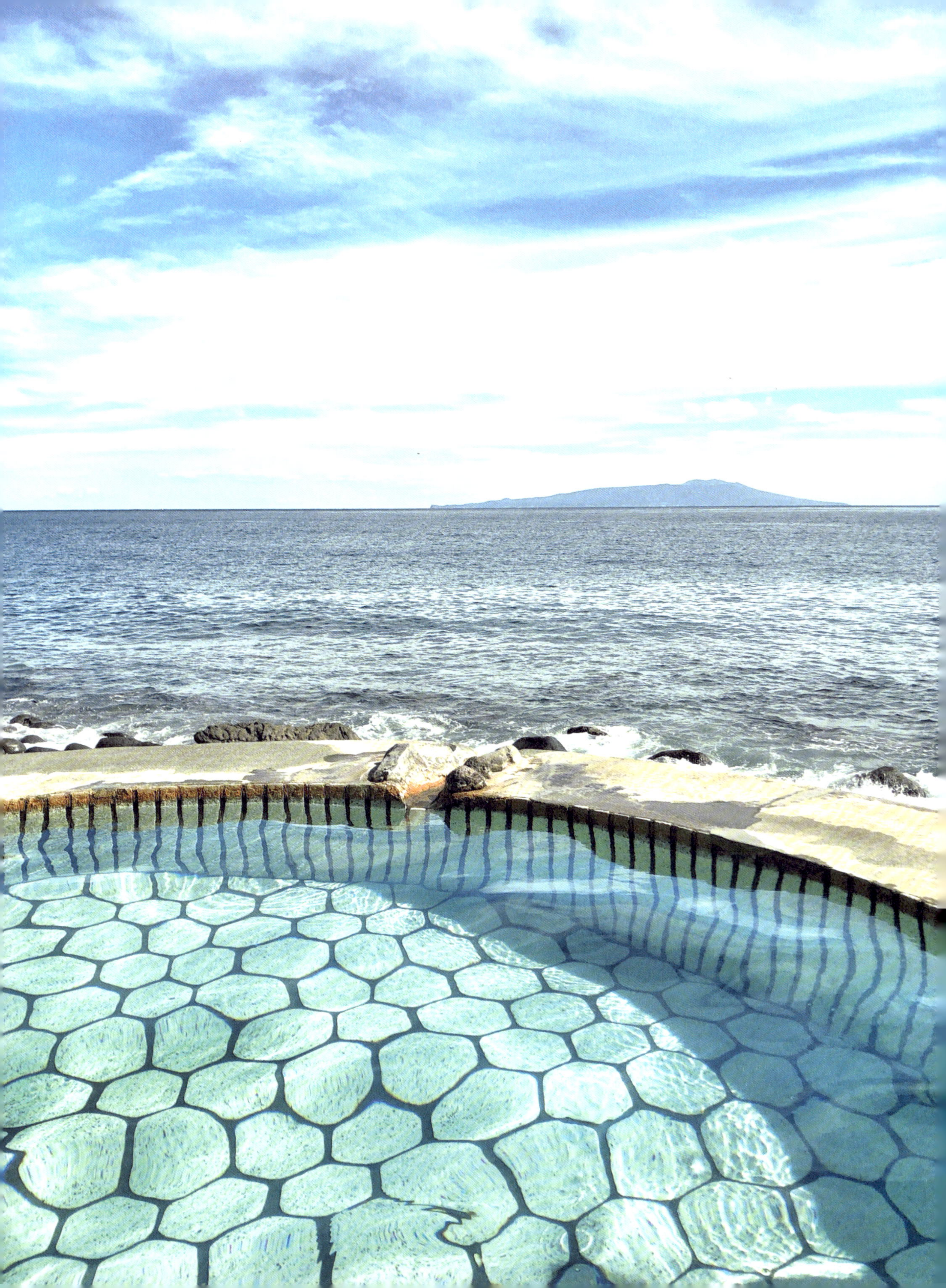

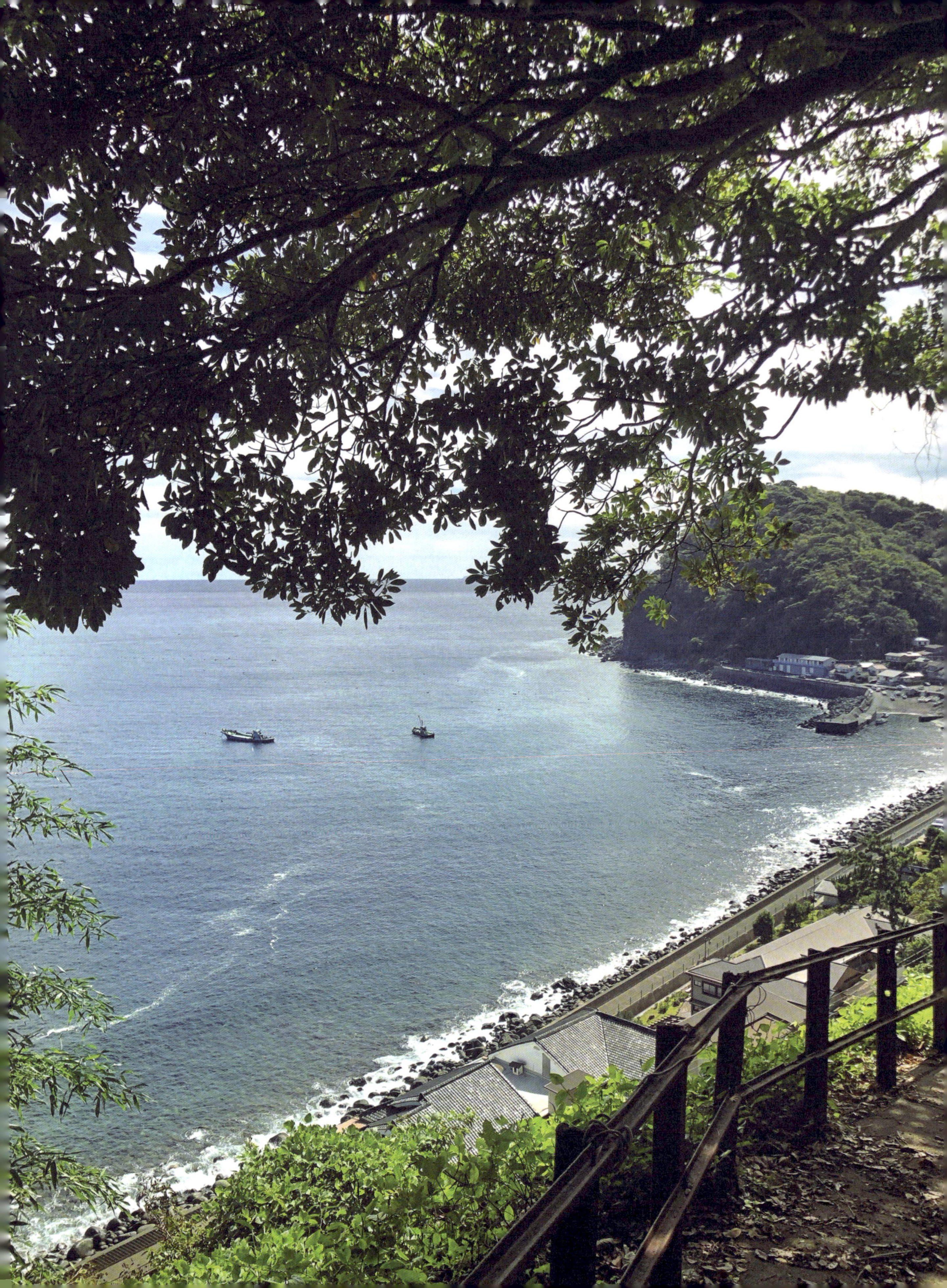

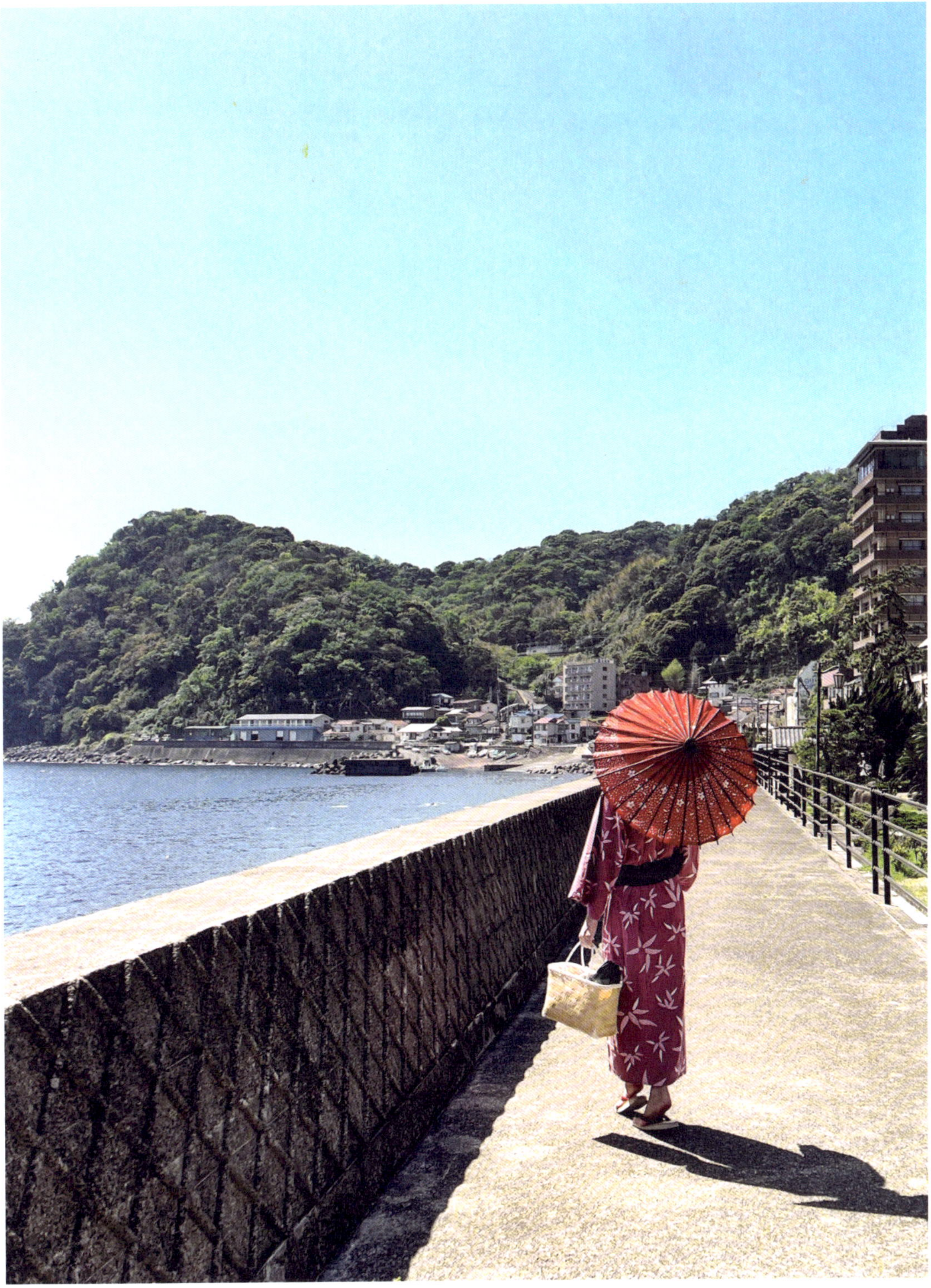

ABOVE Stroll along the "Moon Road" before or after bathing at Kuroneiwaburo.

ONSEN AND RYOKAN OF JAPAN

Traditional Spa and Bathing Culture

This book was conceived, edited, and designed by gestalten.

Edited by Robert Klanten and François-Luc Giraldeau
With Contributing Editor Lia of Ryokanwanderings/ ryokanwanderings.com
Editorial support by Effie Efthymiadi

Text by Lia of Ryokanwanderings
Photography by Lia of Ryokanwanderings
Except for pp. 5–6, 9–11, 55–61, 97–103, 245–251 by Hoshino Resorts; pp. 7–8, 122–129 by Takamiya Ryokan Inc.; pp. 12–18 by Nishimuraya/nishimuraya.ne.jp; pp. 21–25 by Hiroshi Mizusaki/loop-pc.jp, design of Kamenoi Bessou by Koichi Futatsumata and Koichi Furumura for CASE-REAL/ casereal.com; p. 34 by Nagato Yumoto Onsen Machi Co. Ltd./ lyumotoonsen.com; pp. 37–43 by Visit Kinosaki/visitkinosaki.com; pp. 76–77, 79 by Unzen Destination Service/unzen.org; pp. 88–90, 91 bottom by Haiya Ryokan; pp. 137–139 by Nacása & Partners Inc./lnacasa.co.jp, design of Maruhon Ryokan by Kubo Tsushima Architects; pp. 150, 152, 153 top left by Pierre Babin/@pierrebabin; pp. 155–159 by FUFU Japan; pp. 193–199 Courtesy of Jiyujin Inc.; pp. 220–225, 227 by Misasa Onsen Tourism Association; pp. 176–181 by Rankeisou; pp. 229, 230 top left and bottom, 231 by Ryokan Sanga; pp. 234–236 by Kei Sugimoto/sugimoto.lomo.jp and p. 237 by Taku Fukuoka/takufuku.com for Isaribi Corporation

Editorial management by Anna Diekmann

Design and layout by Stefan Morgner
Cover design by Melanie Ullrich and Stefan Morgner

Map by Ataur/iStock/Getty Images Plus
Map design by Stefan Morgner

Photo Editor: Madeline Dudley-Yates

Production management by Vincent Illner

Typefaces: Signifier by Kris Sowersby, Futura by Isabella Chaeva, Paul Renner, Vladimir Andrich, Vladimir Yefimov

Cover image by Lia of Ryokanwanderings
Back cover images by Hoshino Resorts (left) and Nishimuraya/nishimuraya.ne.jp (right)

Printed by aprinta druck GmbH, Wemding
Made in Germany

Published by gestalten, Berlin 2025
ISBN 978-3-96704-197-2

2nd printing, 2026

Die Gestalten Verlag GmbH & Co. KG
Mariannenstrasse 9–10
10999 Berlin, Germany
hello@gestalten.com

Bibliographic information published by the Deutsche Nationalbibliothek. The Deutsche Nationalbibliothek lists this publication in the Deutsche Nationalbibliografie; detailed bibliographic data is available online at www.dnb.de

None of the content in this book was published in exchange for payment by commercial parties or designers; the inclusion of all work is based solely on its artistic merit.

This book was printed on paper certified according to the standards of the FSC®.

FSC www.fsc.org MIX Paper | Supporting responsible forestry FSC® C004592